# ORTHOTICS IN REHABILITATION
## Splinting the Hand and Body

**Pat McKee, MSc, OT(C)**
Assistant Professor
Department of Occupational Therapy
University of Toronto
Toronto, Ontario
Canada

**Leanne Morgan, BSc, OT(C)**

Illustrations by Sarina McKee

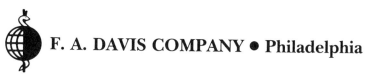

**F. A. DAVIS COMPANY • Philadelphia**

F. A. Davis Company
1915 Arch Street
Philadelphia, PA 19103

Printed in the United States of America

Last digit indicates print number: 10 9 8 7 6 5 4 3 2 1

*Publisher, Health Professions:* Jean-François Vilain
*Senior Editor:* Lynn Borders Caldwell
*Developmental Editor:* Marianne Fithian
*Cover Design by:* Louis J. Forgion

**Library of Congress Cataloging-in-Publication Data**

McKee, Pat.
    Orthotics in rehabilitation: splinting the hand and body / Pat McKee,
Leanne Morgan.
        p.     cm
    Includes bibliographical references and index.
    ISBN 0-8036-0351-7
    1. Splints (Surgery)     I. Morgan, Leanne.     II. Title.
RD757.S67M38   1998
617. 1'06—dc21                                                97-48427
                                                                CIP

# DEDICATION

# FOREWORD

This fine comprehensive book, *Orthotics in Rehabilitation: Splinting the Hand and Body,* should have a place on every rehabilitation specialist's bookshelf. Therapists and physiatrists will find this an indispensable reference in their daily work.

The organization and step-by-step format for client evaluation, orthotic design, material selection, construction, and application of each orthotic requirement are very clear and thoroughly described. The excellent use of graphics enhances the text and makes the book a truly valuable asset for each treating medical facility and outpatient clinic. The thoroughness of each definition used in this book is commendable.

The book is not only for the entry-level therapist, but also for the experienced clinician. The field of rehabilitation is greatly enhanced by this fine reference book. The authors have made a valuable contribution to the field of rehabilitation.

**Maude Malick, OTR, ASHT**
Administrative Consultant
Health South Harmarville
Rehabilitation Hospital
Pittsburgh, Pennsylvania

# PREFACE

This book is intended for students, therapists, and orthotists, bringing together theoretical concepts with fabrication procedures for dozens of orthoses (splints). Unlike other books on this topic, it goes beyond the hand to address the elbow, shoulder, face, head, neck, back, and lower extremities, including many orthoses that therapists have created but never published. The focus is on orthoses that are prevalent in occupational therapy, physical therapy, and hand rehabilitation, as well as less common designs, with an emphasis on custom-fabricated orthoses molded from low-temperature thermoplastics. References to some commonly used pre-formed or prefabricated (mass produced) orthoses are also included.

The theoretical concepts include:

- Objectives of orthotic intervention, design categories, and terminology (Chapter 1)
- Tissue and joint biomechanics, including joint mechanics and considerations for joint positioning, as well as the rationale for orthotic intervention for joint stiffness, carpal tunnel syndrome, inflammation, rheumatoid arthritis, tendon injuries, spasticity, fractures, and scar management (Chapter 2)
- Design and fabrication principles for static and dynamic orthoses, emphasizing features that optimize client comfort and compliance (Chapter 3)
- Criteria for selection of orthotic materials, including thermoplastics, linings and paddings, straps, and outriggers (Chapter 4)
- Equipment and tools for orthotic fabrication (Chapter 5)
- Ergonomic considerations to prevent injuries to the therapist (Chapter 6)
- An in-depth discussion of the orthotic intervention process (Chapter 7)

Chapters 8 through 12 present fabrication procedures for 68 custom orthoses in an easy-to-follow tabular format, with each chapter focusing on a different region. Chapter 8 contains eight orthoses for the midline of the body—head, face, neck, and back. Chapter 9 has 11 orthoses for the axilla, shoulder, elbow, and forearm. Chapter 10 describes 20 forearm-based orthoses. Chapter 11 presents 21 hand or finger/thumb-based orthoses, and Chapter 12 has eight lower extremity orthoses. In each of Chapters 9 through 12, the content is organized from proximal to distal. The well-illustrated fabrication procedures include patterns and step-by-step instructions described in a way that benefits both the beginner and the experienced therapist.

For each orthosis in Chapters 8 through 12, the following components are addressed:

- Name of orthosis
- Common names
- Objectives
- Indications
- Rationale
- Recommended materials
- Equipment and tools
- Positioning of the client and therapist
- Specific joint positioning, where appropriate
- Fabrication procedures
- Wearing regimen
- Precautions
- Options and alternatives
- Pattern

Appendix A has nine tables profiling thermoplastics, linings, and paddings. Throughout the book, terms that are in bold face are defined in the Glossary in Appendix B, or refer to the design categories described in Chapter 1. Appendix C contains 10 case studies to challenge the reader to integrate theory and applications detailed in the book. Addresses and websites for manufacturers and suppliers of orthotic materials, equipment, and tools are provided in Appendix D.

Although this book documents a wide range of orthoses, the possibilities for orthotic designs extend far beyond this book. New challenges and new orthotic materials, combined with the therapist's creative and problem-solving skills and client input, lead to the ongoing development of new designs. The therapist is encouraged to use the fabrication procedures as a guideline and not as strict doctrine. If the recommended materials, equipment, or tools are not available, substitute another thermoplastic or modify the fabrication procedures. Feel free to adapt patterns to meet the individual requirements of the situation. The orthoses described for the various conditions should not be regarded as the only suitable designs to use.

Experienced therapists, orthotists, and physicians may have views that differ from those of the authors. We welcome the opportunity to learn about different perspectives and new ideas. We can be contacted through the publisher's website at www.fadavis.com.

**Pat McKee, MSc, OT(C)**
**Leanne Morgan, BSc, OT(C)**

# ACKNOWLEDGMENTS

We wish to acknowledge the following individuals for their contributions toward the development of this book:

- Colleagues and friends in the Department of Occupational Therapy at the University of Toronto for their support and guidance, especially Judith Friedland, PhD, OT(C), and Rebecca Renwick, PhD, OT(C)
- Sarina McKee for her wonderful illustrations and Janice Marin for her technical assistance
- Godwin Lai for his support, encouragement, and assistance with editing
- Michael London, Andrea Duncan, OT(C), and Melannie Morgan for their assistance with proofreading
- Teachers, mentors, and those who provided opportunities, including Keith Bagnall, Sharon Brintnell, Stephanie Brundle, Gerry Buzzell, Kelly Charlebois, Benita Fifield, Barbara O'Shea, and Annette Rivard
- Occupational therapists who shared their knowledge and expertise, including Barbara Anderson, Dorcas Beaton, Lynn Carter, Sylvia Cooper, Lori Cyr, Susan Ellis, Jennifer Fenton, Debbie Hebert, Carol Hennigar, Louise Kelly, Estera Lackovic, Lisa Lazzarotto, Lonita Mak, Maureen Riley, Barbara Shankland, Jill Stier, Shawna Wade, Lucy Winston, and Terry Wlodarski
- The staff at FA Davis for their patience, guidance, and skills in transforming the manuscript into a published book, including Lynn Borders Caldwell, Glenn Fechner, Marianne Fithian, Ona Kosmos, Herb Powell, Jr., and Jean-François Vilain
- Our production editor, Carol O'Connell at Graphic World Publishing Ser-vices
- Individuals who provided information about orthotic materials and products, including Julie Belkin, John Clark, Mark Durant, John Kirk, Eric Johnson, Gina Johnson, Bob Remington, Steve Repetti, Jane Vaillancourt, and Paul Van Lede
- Occupational therapy students who reviewed the manuscript: Marika Beaumont, Kara Bowman, Joanne Brady, and Cynthia Tam
- Hundreds of students over a 20-year history of teaching orthotics at the University of Toronto and the University of Alberta

We are very especially grateful to the following individuals who reviewed the manuscript and book proposal and provided many helpful suggestions:

Bambi Anderson, OTR
Clinical Sales Consultant
Rehabilitation Division
Smith & Nephew, Inc.
Germantown, Wisconsin

Bruce Curtis, OTR
Clinical Sales Consultant
Rehabilitation Division
Smith & Nephew, Inc.
Germantown, Wisconsin

Patricia L. Davies, PhD, OTR/L
Assistant Professor
Occupational Therapy
SUNY at Buffalo
Buffalo, New York

Christine Denton, COTA
Clinical Education Specialist
Smith & Nephew, Inc.
Rehabilitation Division
Germantown, Wisconsin

Joan Edelstein, MA, PT
Associate Professor/Program Director
Physical Therapy
Columbia University
College of Physicians/Surgeons
New York, New York

Ann Marcolina Hayes, MHS, PT, OCS
Assistant Professor
Physical Therapy
St. Louis University
St. Louis, Missouri

Patricia M. Holz, OTR
Instructor/Coordinator
OTA Program
Fox Valley Technical College
Appleton, Wisconsin

Gwen Klingelhoet, CSC, OTR
Clinical Sales Consultant
Occupational Therapy Department
Smith & Nephew, Inc.
Germantown, Wisconsin

Lili Liu, PhD, OT(C)
Assistant Professor
Department of Occupational Therapy
University of Alberta
Edmonton, Alberta

Margaret Mary Lynn, MS, ORT/L, CHT
Clinical Sales Consultant
Smith & Nephew, Inc.
Germantown, Wisconsin

Maude Malick, OTR, ASHT
Administrative Consultant
Health South Harmarville
Rehabilitation Hospital
Pittsburgh, Pennsylvania

Janet A. McArdle, OTR
Technical Support Coordinator
Marketing Department
Smith & Nephew, Inc.
Germantown, Wisconsin

Susan Nowell Moore, MS, OTR
International Business Manager
Smith & Nephew, Inc.
Germantown, Wisconsin

Donna Sullivan Niswander, MS, OTR, CHT
Clinical Instructor/Senior Hand Therapist
Occupational Therapy
SUNY at Buffalo
Buffalo, New York

Terry Rex, PT
Clinical Research Manager
Research and Development
Smith & Nephew, Inc.
Germantown, Wisconsin

Angela S. Sajdyk, OTR/L, CHT
Clinical Sales Consultant
Rehabilitation Department
Smith & Nephew, Inc.
Germantown, Wisconsin

Fred Sammons, PhD, OTR, FAOTA
Sammons Preston
Holingbrook, Illinois

Melinda Dean Sissel, COTA/L
Instructor, OTA Program
Shawnee State University
Portsmouth, Ohio

Catherine Anne Trombly, SCD, OTR, FAOTA
Professor
Occupational Therapy
Boston University
Sargent College
Boston, Massachusetts

Kim Waldvogel, OTR/L
Senior Product Manager
Sammons Preston
Holingbrook, Illinois

# CONTENTS

CHAPTER **9**

*Orthoses for Shoulder and Elbow*   165

CHAPTER **10**

*Forearm-Based Orthoses*   195

## CHAPTER 11

### *Hand-, Finger-, Thumb-Based Orthoses   239*

## CHAPTER 12

### *Lower Extremity Orthoses   275*

CHAPTER **1**

# Objectives, Design, and Terminology

**Orthotics** is the science or field of practice pertaining to orthoses (pronounced or-*tho*-seas). An **orthosis** is a device applied to the body to stabilize or immobilize, prevent or correct deformity, protect against injury, promote healing, or assist function.[1] It can be applied to any part of the body—hand, elbow, shoulder, head, neck, back, hip, knee, ankle, and foot. Orthoses are designed to promote function when it is compromised by acute injury, cumulative trauma, disease, surgical intervention, congenital anomaly, or degenerative changes.

An orthosis can be regarded as

- An intervention modality
- An environmental adaptation
- A component of the individual's microenvironment
- An interface between the individual and the environment

Orthotic intervention is both an art and a science. The art is the therapist's creativity and skill in design and fabrication. The science is the sound base of knowledge in anatomy, histology, physiology, joint and tissue biomechanics, pathology, and wound healing. Without this foundation, the therapist may inadvertently overstress tissues and promote inflammation or injury. Understressing tissues is also undesirable because it can cause atrophy or contracture. To lend support to this foundation, Chapter 2 contains an in-depth discussion of joint and tissue biomechanics. Design and fabrication principles are explained in Chapter 3.

Therapists are perpetually challenged to apply theory, creativity, and problem-solving skills to meet the unique requirements and preferences of each client. Consequently, adaptations and innovations in orthotic designs and techniques often appear in rehabilitation journals and texts. The intent of this book is to provide the foundation and rationale for orthotic intervention. This is followed by a presentation of orthoses that are prevalent in occupational therapy and hand rehabilitation, as well as some less common designs. The focus will be on custom-fabricated orthoses molded from **low-temperature thermoplastics (LTTs).** References to some commonly used preformed or prefabricated (mass-produced) orthoses are also included.

Low-temperature thermoplastics (LTTs) are rubber- or plastic-based materials that are commonly supplied in sheets ranging in thickness from 1/16 to 1/8 in. (1.6 to 3.2 mm). When heated in water between 135° and 180°F (57° and 82°C), these sheets soften and become pliable, allowing for molding directly to the body part. After a few minutes, they harden and return to their previous rigid state. Less commonly, therapists use high-temperature thermoplastics, which are usually molded over a positive plaster replica of the body part. One exception is polyethylene, which can be directly molded to the body if it is lined with Plastazote. The technique is described in Chapter 10. A complete description of orthotic materials is provided in Chapter 4.

Orthoses are dispensed by therapists in one of three forms:

1. Custom-fabricated orthoses
   ○ From a pattern, made to the client's specifications, that is transferred to and cut and molded from LTT, neoprene, foam thermoplastic (e.g., Plastazote), or other materials
   ○ From a precut "splint blank" of LTT
2. Preformed LTT orthoses, which are mass produced and adjustable to customize the fit
3. Prefabricated orthoses, which are mass produced and ready to wear

Chapter 5 discusses the equipment and tools required for orthotic fabrication. This process can be stressful to the therapist's hands and back if body mechanics are poor or tools are not well maintained. Useful suggestions to minimize the harmful effects of orthotic fabrication are addressed in Chapter 6.

Only a few orthotic instructional textbooks or book chapters for occupational therapists address orthoses for all parts of the body.[2-6] The majority focuses on devices for the hand.[7-26] As the title of this book indicates, the orthotic interventions deal principally with the hand but also address other parts of the body—head, neck, shoulder, elbow, hip, knee, ankle, and foot. The therapist who manages complex hand trauma is strongly urged to supplement the information in this book with a comprehensive hand rehabilitation text.[4]

## ● Orthosis vs. Splint– What's in a Name?

Most rehabilitation literature refers to an LTT device as a **splint** and the field of practice as **splinting.**[7-24] Less commonly, the device is referred to as an **orthosis,**[25-28] derived from the Greek term *orthos,* which means to correct or make straight. Sometimes the term *brace* is used, but generally this term denotes a device made from high-temperature thermoplastic or metal for long-term use. Orthoses fabricated from LTTs can have a short- or long-term requirement.

The term *orthosis* originated after World War II. At the time there was debate over whether the term should be *orthosis* or *orthesis* to match the sound of *prosthesis,* which refers to the artificial replacement for a missing body part.[29] There was also some objection to "osis" as the ending of the word because, in medical usage, it means "condition" or denotes a morbid or disease process.[30]

An alternate term for an orthosis is **orthotic device.** As used here, the word *orthotic* is an adjective.[1] It is commonly used as a synonym for orthosis, for example, "foot orthotic." However, dictionaries do not recognize orthotic as a noun, and to use it as such is grammatically incorrect.

The term *splint,* originating from Middle Dutch *splinte,* is likely to conjure up an image of two pieces of wood lashed to an injured leg on a ski slope by an untrained person. Dictionaries reinforce the limited view of splints as devices that immobilize injuries.[1,30–33]

Similarly, the verb *to splint,* which means "to support and immobilize as if with a splint or splints,"[33] emphasizes the immobilizing outcome of the device. Although immobilization is the intended outcome of some devices, the objective of many is to restore mobility.

Because there is no consensus among therapists as to which term is more appropriate, it is a matter of personal choice whether to use splint or orthosis. It is difficult to argue against the common use of the term *splint.* It is a shorter word, is easier to say, and has a long history in rehabilitation. Furthermore, there is no verb to correspond directly with the term *orthosis.* However, the term *splint,* as either a noun or a verb, has a narrow scope, is perhaps misleading, and does not adequately reflect the professional training and skill required for orthotic intervention. In contrast, the definition of orthosis found in medical dictionaries better describes the broad spectrum of sophisticated devices currently fabricated by therapists.[1,30–32]

# ● Objectives of Orthotic Intervention

The objectives of orthotic intervention are to protect, correct, and assist. Orthoses *protect* against forces that cause pain, injury, or deformity or stresses that interfere with healing. They *assist* weak, paralyzed, or spastic muscles to promote functional use of the limb, and they *correct* deformity. In doing so, most orthoses affect joint mobility, as explained below.

- **Protective** orthoses
  - Immobilize the joint, preventing any motion and promoting optional joint alignment
  - Block the motion at a certain point, restricting the permitted range of the joint

  - Prevent deformity by maintaining joint mobility
  - Stabilize an unstable joint or tendon or a fractured bone
  - Protect vulnerable or healing structures (e.g., bone, joint, tendon, blood vessel, nerve, skin) to promote healing, prevent (re)injury, and prevent subluxation of joints or tendons
  - Exert traction force on a joint with damaged cartilage while permitting joint motion
  - Continuously move the joint through a flexion-extension arc of movement
- **Corrective** orthoses
  - Correct joint contracture
  - Correct subluxation of joints or tendons
- **Assistive** orthoses
  - Assist movement of joints during functional activities when muscles are weak or paralyzed
  - Reduce muscle tone of spastic muscles to promote joint mobility

A single orthosis may be designed to meet more than one objective, and more than one orthosis may be required for an individual to meet all the objectives. If the condition changes, the objectives should be revised, and alterations to the orthosis may be necessary.

The device may be required for short-term use, as in a postsurgical application; for an extended period, such as during the regeneration of a peripheral nerve; or on an intermittent but ongoing basis for a chronic condition such as rheumatoid arthritis. These various considerations influence choices in the design of the orthosis and the optimal LTT for the circumstances.

For some clients, orthoses reduce pain and enhance current *function.* In other circumstances, the orthosis may actually limit function while it is used because it has been designed to prevent deformity or injury or promote healing to ensure optimal future function. When function is temporarily compromised, the client or caregiver must clearly understand the merit of orthotic intervention and the consequences of noncompliance. Strategies to promote compliance are discussed in Chapter 3 under "Optimizing Compliance."

# ● Orthotic Design Categories and Their Objectives

The simplest orthotic design consists of a plastic shell molded to the body, providing **static** support to one or more joints. Alternatively, the simple shell orthosis can be **nonarticular,** stabilizing a bone such as the humerus, without crossing any joints. Orthoses that are more complex begin with a shell, which acts as a base to which outriggers or motors can be attached. **Outriggers** apply force in one direction to a joint, usually pulling it into flexion or extension. If the outrigger uses energy-storing materials, such as elastic, springs, or spring wire, the force will be dynamic, allowing active-resisted movement in the opposite direction of the dynamic force. Orthoses that use this type of outrigger are called *dynamic orthoses.* Alternatively, the outriggers can use passive components such as

screws, hook and loop Velcro, nylon line, or hinges to apply a static corrective force that can be adjusted as the condition progresses. Orthoses that use passive outriggers are called *static-progressive orthoses.* The essential difference between dynamic and static-progressive orthoses is that joint movement can occur in the former but not the latter.

In this book, orthoses are categorized according to their basic design as it relates to their influence over joint mobility (Table 1-1). The rationale for this categorization is that orthoses have an immediate or delayed impact on joint mobility, with the exception of nonarticular designs. The examples provided for each category are not comprehensive.

## SIMPLE SHELL ORTHOSES

**Nonarticular** orthoses do not cross any joints and have no direct influence on joint mobility. They protect or correct a body segment or bone, rather than targeting a joint as all other categories do. This category includes the following:

- Circumferential stabilizing orthoses (commonly called fracture braces), used to stabi-

| TABLE 1-1.   Orthotic Design Categories and Their Impact on Joint Mobility | |
| --- | --- |
| **Design Category** | **Impact on Joint Mobility** |
| Nonarticular | Crosses no joints, therefore has no direct influence on joint mobility; however, may stabilize joints (e.g., buddy straps) |
| Static | Completely immobilizes joint(s) |
| Static motion-blocking | Permits full active range of motion in one direction and restricted active motion in the opposite direction |
| Serial-static; static-progressive | Applies force on joint(s) to increase passive range of motion—no joint motion permitted |
| Dynamic | Applies a passive pulling force in one direction while permitting active-resisted motion in the opposite direction |
| Dynamic motion-blocking | Applies a passive pulling force in one direction while permitting restricted active-resisted motion in the opposite direction |
| Dynamic traction | Permits full active range of motion while applying a constant traction force to the joint |
| Tenodesis | Links active wrist extension with passive finger flexion |
| Continuous passive motion | Continuously moves targeted joint(s) through controlled arc of passive motion to promote optimal healing of joint cartilage and maintain joint mobility |

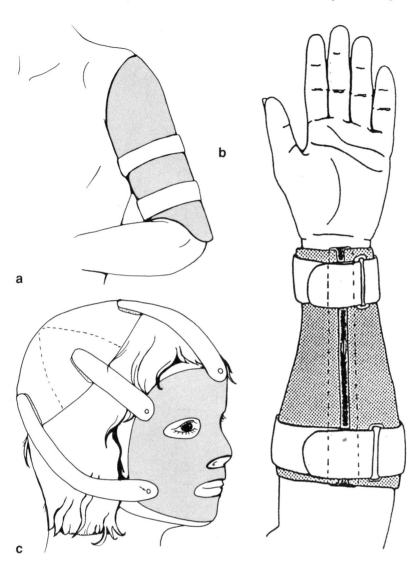

**FIGURE 1-1.** Nonarticular orthoses. *(a)* Circumferential nonarticular humerus-stabilizing orthosis. *(b)* Circumferential nonarticular ulna-stabilizing orthosis. *(c)* Nonarticular scar-controlling face mask. The thermoplastic face mask is secured by elastic straps, which are attached by Velcro to a skullcap or beanie.

lize and promote healing of **fractures** of long bones when joint immobilization is neither required nor beneficial. Midshaft fractures of the humerus (Fig. 1-1*a*), ulna (Fig.1-1*b*), metacarpal, phalanx, or tibia lend themselves well to this type of orthosis.

- Face masks to control **hypertrophic** scar tissue (Fig. 1-1*c*)

**Static** orthoses immobilize one or more joints and are designed to do the following:

- Maintain tissue length to prevent **contractures** (Fig. 1-2)

- Rest injured or inflamed tissues to reduce **inflammation** and pain (Fig. 1-3)
- Stabilize injured structures to promote healing (Fig. 1-4)
- Unload tissues to promote resorption of lax structures such as ligaments or capsules to correct joint instability (Fig. 1-5)
- Reduce **muscle tone** of spastic muscles (Fig. 1-6)
- Position the lower extremity joints to enhance joint alignment and promote pain-free gait (Fig. 1-7)

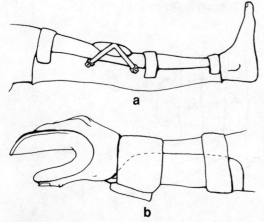

**FIGURE 1-2.** Static or serial-static orthoses. The objectives of these orthoses have not been identified by name because they can be used to meet various goals. *(a)* Posterior static (or serial-static) knee orthosis secured by three straps and a contoured Plastazote kneepad. *(b)* Volar forearm-based static (or serial-static) wrist-hand orthosis secured by a wrist and proximal strap. An additional strap over the proximal phalanges (not shown) is optional.

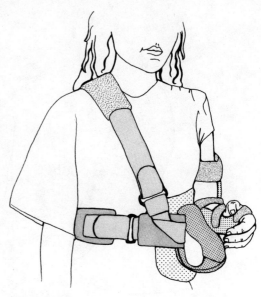

**FIGURE 1-4.** Lateral trunk-based static shoulder-elbow-wrist orthosis. This orthosis, designed to immobilize the shoulder, consists of three plastic components: a body shell, a forearm trough, and a stay that attaches them together. A waist belt and shoulder strap secure the orthosis to the body.

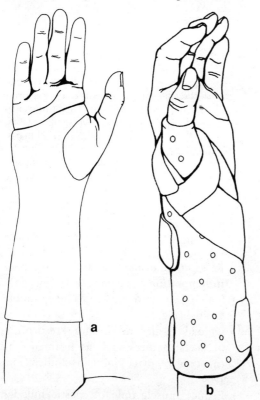

**FIGURE 1-3.** The objectives of these orthoses have not been identified by name because they can be used to meet various goals. *(a)* Volar forearm-based static thumb-hole wrist orthosis (straps not shown). *(b)* Radial forearm-based static, wrist-thumb orthosis (prefabricated Rolyan® Cool Flo™ Splint[34]); Cool Flo™ is a trademark of Smith & Nephew, Inc.).

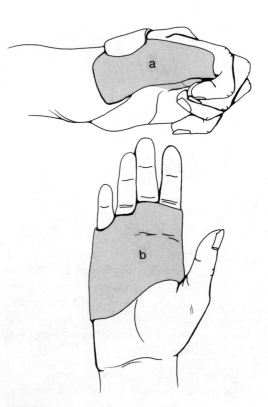

**FIGURE 1-5.** Volar hand-based static metacarpophalangeal (MCP) stabilizing orthosis. *(a)* Ulnar view. *(b)* Volar view.

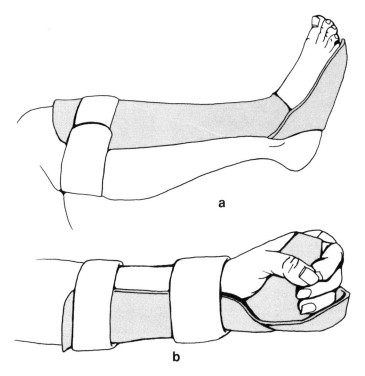

a

b

**FIGURE 1-6.** *(a)* Bisurfaced static (or serial-static) tone-reducing ankle-foot orthosis. This orthosis can also be used when muscle tone is unimpaired, to immobilize the ankle, in which case the objective *tone-reducing* would not be included. *(b)* Ulnar forearm-based static (or serial-static) tone-reducing, cone-style wrist-hand orthosis. (Roland® Static Progressive Finger Extension Splint: U.S. patent pending.)

**Static motion-blocking** orthoses permit full motion in one direction but limit (or block) motion in the opposite direction. They are commonly used to do the following:

- Protect against **swan-neck deformity,** which may develop with rheumatoid arthritis, or **trigger finger,** to help promote restabilization or healing (Fig. 1-8*a*)
- Help correct elbow flexion contractures, maintaining elbow extension to the limit of the soft tissue length, but allowing the triceps to actively stretch the contracted tissues (Fig. 1-8*b*)

**Serial-static** orthoses immobilize one or more joints and are designed to do the following:

- Reduce muscle tone of **spastic** muscles
- Correct contractures by applying a gentle, prolonged stretch to promote growth of contracted soft tissues

In this category, a static orthosis is reheated and remolded several times as the tissues grow. Thus the contracture is reduced by a "series" of orthoses (Fig. 1-9). Those LTTs with "memory" are best suited for this orthotic design (see Chapter 4). These thermoplastics recover their original shape when reheated, allowing repeated remolding of the orthosis to gradually increase the range of motion of a stiff joint.

Before the introduction of low-temperature thermoplastics in the mid-1960s, plaster of Paris was used to create a series of casts or splints, using a technique called *serial casting.*

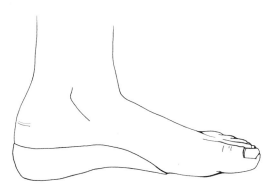

**FIGURE 1-7.** Plantar static foot orthosis.

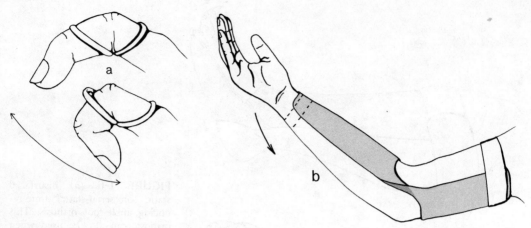

**FIGURE 1-8.** *(a)* Figure-8 finger-based static proximal interphalangeal (PIP) extension-blocking orthosis (Siris Swan-Neck Silver Ring Splint[35]). Upper: The PIP is extended to the limit of extension block. Lower: PIP flexion is unrestricted. *(b)* Bisurfaced static elbow flexion-blocking orthosis. The distal strap at the wrist is optional (broken line). When it is absent, the elbow is free to extend out of the orthosis in the direction of the arrow.

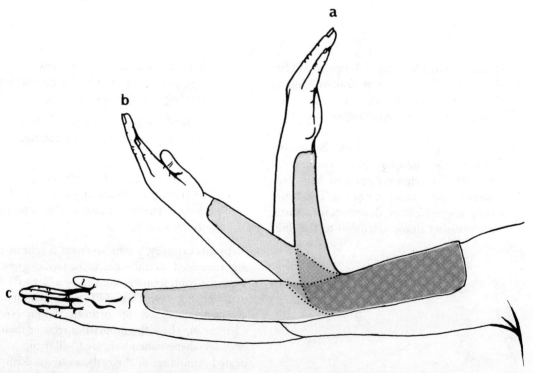

**FIGURE 1-9.** Anterior serial static elbow corrective-extension orthosis. *(a)* First orthosis in a series, at outset of orthotic intervention when the elbow flexion contracture is about 90°. *(b)* Fifth orthosis in a series, at week five. The flexion contracture has been reduced to about 45°. *(c)* Tenth orthosis in a series, at week 10 of intervention. The flexion contracture has completely resolved. This orthosis may be used to maintain elbow extension if there is a possibility to contracture recurrence.

When thermoplastics replaced plaster of Paris, the technique was renamed *serial splinting.* In recent years, the use of circumferential serial plaster casts to soften scar tissue while correcting joint contractures has regained popularity, especially for interphalangeal joint contractures.[36]

## ORTHOSES WITH OUTRIGGERS

**Static-progressive** orthoses are designed to correct contractures by applying a gentle prolonged stretch to promote growth of contracted soft tissues. Unlike serial-static orthoses, the thermoplastic is not remolded as the tissues grow. Instead, a nonelastic component, attached to a thermoplastic base, is adjusted by small increments as the contracture is reduced. This component could be a turnbuckle, hook and loop Velcro, a nylon line, an adjustable hinge, or a screw. Many completely prefabricated (mass-produced) orthoses are designed specifically for this purpose (Fig. 1-10). Alternatively, the therapist can mount a prefabricated progressive component to a custom-molded static orthosis. No joint motion occurs when this type of orthosis is in place.

**Dynamic** orthoses apply a passive pulling force in one direction while permitting active motion in the opposite direction, using energy-storing materials such as rubber bands, Theraband, elastic, springs, or spring wire. This category is commonly used to do the following:

- Provide a passive assist to substitute for weak or absent motor function due to a peripheral nerve lesion (Fig. 1-11*a* through *c*)
- Apply gentle, prolonged stretch to correct contractures by promoting tissue growth, similar to serial-static and static-progressive orthoses (Fig. 1-11*d* through *f* )

Dynamic orthoses differ from static-progressive orthoses, (which use nonelastic force components) in that they allow active-resisted movement in the direction opposite to the assistive or corrective force.

**Dynamic motion-blocking** orthoses are modified dynamic orthoses that incorporate a motion-blocking component. They apply passive pulling force in one direction using energy-storing materials while permitting active motion in the opposite direction, up to the limit of the blocking component, to facilitate controlled, protected tendon excursion after flexor or extensor tendon injury (Fig. 1-12).

**Dynamic traction** orthoses have a thermoplastic base with a hinged outrigger, which permits a full active range of motion of the target joint while applying a contrast distraction force to the joint. A motion-blocking component can be incorporated into this design. This orthotic design is used to help promote healing of intra-articular fractures of the finger interphalangeal (IP) joints (Fig. 1-13) and to help maintain tissue length and promote tendon glide.

**Tenodesis orthoses** are pseudodynamic orthoses that use active wrist extension to bring about passive flexion of the metacarpophalangeal joints (MCPs) and IPs when the muscles to the distal joints are weak or paralyzed

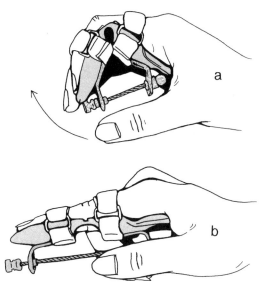

**FIGURE 1-10.** Volar finger-based static-progressive screw D2 PIP-extension orthosis (prefabricated Rolyan® Static Progressive Finger Extension Splint.[34] *(a)* At the beginning of intervention for PIP flexion contracture. Orthosis applies gentle extension force. The screw can be adjusted in small increments as the contracture reduces. *(b)* At the end of intervention, the PIP flexion contracture has been fully reduced, achieving full PIP extension. (Rolyan® Static Progressive Finger Extension Splint: U.S. patent pending.)

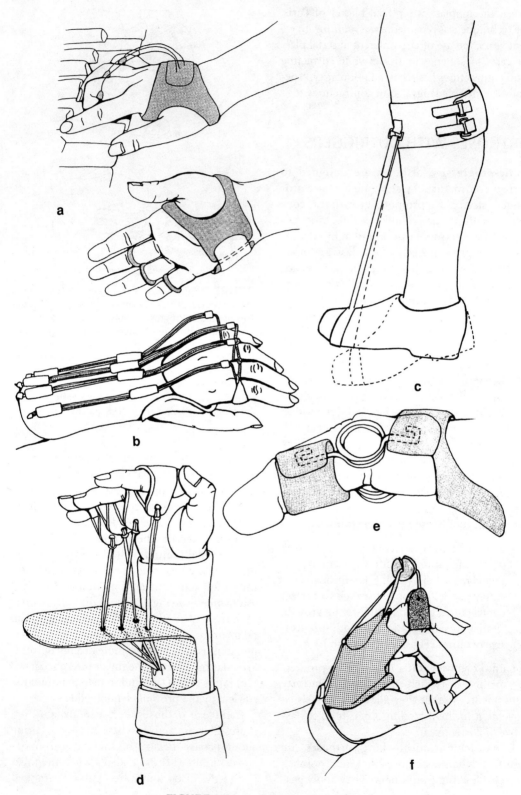

**FIGURE 1-11.** See legend on facing page.

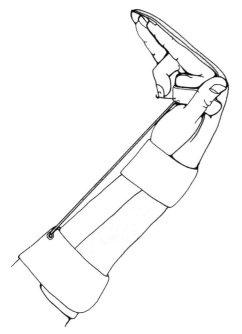

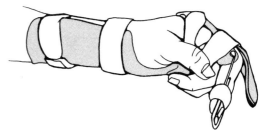

**FIGURE 1-13.** Volar forearm-based dynamic lateral-hinge D2 PIP-traction and extension-blocking orthosis. (Redrawn from Byrne, A, et al: A modified dynamic traction splint for unstable intra-articular fractures of the proximal interphalangeal joint. J Hand Ther 8:216, 1995.)

**FIGURE 1-12.** Dorsal forearm-based dynamic D3 MCP-IP protective-flexion and MCP extension-blocking orthosis. An elastic thread is secured to the proximal strap, passes through a pulley on the palmar bar, and loops over a hook glued to the fingernail. The interphalangeal (IP) joints can extend against the resistance of the elastic thread to the limit of the extension block over the fingers.

(Fig. 1-14). Individuals with C6 quadriplegia can use this type of assistive orthosis.

## ORTHOSES WITH MOTORS

**Continuous passive motion (CPM)** orthoses have a base with a battery-powered motor that continuously moves the targeted joint or joints through a controlled arc of movement. CPM orthoses are most commonly provided for the hand (Fig. 1-15*a*), elbow (Fig. 1-15*b*), wrist, shoulder, knee, and ankle to promote healing of the articular cartilage[38] and to prevent ligamentous or tendinous contracture.

## ● **Terminology**

A lack of consistency in terminology for orthoses presents a communication barrier among health professionals. In the literature, an orthosis may be named for

- The incorporated joint(s) (e.g., wrist)
- The condition it is commonly used for (e.g., carpal tunnel syndrome)
- The goal of the orthosis (e.g., immobilization, resting)

---

**FIGURE 1-11.** Dynamic orthoses. (*a*) Circumferential hand-based dynamic arching-spring-wire MCP assistive-extension orthosis. (*b*) Dorsal forearm-based dynamic tube-outrigger MCP assistive-extension orthosis. Each tube mounted to the base transmits an elastic cord, which is attached to a finger loop, to pull the MCP into extension. (*c*) Calf-based dynamic ankle assistive-extension orthosis. An elastic spans between the calf strap and the shoe strap to pull the ankle into extension (solid line) and allow active-resisted ankle flexion (broken line). (*d*) Volar forearm-based dynamic MCP corrective-flexion orthosis. Rubber bands are anchored to the proximal end of the forearm base, pass through a pulley of perforated thermoplastic bonded to the base, and are attached to finger loops. (*e*) Three-point finger-based dynamic joint-aligned coil-spring D2 PIP-corrective extension orthosis. (*f*) Circumferential hand-based dynamic low-profile, D2 PIP corrective-extension orthosis (prefabricated Phoenix® Single Finger Outrigger—Phoenix is a trademark of Human Factors Engineering, Wickenberg, Arizona). In (*b*) and (*d*), the wrist is included in the orthosis by virtue of the forearm base, but it is not a target joint; therefore it is not listed in the description. In (*f*), the low-profile outrigger serves as a pulley to redirect the nylon line, which is attached to a rubber band secured to the hand base.

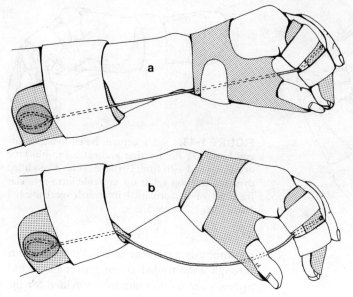

**FIGURE 1-14.** Volar forearm-based tenodesis wrist-hand orthosis. This orthosis has three separate components: a forearm base, a hand component to position the thumb, and a dorsal finger component for the index and long fingers. Tenodesis is explained in Chapter 2. *(a)* Active wrist extension creates tension in the cord, pulling the MCPs of the index and long fingers into flexion, to oppose the thumb. *(b)* Relaxation of the wrist extensors allows the wrist to flex, slackening the cord and releasing the grasp so that the fingers can open.

**FIGURE 1-15.** Continuous passive motion (CPM) designs. *(a)* Volar forearm-based CPM D2-5MCP-IP orthosis (Hand-H3[37]). *(b)* Trunk-based CPM elbow orthosis (Elbow-E2[37]), which moves the elbow through an adjustable range of flexion and extension.

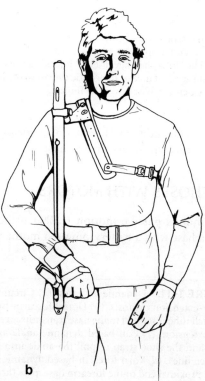

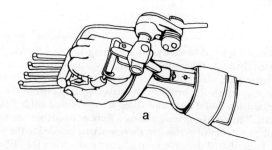

- The body surface in contact with the orthosis (e.g., volar or palmar)
- The individual who pioneered the design (e.g., Kleinert, Sarmiento, Denis Browne)
- Its appearance (e.g., clamdigger, banjo, cock-up)

For example, consider the many terms for a wrist orthosis (see Fig. 1-3*a*) that follow. In most cases, the design is unclear.

- Wrist splint[6]
- **Cock-up splint**[14]
- Wrist cock-up splint[26]
- Simple cock-up splint[18]
- Volar wrist cock-up splint[11,21]
- Palmar wrist cock-up splint[4]
- Palmarly based, static, wrist cock-up splint[20]
- Work splint[39]
- Wrist splint—**volar**[17]
- Volar splint, type 1[3]
- Wrist orthosis, volar type[27]
- Wrist immobilization splint[10,23]
- Simple wrist immobilization splint[13]
- Wrist extension immobilization; Type O[1]22

Various authors and organizations have proposed classification systems. The simplest system identifies only the incorporated joints or anatomic regions[40] (Table 1-2). The orthoses are often identified by their acronyms, for example, WHO, meaning wrist-hand orthosis, or AFO, meaning ankle-foot orthosis. This system has been adopted by orthotists. Although we find that this classification lacks sufficient description, it serves well as the basis for the organization of Chapters 8 through 12.

In 1987 Fess and Philips[13] proposed a splint classification system, designed to describe hand orthoses according to "how," "where," and "why." In 1991 the American Society of Hand Therapists[22] published the *Splint Classification System* to provide a standard nomenclature for upper extremity orthoses that is based on the function of the orthosis. However, because the scope of this textbook goes beyond the upper extremity, we have devised our own terminology to describe the form and function of orthoses for all parts of the body.

---

**TABLE 1-2. Names of Orthoses Based on Incorporated Joints or Regions**

| Acronym | Single-Joint/ Single-Region Orthoses | Acronym | Multiple-Joint/ Multiple-Region Orthoses |
|---|---|---|---|
| ***Upper Limb Orthoses*** | | | |
| HO | Hand orthosis | | |
| WO | Wrist orthosis | WHO | Wrist-hand orthosis |
| EO | Elbow orthosis | EWHO | Elbow-wrist-hand orthosis |
| SO | Shoulder orthosis | SEWHO | Shoulder-elbow-wrist-hand orthosis |
| ***Spinal Orthoses*** | | | |
| CO | Cervical orthosis | CTLSO | Cervical-thoracic-lumbosacral orthosis |
| TO | Thoracic orthosis | TLSO | Thoracic-lumbosacral orthosis |
| LO | Lumbar orthosis | LSO | Lumbosacral orthosis |
| | | SIO | Sacroiliac orthosis |
| ***Lower Limb Orthoses*** | | | |
| FO | Foot orthosis | AFO | Ankle-foot orthosis |
| KO | Knee orthosis | KAFO | Knee-ankle-foot orthosis |
| HO | Hip orthosis | HKAFO | Hip-knee-ankle-foot orthosis |

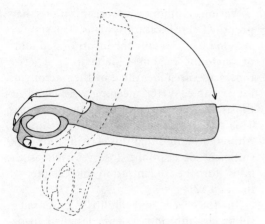

**FIGURE 1-16.** Using a bisurfaced static wrist-hand orthosis to lever the wrist into extension.

## A SYSTEM FOR NAMING ORTHOSES

This nomenclature is designed to describe the basic form and function of each orthosis such that its appearance is clearly understood without the need of an illustration. Furthermore, the terms are intended to be self-explanatory to health professionals, without the need of a key to decipher the meaning of descriptors. This system of naming has been used for Figures 1-1 through 1-16 and is summarized in Table 1-3.

The seven descriptors used in this terminology are as follows:

1. Surface
2. Base
3. Design category
4. Target joint, region, or bone
5. Objective
6. Variables
7. Concluding term

### Surface

To apply this system, begin by describing the basic form of the orthotic base, which can have different degrees of surface contact with the body part and contact on different surfaces. The most common base design is the **half-shell** or **trough**, enclosing about half the circumference of the limb. In the upper limb, the half-shell design can be

- Volar (Figs. 1-2*b*, 1-3*a*, 1-11*d*) or anterior (Fig. 1-9)
- Dorsal (Figs. 1-11*b* and 1-12) or posterior
- Lateral (Fig. 1-4)
- Radial (Fig. 1-3*b*)
- Ulnar (Fig. 1-6*b*)

In the lower limb, the half-shell design can be

- Anterior or dorsal
- Posterior (Fig. 1-2*a*) or plantar (Fig. 1-7)
- Medial
- Lateral

A variation of this style is the **bisurfaced** design, which contacts one surface on one side of the joint and the opposite surface on the other side of the joint (Figs. 1-6*a* and 1-8*b*). This design uses leverage to position the joint (Fig. 1-16).

Two styles with little contact are the **figure-eight** design (Fig. 1-8*a*) and the **three-point** design (Fig. 1-11*e*). In contrast, **circumferential** orthoses enclose the body part (Figs. 1-1*a*, 1-1*b*, and 1-11*a*) and provide more stabilization than other designs. A variation of the circumferential design is the **bivalved** orthosis, which encircles the body part with two half-shells that overlap slightly at the sides.

In the literature, the term **gutter** is sometimes used to refer to radial or ulnar half-shell designs. An alternate term for circumferential upper extremity design is **gauntlet.**

### Base

Identify the body segment of the most proximal part of the orthotic base. With the exception of nonarticular designs, the base of an orthosis is located at least one body segment proximal to the target joint(s). An orthosis acting on the hand can have its base located on the forearm, hand, or finger. For example, the orthosis in Figure 1-11*a* provides dynamic assistive-extension force to the MCPs with its base located in the hand. Figure 1-11*b* shows a similar orthosis, but its base is proximal to the wrist

**TABLE 1-3.  System for Naming Orthoses**

| Surface | Location of Base | Design Category | Target | Objective | Examples of Variables |
|---|---|---|---|---|---|
| *Circumferential* | *N/A* | *Nonarticular* | Bone:<br>  Phalanx*<br>  Metacarpal* | Protective<br>Scar-controlling<br>Stabilizing | C-bar<br>Cone-style<br>Plastazote<br>Plaster of Paris<br>Thumb-hole |
| Anterior<br>Bisurfaced<br>Bivalved<br>Circumferential<br>Dorsal<br>Figure-eight<br>Lateral<br>Medial<br>Plantar<br>Posterior<br>Radial<br>Spiral<br>Three-point<br>Ulnar<br>Volar | Calf-based<br>Finger-based<br>Forearm-based<br>Hand-based<br>Leg-based<br>Thumb-based<br>Trunk-based | Static | Ulna<br>Humerus<br>Tibia<br>Femur | Stabilizing<br>Tone-reducing | |
| | | Static<br>  (motion-blocking) | Joint:<br>  IPs*<br>  PIP*<br>  DIP*<br>  MCP*<br>  Wrist<br>  Elbow<br>  Shoulder<br>  Hip<br>  Ankle<br>  Knee | Extension-<br>  blocking<br>Flexion-blocking | |
| | | | | Corrective-<br>  extension<br>Corrective-<br>  flexion<br>Tone-reducing | |
| | | Serial-static | | (Corrective)<br>  extension<br>(Corrective)<br>  flexion<br>Tone-reducing | Style of<br>  Outrigger:<br>Arching<br>  spring-wire<br>Joint-aligned<br>  coil-spring<br>High-profile<br>Lateral-<br>  hinge<br>Low-profile<br>Screw<br>Tube-<br>  outrigger |
| | | Static-progressive | Region:<br>  Thumb<br>  Finger<br>  Hand<br>  Neck<br>  Face<br>  Lumbar<br>  Calf<br>  Foot | Assistive-<br>  extensive<br>Assistive-flexion<br>Corrective-<br>  flexion<br>Corrective-<br>  extension<br>Tone-reducing | |
| | | Dynamic | | Corrective-<br>  flexion<br>Corrective-<br>  extension<br>Extension-<br>  blocking<br>Flexion-blocking<br>Protective-<br>  flexion<br>Protective-<br>  extension | |
| | | Dynamic<br>  (motion-blocking) | | | |
| | | Dynamic (traction) | PIP*<br>DIP* | Extension-<br>  blocking<br>Traction | |
| | | Continuous<br>  passive motion | See joints<br>above | (Continuous<br>  motion) | |
| Volar | Forearm-based | Tenodesis | N/A | (To facilitate<br>  tenodesis<br>  grasp) | |

Shading indicates that the descriptor is not required for that particular design category. Terms in parentheses are excluded from the list of descriptors.
*For these bones or joints, identify the specific digit(s): thumb/D1, index/D2, long/D3, ring/D4, little/D5.

joint on the forearm. Comparison of these two orthoses illustrates the value of designating the orthosis as hand-based (Fig. 1-11*a*) or forearm-based (Fig. 1-11*b*). Similarly, identifying the hand base of Figure 1-5 and the forearm base of Figure 1-11*d* helps distinguish the designs because both orthoses act on the MCPs. The orthosis in Figure 1-11*e* is finger based, applying dynamic corrective-extension force to a stiff PIP. However, the same orthotic objective can be achieved by a hand-based orthosis (Fig. 1-11*f*).

In summary, for orthoses acting on the hand, identify the base location proximal to the target joint or region as follows:

- Forearm-based
- Hand-based
- Finger-based
- Thumb-based

Sometimes an orthosis acting outside the hand also needs to have its base identified as in Figures 1-4, 1-11*c*, and 1-15*b*.

## Design Category

Identify the design category as discussed previously in this chapter as follows:

- Nonarticular
- Static
- Static (motion-blocking)
- Serial-static
- Static-progressive
- Dynamic
- Dynamic (motion-blocking)
- Dynamic traction
- Tenodesis
- Continuous passive motion

In the case of static or dynamic orthoses with a motion-blocking component, it is not necessary to include the term *motion-blocking* because this is indicated in the objective (e.g., flexion-blocking or extension-blocking).

## Target Joint, Region, or Bone

Identify the target joint, body region, or bone. For example, target joints include wrist (Fig.

1-3*a*), MCPs (Figs. 1-5, 1-11*a*, *b*, and *d*), PIPs (Fig. 1-11*e* and *f*), elbow (Figs. 1-8*b* and 1-9), and shoulder (Fig. 1-4), to name a few. If more than one joint is targeted, for example the MCPs and IPs of all fingers and the thumb, it is sometimes easier to identify a target body segment or region, which in this case would be the hand (Fig. 1-2*b*). Other target regions include the face (Fig. 1-1*c*), neck, back, and axilla. Descriptors identifying the target bone include humerus (Fig 1-1*a*), tibia, metacarpal, phalanx, and ulna (Fig. 1-1*b*) and are used when joints are excluded from an orthosis. For a complete list of joints, regions, and bones, refer to Table 1-3.

If a hand-based dynamic orthosis stabilizes the MCP joint of a finger to direct its extension force to the targeted PIP joint, it is not necessary to incorporate *MCP* in the name because its inclusion is implied by identifying the hand base and the target PIP joint (Fig. 1-11*f*).

For bones and joints in the hand, identify the specific digits:

- Thumb/D1 (Fig. 1-3*b*)
- Index/D2 (Figs. 1-10, 1-11*e* and *f*)
- Long/D3 (Fig. 1-12)
- Ring/D4
- Little/D5

If multiple digits are acted on, this is indicated as, for example, D2-5 (Fig. 1-15*a*). For a hand orthosis that acts on all the digits, it is not necessary to specify D1-D5 (Fig. 1-2*b*).

## Objective

Identify the orthotic objective using the following descriptors:

- Stabilizing (Fig. 1-1*a* and *b*)
- Scar-controlling (Fig. 1-1*c*)
- **Tone-reducing** (Fig. 1-6)
- **Protective** (Fig. 1-12)
- Assistive-extension (Fig 1-11*a* to *c*)
- Assistive-flexion
- Corrective-flexion (Fig. 1-11*d*)
- Corrective-extension (Fig. 1-11 *e* and *f*)
- Flexion-blocking (Fig. 1-8*b*)
- Extension-blocking (Figs. 1-8*a*, 1-12, and 1-13)

Identifying the objective is not required when the design category is static-progressive because it can be only corrective. Similarly, dynamic traction and continuous passive motion orthoses do not require description of their objectives. Note that some orthoses have more than one objective (Figs. 1-12 and 1-13).

## Variables

Additional optional descriptors help clarify the design. The list in Table 1-3 provides examples and is not comprehensive. Therapists can add variables at their discretion, and the variable can be positioned wherever it fits best in the name.

The concluding term is usually *orthosis,* which indicates that the device is primarily thermoplastic. However, some devices are constructed from elastic or webbing and are termed *strap* or *harness,* depending on the design. Another exception is the circumferential cervical orthosis, which is termed *collar.*

## ● **References**

1. Thomas, CL (ed): Taber's Cyclopedic Medical Dictionary, ed 18. FA Davis, Philadelphia, 1997.
2. Chan, SYC, et al: Splint Manual. Hong Kong, undated.
3. Logghe, R: Turbocast Thermoplastic Material: Guide to the Most Frequent Applications. T. Tape company B.V., The Netherlands, undated.
4. Malick, MH, and Carr, JA: Manual on Management of the Burn Patient. Harmarville Rehabilitation Center, Pittsburgh, 1982.
5. Orfit Industries: Orfit Splinting Guide, Antwerp, 1990.
6. Smith & Nephew Inc.: Smith & Nephew: Splinting Guidelines. Smith & Nephew Inc., Quebec, 1986.
7. Barr, NR, and Swan, D: The Hand: Principles and Techniques of Splintmaking, ed 2. Butterworth, London, 1988.
8. Balkan, J, and Blackmore, SM: Injury prevention through splinting. In Roth, J, and Levine, R: Prevention Practice—Strategies for Physical Therapy and Occupational Therapy. WB Saunders, Philadelphia, 1992.
9. Balkan, J, and English, CB: Hand splinting: principles, practice, and decision-making. In Pedretti, LW: Occupational Therapy—Practice Skills for Physical Dysfunction, ed 4. Mosby, St. Louis, 1996.
10. Cannon, NM, et al: Manual of Hand Splinting. Churchill Livingstone, New York, 1985.
11. Coppard, BM, and Lohman, H: Introduction to Splinting: A Critical Problem-Solving Approach. Mosby, St. Louis, 1996.
12. Fess, EE, and Kiel, JH: Upper-extremity splinting. In Hopkins, HL, and Smith, HD: Willard and Spackman's Occupational Therapy, ed 8. JB Lippincott, Philadelphia, 1993.
13. Fess, EE, and Philips, CA: Hand Splinting Principles and Methods. Mosby, St. Louis, 1987.
14. Kiel, JH: Basic Hand Splinting: A Pattern-Designing Approach. Little, Brown, Boston, 1983.
15. Malick, MH: Manual on Dynamic Hand Splinting with Thermoplastic Materials, ed 2. Harmarville Rehabilitation Center, Pittsburgh, 1982.
16. Malick, MH: Manual on Static Hand Splinting: New Materials and Techniques, ed 5. AREN Publications, Pittsburgh, 1985.
17. Malick, MH: Upper limb orthotics. Current Opinion in Orthopedics 1(3):450, 1990.
18. Malick, MH, and Kasch, MC (eds): Manual on Management of Specific Hand Problems. AREN Publications, Pittsburgh, 1984.
19. Moran, CA: Hand Rehabilitation. Churchill Livingstone, New York, 1986.
20. Schultz-Johnson, K: Splinting: A problem-solving approach. In Stanley, BG, and Tribuzi, SM: Concepts in Hand Rehabilitation. FA Davis, Philadelphia, 1992.
21. Tenney, CG, and Lisak, JM: Atlas of Hand Splinting: Little, Brown, Boston, 1986.
22. American Society of Hand Therapists (ASHT), Splint Nomenclature Task Force: Splint Classification System. ASHT, Garner, NC, 1991.
23. Mannarino, SL: Skeletal injuries. In Stanley, BG, and Tribuzi, SM: Concepts in Hand Rehabilitation. FA Davis, Philadelphia, 1992.
24. Stanley, BG, and Tribuzi, SM: Concepts in Hand Rehabilitation. FA Davis, Philadelphia, 1992.
25. Linden, CA, and Trombly, CA: Orthoses: Kinds and purposes. In Trombly, CA: Occupational Therapy for Physical Dysfunction, ed 5. Williams & Wilkins, Baltimore, 1995.
26. Zeigler, EM: Current Concepts in Orthotics: A Diagnosis Related Approach to Splinting. Rolyan Medical Products, Menomenee Falls, 1984.
27. Melvin, JL: Rheumatic Disease in the Adult and Child, Occupational Therapy and Rehabilitation, ed 3. FA Davis, Philadelphia, 1989.
28. Merritt, JL: Advances in orthotics for the patient with rheumatoid arthritis. J Rheumatol 14:62, 1987.
29. Licht, S (ed): Orthotics Etcetera. Elizabeth Licht, New Haven, 1966.
30. Dorland's Illustrated Medical Dictionary, ed 28. WB Saunders, 1994, p 1562.
31. Glance, WD, Anderson, KN, and Anderson, LE (eds): Mosby's Medical, Nursing and Allied Health Dictionary, ed 4. Mosby, St. Louis, 1994, p 1469.
32. Stedman's Medical Dictionary, ed 26. Williams & Wilkins, Baltimore, 1995, p 1655.
33. Webster's New Encyclopedic Dictionary, new revised ed. Black Dog and Leventhal Publishers, New York, 1995.
34. Smith & Nephew, Inc.: Rehabilitation Division Catalogue, 1997. Rolyan® is a trademark of Smith & Nephew, Inc.
35. Silver Ring Splint Company Catalogue, 1994. Siris and Silver Ring Splint are trademarks of Silver Ring Splint Company.
36. Bell, J: Plaster casting for the remodeling of soft tissue.

In Fess, EE, and Philips, CA: Hand Splinting Principles and Methods. Mosby, St. Louis, 1987.

37. Toronto Medical Orthopaedics Ltd. brochure, 1997.

38. Coutts, RD, et al: The use of continuous passive motion in the rehabilitation of orthopaedic problems. Contemporary Orthopaedics 16:75, 1988.

39. Hanes, B: Orthotics, splinting, and lifestyle factors. In Walker, JM, and Helewa, A: Physical Therapy in Arthritis. WB Saunders, Philadelphia, 1996.

40. Shurr, DG, and Cook, TM: Prosthetics and Orthotics. Appleton & Lange, Norwalk, Conn, 1990.

## CHAPTER 2

# Tissue and Joint Biomechanics

## Chapter Outline

# Histology and Nourishment of Connective Tissues

## DENSE CONNECTIVE TISSUES

Tendon, ligament, joint capsule, and dermis are dense connective tissues, composed primarily of **collagen** fibers, with small amounts of elastic fibers. Resident cells called fibroblasts synthesize both types of fiber. The orientation of the collagen fibers is **tension** dependent; that is, the collagen fibers become aligned with the tensile forces exerted on the tissues (Fig. 2–1). Habitual stress influences structure, which in turn defines the function of the structure. **Tendons** are exposed to unidirectional tensile forces; consequently, their fibers develop a parallel orientation, endowing the tendons with high tensile strength. **Ligaments** and **joint capsules** must withstand tensile loads in one predominant direction, as well as smaller tensile loads in other directions; as a result, their fibers are largely but not entirely parallel.[1] The fibers of the dermis have the least parallel orientation because of the application of multidirectional tensile forces.

Between the fibers and cells is amorphous material or ground substance. It permits the diffusion of **tissue fluid,** which transports oxygen and other nutrients from the bloodstream to the cells and waste products from the cells back to the bloodstream (Fig. 2-2). In this way, connective tissues are nourished.[2] Joint movement, either passive or active, facilitates the circulation of tissue fluid, whereas inactivity or immobilization promotes stasis and, consequently, poor nutrition of the tissues.[3]

Tissue fluid, also called interstitial fluid, is a filtrate of blood plasma that leaks naturally

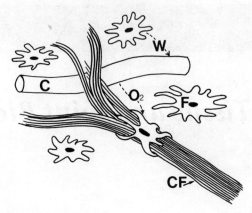

**FIGURE 2-2.** Schematic representation of how connective tissues are nourished by oxygen ($O_2$) and wastes (W) are removed. CF = collagen fibers; F = fibroblast; C = capillary.

from the capillaries. When tissues become injured or inflamed, resident cells release histamine, which causes vasodilation and increased capillary permeability.[2] Large amounts of tissue fluid leak into the injured or inflamed site, creating local swelling called **edema.** In the early stages, the edema is reversible. However, if it is allowed to persist for an extended period, the protein-rich tissue fluid will set like glue, becoming fibrotic and creating adhesions between the collagenous structures it surrounds.[4] Therefore, early intervention is important. Edema poses a serious threat to joint mobility and tendon excursion, and efforts to control it are a fundamental component of occupational therapy and physical therapy. See Chapter 3 for a discussion of implications of edema in orthotic intervention.

In many areas of the body, tendons have a dual source of nourishment, from blood vessels among the collagen fibers and from surrounding synovial sheaths. For example, the tendons of the long finger flexors receive a blood supply through the vinculi. However, sections of the tendon that are distant from the vinculi are avascular (Fig. 2-3). These sections are nourished by synovial fluid diffusion from the surrounding synovial sheaths.[5] As a result, nourishment of these **avascular** regions of the tendons depends on movement to help circulate the synovial fluid.

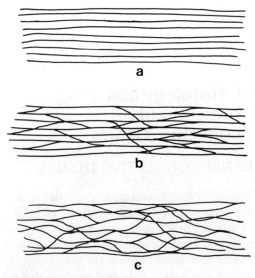

**FIGURE 2-1.** Orientation of collagen fibers in *(a)* tendon, *(b)* ligament, and *(c)* dermis.

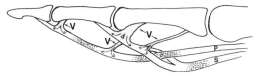

**FIGURE 2-3.** Blood vessels in the four vinculi (V) transmit oxygen (curved arrows) to the tendons of flexor digitorum superficialis (S) and profundus (P). Avascular regions of the tendons (stippled) rely on synovial fluid diffusion for nourishment.

## ARTICULAR CARTILAGE

Articular cartilage is a specialized connective tissue. In contrast to other connective tissues, it is avascular, nourished by nutrients that are absorbed through the surface of the cartilage from the synovial fluid.[3,6,7] Similar to tissue fluid, synovial fluid is a filtrate of blood plasma. It is produced by the richly vascular synovial membrane that lines the joint and, like tissue fluid, provides a two-way transport of nutrients from the bloodstream to the cartilage and waste products from the cartilage back to the bloodstream (Fig. 2-4a). The synovial membrane releases nutrient-rich synovial fluid into the joint cavity and removes waste-laden synovial fluid from the cavity. This transport is highly dependent on joint movement, which circulates the fresh synovial fluid to the surface of the cartilage, and is impaired by immobilization.[7]

The matrix of cartilage contains a proteoglycan gel that is strongly hydrophilic. Consequently, cartilage is a superhydrated, porous medium that behaves like a wet sponge, absorbing fluid from its surroundings when unloaded and expelling fluid when loaded.[6] To effectively absorb nutrients and expel wastes, cartilage requires cyclic loading and unloading through weight bearing and joint movement[6] (Fig. 2-4b and c). In the absence of loading and unloading, nutrition of the cartilage is impaired. Cartilage responds favorably to an optimal level of stress; conversely when it is under-

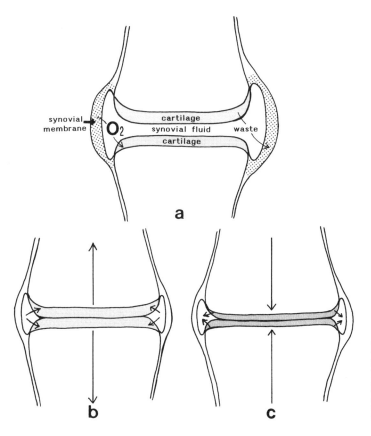

**FIGURE 2-4.** *(a)* Schematic representation of how articular cartilage is nourished. *(b)* Cyclical unloading and *(c)* loading of cartilage promotes absorption of nutrients *(b)* and emission of wastes *(c)*.

stressed, it begins to degenerate as a result of malnourishment.[8]

## CONTINUOUS PASSIVE MOTION ORTHOSES

Because of the absence of vascularity, adult cartilage has a slow turnover rate and consequently limited capacity for repair or regeneration when it degenerates (as in osteoarthritis) or becomes injured (as in an intra-articular fracture). Beginning in 1970, research by Coutts, Salter, and Mooney[8] drew attention to the harmful effects of immobilization and the benefits of motion to improve the nutrition and metabolic activity of cartilage. They also found that movement accelerated the healing of tendons and ligaments. Even adult cartilage, which was thought to be inert and lacking in regenerative capacity, healed after experimentally induced defects in animals were treated by continuous passive motion (CPM) orthoses. These devices have motors that passively move the target joints through a controlled arc of motion. Continuous passive motion orthoses have been created for the hand, wrist, elbow, shoulder, knee, and ankle (see Fig. 1-15).

Continuous passive motion orthoses maintain mobility, promote cartilage and tendon healing, and control edema and pain after a wide range of injuries or surgeries. However, there is controversy regarding whether CPM can overcome an established contracture.[8,9]

## ● How Connective Tissues Respond to Stress

### THE LOAD-DEFORMATION CURVE

Loading, through the application of a force, causes deformation within the structure being stressed. Figure 2-5*a* depicts a load-deformation curve (or stress-strain curve), which demonstrates how a structure, such as bone, deforms (or shows strain) in response to the application of a single load (or stress) of gradually increasing magnitude.

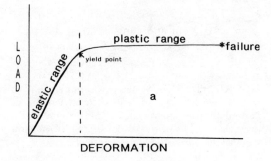

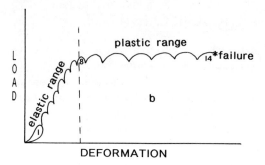

**FIGURE 2-5.** (*a*) Load-deformation curve for a semipliable material such as bone when a single load of increasing magnitude is applied. (Redrawn from Nordin and Frankel,[10] p 8.) (*b*) Diagram of the cumulative effect of repeated application of low stress when tissues are not allowed sufficient time to recover. As a one-time application (1), the load is within the elastic range. However, as successive loads are applied before the tissue has time to fully recover, each new deformation is added to the residual, unresolved deformation until, for example, after the application of 8 loads, when the deformation exceeds the yield point and enters the plastic range. In this case, during the 14th application of a low load, the deformation exceeds the plastic limit of the tissue, causing it to fail.

When a low load is applied, temporary deformation occurs within the elastic range of the structure. If the load is removed before the deformation exceeds the elastic limit of the tissue, the structure will return to its original shape. The deformation will immediately resolve and the structure will fully recover and return to its original state.[10] To illustrate this phenomenon, inflate a balloon slightly with air. As long as the deformation in the balloon remains within the elastic range, when it is deflated it will return to its original shape without any permanent distortion.

When the load exceeds the elastic limit, or **yield point,** plastic change occurs. When the load is removed, the structure will not return to its original form and some residual deformation will persist.[10] The balloon that is inflated beyond its elastic limit into its plastic range will not return to its original shape when deflated. The plastic change will have caused internal disruption and permanent deformation. Similarly, if living soft tissue is stretched beyond its yield point into its plastic range, microscopic injury in the form of fiber rupture and slippage occurs.[5] However, unlike the balloon, given time to recover in the absence of a stressful load, living tissues can repair themselves and remodel to eliminate the deformation.

If the load exerted on a structure exceeds its plastic limit, the structure will fail.[10] The overinflated balloon will burst; the overstressed bone will fracture; and the overstretched tendon or ligament will rupture.

## SUDDEN TRAUMA COMPARED WITH CUMULATIVE TRAUMA

The load-deformation model in Figure 2-5a depicts the response of a structure or tissue to the one-time application of a load of increasing magnitude. When a structure fails because of excessive loading, the injury is attributed to sudden trauma (i.e., a single excessive load). For example, when a fall on the outstretched hand causes a wrist fracture, the bone fails because it is subjected to a sudden stress that exceeds the plastic range. Similarly, when the ankle is forcefully inverted, sudden tensile forces that exceed its plastic range will cause the calcaneofibular ligament to tear, causing a sprain.

Tissue injury also occurs when the remodeling process is outpaced by the fatigue process.[10] As shown in Figure 2-5b, even if the repetitive stress is initially within the elastic range, if there is insufficient time for the deformation to resolve and the tissues are not allowed to fully recover, the cumulative effect of the repeated low stress will enter the plastic range. This is referred to as **cumulative trauma,** overuse injury, or repetitive strain injury. Examples include **tendinitis, tenosynovitis,** shinsplints, and nerve compression. If the stress is removed or

reduced, most connective tissues will repair themselves if given time to recover. However, if stress within the plastic range is reapplied before the repair is complete, additional microinjury will be added to the residual microinjury. The cumulative effect of the microtrauma will eventually exceed the plastic limit of the tissue, causing it to fatigue to the point of failure (e.g., tendon rupture, stress fracture).[10]

The interplay between load and repetition is summarized in the fatigue curve depicted in Figure 2-6. Tissue failure occurs either when a single, high-magnitude load exceeds the ultimate strength of the tissue or by repeated applications of a lower-magnitude load.[10] The lower the magnitude of the load, the more repetitions the tissue can withstand before it fatigues.

Most living tissues are self-repairing. The more vascular they are, and the younger they are, the more rapidly they can remodel. The key to minimizing the injurious effect of repetitive motions or stress is to keep the combined effect of load and repetition below the threshold injury line shown in Figure 2-6. This can be achieved by reducing the load; reducing the number of repetitions; or ensuring sufficient

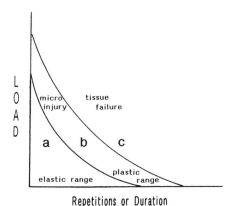

**FIGURE 2-6.** Fatigue curve. For example, clapping your hands repeatedly for 1 minute may stress the tissues within the elastic range *(a)*, causing no residual deformation once the clapping has ceased. Clapping your hands together for 10 minutes may elevate the tissue deformation into the plastic range *(b)*. Continued hand clapping will eventually exceed the limits of the plastic range and tissues will fatigue to the point of failure *(c)*. (Adapted from Nordin and Frankle,[10] p 19.)

recovery time to eliminate the injurious, cumulative effect of microstress.

## TISSUE GROWTH AND RESORPTION

Brand[11,12] was perhaps the first to describe how gentle, prolonged stress promotes growth of soft tissues whereas reduction or removal of tension promotes resorption of soft tissues. Therapists should have a good understanding of these reciprocal principles because they are often used when designing an orthosis and developing a wearing schedule.

When living tissue (skin, ligament, joint capsule, or tendon) is held in a slightly lengthened position (i.e., gentle, prolonged stretch) for a period of days, the fibroblasts will sense the tendon and synthesize more collagen, causing growth.[11,13] This phenomenon is clearly demonstrated in the abdominal wall of the pregnant woman. The gradual growth of the fetus exerts constant, gentle tension within the abdominal wall. The fibroblasts within the connective tissue sense the tension and respond by producing more collagen, causing tissue growth to accommodate the growing fetus.[12] Plastic surgeons have replicated this phenomenon to create extra skin for individuals with deep burns or other skin injuries, using a process called tissue expansion.[14–17]

Sometimes the fetus grows so quickly that tensile forces within the abdominal wall exceed the elastic limit of the skin and enter the plastic range. The resulting tissue injury is seen as stretch marks. However, not every pregnant woman develops stretch marks; the elastic limit of abdominal skin appears to vary among individuals, which is likely the case for all connective tissues.

After childbirth, the tissue of the abdominal wall becomes slack and redundant. The absence of tension (previously caused by the growing fetus) signals the body to **resorb** the excess tissue, restoring tissue length to the prepregnancy condition. The body does not maintain a range of motion or a redundancy of connective tissue that is not being used.[11] Because the body is not

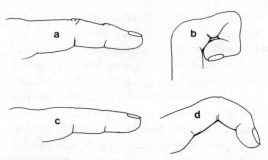

**FIGURE 2-7.** *(a)* Redundant skin over the interphalangeal (IP) joints that unfolds during flexion *(b)* to permit a full range of motion. *(c)* After immobilization in extension, the body has resorbed the redundant skin and the creases over the IP joints are lost. *(d)* As a result, IP flexion is limited.

using the redundant skin, it interprets that it is not needed, so the body resorbs it.

Tissue **resorption** is not always desirable. For example, when finger interphalangeal (IP) joints are immobilized in extension, the naturally occurring, slack skin over the extensor surface of these joints will not be subjected to the usual tensile forces that are exerted during IP joint flexion. After a few weeks of immobilization, the skin creases will disappear because of resorption of the underused slack skin.[11] Consequently, IP joint flexion will be restricted (Fig. 2-7). Internally, tendons, ligaments, and joint capsules will also shorten in the absence of habitual tensile forces.

## CONNECTIVE TISSUE REMODELING IN RESPONSE TO STRESS

Bone, tendon, ligament, joint capsule, and dermis are dynamic tissues in which there is a constant turnover of connective tissue, achieved by perpetual resorption and resynthesis of collagen by fibroblasts. The more **vascular** the tissue, the higher its metabolism and the faster its turnover rate. For example, bone is more vascular than ligaments and tendons, and thus repairs itself faster and regains its strength sooner after injury.[7]

The process of tissue remodeling is also greatly influenced by the frequency and magnitude of forces placed on the tissues, as shown in Figure 2-8. When the demands of habitual activity remain fairly constant, resorption and synthesis are balanced, thus maintaining the strength and length of the tissues and creating **homeostasis**.[7,18] When the tissues are challenged by stress that exceeds habitual levels, they will respond in one of two ways. Ideally, they will remodel and grow stronger or longer to accommodate the increased demands, provided that the stress is gradually increased and spread over time to allow the tissues to adapt. This is seen in a well-designed athletic training program. However, if the applied stress is too great or the demands are increased too quickly without sufficient time for them to adapt, the tissues will become fatigued and injured, and they may fail. At the other extreme, when tissues are understressed, they will **atrophy** and weaken. In conclusion, connective tissues need to be optimally stressed to either maintain their status or promote growth and strengthening. They respond adversely to both stress deprivation and stress overload.[11]

**Stress deprivation** occurs when activity levels are reduced below habitual levels; immobilization imposes the most severe form of stress deprivation, leading to decreased collagen strength. Prolonged immobilization of a synovial joint deprives it of essential stress, causing cartilage degeneration and joint adhesions.[19] Animal studies have shown that the tensile strength of connective tissue diminishes to about 40 percent after 6 weeks of immobilization; 9 months after restoration of activity, the tissues had regained only 80 percent of their original strength.[7]

## IMPLICATIONS IN ORTHOTIC INTERVENTION

Rehabilitation should focus on efforts to prevent or minimize the effects of stress deprivation. Prolonged joint immobilization is generally undesirable because of the rapid loss of tissue strength. Whenever possible, provide orthoses that promote movement and do not unnecessarily restrict joint motion. Immobilize only the joints that require stabilization to achieve the orthotic objectives. If the objective is to control joint position, as in carpal tunnel syndrome, consider a semiflexible orthosis rather than a rigidly immobilizing orthosis. Similarly, select dynamic rather than static designs when options are available.

In tendons and ligaments, movement helps the collagen fibers to orient themselves along the lines of greatest tensile force. As a result, orthoses for tendon injuries are designed to apply a controlled amount of stress to healing tendons.[20]

Where immobilization is warranted to promote healing, it is important to reintroduce movement as soon as possible. Therefore, a removable orthosis is generally preferable to a nonremovable cast. In addition, guidelines for discontinuing an orthosis should be clarified in the wearing regimen.

If joint stiffness has resulted from stress deprivation associated with immobilization, tissue strength is compromised and the threshold for failure is much lower. As a result, stressing the tissues with an orthosis to restore tissue length should be conducted with extreme caution.

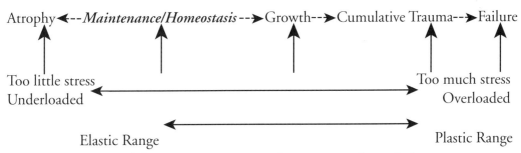

**FIGURE 2-8.**  How varying amounts of stress promote changes in tissues.

## ● How Orthoses Can Influence Tissue Length and Range of Motion

As discussed in Chapter 1, objectives of orthotic intervention include the following:

- Maintaining range of motion by preserving tissue length and tendon excursion
- Increasing range of motion by promoting soft tissue growth to reduce contractures
- Restabilizing a lax joint by promoting soft tissue resorption

### MAINTAINING TISSUE LENGTH AND RANGE OF MOTION

The objective of an orthosis may be to maintain the optimal length of tissues and prevent the loss of range of motion. For example, when the adult hand is injured, it is important to preserve the length of the metacarpophalangeal (**MCP**) and IP collateral ligaments by keeping these tissues taut. This is achieved by positioning the MCP joints in full flexion and the IP joints in full extension (Fig. 2-9*a*). These

positions also represent the close-packed position of the respective joints. (See *Joint Mechanics* later in this chapter.) To maintain the length of the flexor tendons, MCP flexion should be balanced with wrist extension to take up the slack in the flexor tendons (Fig. 2-9*b*), or they will resorb and shorten. Children are less susceptible to developing MCP collateral ligament contractures than adults; as a result, it is not necessary to position the child's MCP joints in flexion to preserve collateral ligament length.

Maintenance of tissue length is particularly important in the management of burns to prevent joint deformities. During the acute stage, the client who is in pain tends to adopt the position of comfort, which is fetal-like flexion of the extremities, while a hand adopts a **clawhand** posture (Fig. 2-10*a*). Perpetual malpositioning results in severe contractures of the involved joints; therefore during the acute stage it is essential to position the hand, as shown in Figure 2-10*b*, to maintain the length of the ligaments and flexor tendons and oppose the deforming position of comfort. Similarly, flexion deformities of other joints are prevented by ju-

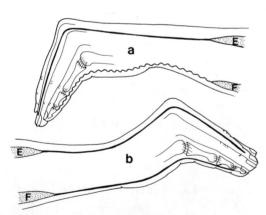

**FIGURE 2-9.** (*a*) Positioning the MCP joints in flexion and the IP joints in full extension keeps the respective collateral ligaments taut, exerting length-preserving tension to prevent contractures. The combination of wrist neutral (as shown here) and MCP flexion slackens the extrinsic finger flexors (F) and could cause them to resorb and shorten, limiting extension range. (*b*) Length-preserving tension is restored to the extrinsic finger flexors (F) by combining the MCP flexion with wrist extension. E = finger extensors.

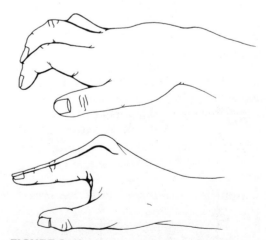

**FIGURE 2-10.** (*Top*) Dorsal hand edema creates tension in the dorsal skin, pulling the MCPs into hyperextension and the IPs into flexion, which causes a clawhand posture. (*Bottom*) The corrected position to prevent contractures that would develop with prolonged positioning in the clawhand posture: MCPs in 50 to 70° of flexion; IPs in extension (or slight flexion) and thumb well abducted, with a well-rounded web space.

dicious positioning that may need the support of an orthosis.

## PROMOTING TISSUE GROWTH TO REDUCE CONTRACTURES

Soft tissue contractures are resolved most effectively when a constant tensile force within their elastic range gently stretches the contracted tissues. The fibroblasts will sense the tension and synthesize more collagen so that the fibers will become elongated through growth. In contrast, lengthening that occurs because of tension within the plastic range of deformation is referred to as *creep*.[11] This is undesirable because elongation that has been achieved through trauma will give rise to inflammation, and the resulting scar tissue will probably restrict motion. If further tension is used, the tissue will eventually fail (i.e., tear or rupture).[10]

A study by Flowers and LaStayo[21] demonstrated that improvement in range of motion is directly proportional to the length of time a joint is held at its end range, which they called *total end range time* (TERT). The longer the TERT, the more quickly a contracture resolves. They also emphasized that there is a very narrow range of a clinically safe amount of force.

According to Cummings and Tillman,[18] 3° of gain in joint range of motion per week (with a range of 1° to 10° per week) is an acceptable standard for remodeling connective tissue. High-intensity short-term stretching, as occurs in manual therapy or a few minutes of traction, should be avoided. The resulting short-term strain of 4 to 6 percent will lengthen the tissue but at the expense of denaturing the collagen and tearing the fibers. Furthermore, high-intensity short-term stretching elicits a counterproductive painful inflammatory reaction that actually promotes stiffness.[11,18,22] Even a lower strain of 1½ to 2 percent is contraindicated if sustained for 1 hour or longer. It can cause occlusion of the circulation, **ischemic** trauma, and inflammation. Chronic inflammation produces pain and stimulates myofibroblast production, which in turn accelerates contracture by active contraction, favoring loss rather than

gain in motion[18] (see "Scar Management" later in this chapter).

A **torque-angle measurement** can demonstrate how responsive the tissues will be to tensile forces and the optimal joint angle to achieve the desired tissue tension within the elastic range.[11,12] The technique is described in Chapter 7.

Orthoses can offer a safe, effective medium for applying gentle, prolonged stretch.[23] However, therapists must ensure that the tension exerted by the orthosis is low and that the orthosis does no harm. Furthermore, one should also be cautious when prescribing a prefabricated corrective orthosis. According to Fess,[23] the amount of torque applied by some commercial orthoses is up to six times greater than the range advocated for soft tissue remodeling.

To ensure a safe amount of stress, one should use the client's feedback regarding the degree of comfort with the tension generated by the orthosis. The client should sense tension in the tissues but feel no pain. The adage "no pain, no gain" does not apply in contracture reduction. If the client feels pain, the tissues are being stretched in their plastic range, causing microinjury that obstructs tissue growth.

Hepburn[24] suggested the following guidelines for nontraumatic, effective stress applied by a dynamic orthosis. The stress should not be perceived as a "stretching" force until at least 1 hour has passed, and the client should remain comfortable with the orthosis for up to 12 hours.[24] After orthosis removal, the client should feel no more than a feeling of stiffness or a mild ache, which quickly resolves. This subjective feedback from the client helps guide the therapist to keep the stress below 1½ percent.

## PROMOTING TISSUE RESORPTION

When a joint has become unstable because of laxity of ligaments and tendon restraints (e.g., secondary to arthritic joint **effusion**), it readily subluxes (Fig. 2-11). Orthotic intervention can promote resorption of the redundant soft tis-

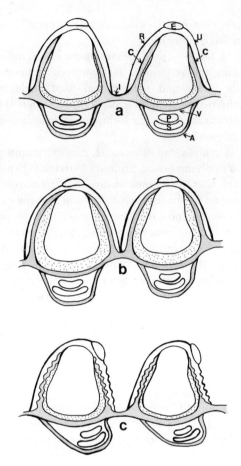

**FIGURE 2-11.** Cross section through the metacarpal (MC) heads showing flexor and extensor tendon restraints. *(a)* The unimpaired hand with good tendon alignment. On the volar side, the strong restraining fibers of the annular ligament (A) keep the tendons of flexor digitorum superficialis (S) and profundus (P) close to and centered across the MCP joint. Dorsally, equal tension through the radial (R) and ulnar (U) sagittal bands, which are anchored to the intermetacarpal ligament (I), keeps the central slip (E) of the extensor mechanism centered on top of the MC head. The collateral ligaments (C) span from the MC head to the proximal phalanx (not shown) and the volar plate (V). *(b)* MCP effusion (increased synovial fluid) resulting from joint inflammation is stretching the collateral ligaments, the sagittal bands, and the annular ligament. *(c)* After effusion has subsided, laxity in the collateral and annular ligaments promotes ulnar subluxation of the flexor tendons. Similarly, laxity in the sagittal bands promotes ulnar subluxation of the extensor tendon. Subluxation of the flexor and extensor tendons leads to MCP ulnar drift. (Adapted from Kapandji,[82] p 183.)

sues to restabilize the joint. This is achieved by underloading the lax joint tissues by positioning the joint in its loose-packed position, thereby neutralizing any potential malaligning forces (see "Joint Mechanics" later in this chapter). For example, when the MCPs become unstable and begin to sublux ulnarly (i.e., ulnar drift) or volarly (Fig. 2-12), the orthosis should position the MCPs in neutral deviation and slight flexion.[25] This slackens the annular ligaments, radial sagittal bands, and radial MCP collateral ligaments; under ideal circumstances, the body will resorb the redundant soft tissue, the ligaments will shorten, and joint stability will improve.

The efficacy of this approach is enhanced by early intervention, before joint subluxation progresses too far and before the articular structures become irreversibly damaged. For example, a young woman with rheumatoid arthritis of 5 years' duration had the early stages of MCP ulnar drift in the ring and little fingers. Whenever she made a fist, the extensor tendons over the fourth and fifth MC heads would sublux ulnarly because of lax radial sagittal bands (Fig. 2-13a). She was fitted with an orthosis (Fig. 2-13b, c, and d) that prevented ulnar deviation and blocked the MCPs in slight flexion so that the extensor tendons would not be allowed to sublux. After 5 months of continuous orthotic use, the ulnar drift had been corrected and the tendons no longer subluxed when the MCPs were flexed. In the absence of stressful MCP flexion, the integrity of the sagittal bands had been restored and they were once again able to keep the extensor tendons centralized over the MC heads (Fig. 2-11a). Because of the recurring cycle of joint inflammation, the client was advised to wear the orthosis whenever the joints became effused, whenever tendon subluxation recurred, or when she engaged in strenuous hand activities. A follow-up 5 years later found that joint subluxation had not recurred.

For individuals with C6 quadriplegia, orthoses are used to help promote functional contractures of the finger flexors to develop tenodesis grasp (see Chapter 10). Tenodesis is described later in this chapter.

**FIGURE 2-12.** MCP malalignment that can develop when MCP joint effusion causes ligamentous laxity. *(a)* Lateral view demonstrates MCP volar subluxation. (From Melvin,[25] p 276, with permission.) *(b)* Dorsal view demonstrates MCP ulnar drift. (From Melvin,[25] p 281, with permission.)

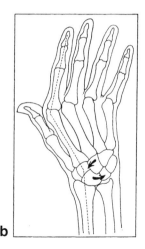

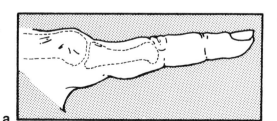

## ● Joint Mechanics and Considerations for Positioning Hand Joints

With the exception of nonarticular designs, orthoses cross at least one joint, affecting joint mobility and influencing tissue tension within the joint capsule, ligaments, tendons, and skin.

To a large extent, joint positioning controls tissue tension.

### TENSION IN JOINT TISSUES

Joint positioning may be either close- or loose-packed, and the articular capsule and ligaments will be correspondingly taut or slack. Close-

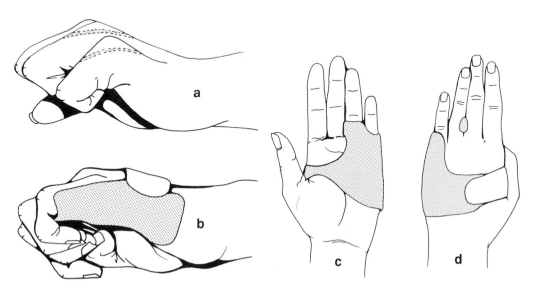

**FIGURE 2-13.** *(a)* Ulnar subluxation of the extensor tendons off the fourth and fifth MC heads occurring when the fingers are flexed, due to laxity of the radial sagittal bands. *(b, c, d)* Circumferential hand-based static D4/5 MCP-stabilizing orthosis fabricated from 1/16 in. (1.6 mm) thick thermoplastic.

**TABLE 2–1. Close-Packed and Loose-Packed Joint Positions and Positions of Least Intra-articular Pressure and Implications for Orthotics**

| Joint | Close-Packed Position[37] | Implication for Orthoses | Loose-Packed Position (Resting Position)[37] | Implication for Orthoses | Position of Least Intra-articular Pressure[39] | Implication for Orthoses |
|---|---|---|---|---|---|---|
| Facet | Extension | Contraindicated due to articular cartilage compression | Midway between flexion and extension | Appropriate positioning for cervical collar | | Spontaneous position of effused joints |
| Glenohumeral | Abduction and lateral rotation | | 55° abduction, 30° horizontal adduction | Postsurgical positioning to prevent capsular tension | 30° to 65° abduction, 0° external rotation, 0° flexion | Recommended positioning when providing orthoses to rest inflamed joints |
| Elbow (ulnohumeral) | Extension | | 70° flexion, 10° supination | Resting position when joint is inflamed | 30° to 75° flexion | |
| Wrist (radiocarpal) | Extension with radial deviation | | Neutral with slight ulnar deviation | | Neutral flexion and deviation | |
| Thumb Carpometa- carpal (CMC) | Full opposition | | Midway between abduction/adduction Midway between flexion/extension | | | |
| Finger MCPs | Full flexion | Preserves length of adult MCP collateral ligaments | Slight flexion | Promotes resorption of lax MCP collateral ligaments | | |

| | | | | | |
|---|---|---|---|---|---|
| Thumb MCP | Full operation | | Slight flexion | | |
| Finger IPs | Full extension | Preserves length of adult IP collateral ligaments | Slight flexion | Promotes resorption of lax IP collateral ligaments | |
| Hip | Full extension, medial femoral rotation | | 30° flexion, 30° abduction, slight lateral rotation | | 30° to 65° flexion, 15° abduction, 15° lateral rotation |
| Knee | Full extension with lateral rotation of the tibia | | 25° flexion | | 15° to 60° flexion |
| Ankle | Maximum dorsiflexion | Maintains length of calcaneal tendon | 10° plantar flexion, midway between maximum inversion and eversion | | 15° plantar flexion |
| Subtalar | Supination | | Midway between extremes of range of movement | | Midposition |
| Midtarsal | Supination | | Midway between extremes of range of movement | | |

packed and loose-packed refer to the amount of joint play, or accessory movement available as a result of joint position and resulting tension in the capsule and ligaments. Accessory movements are the small amount of passive range of motion that is not under voluntary control. A comprehensive list of close- and loose-packed joint positions is found in Table 2-1.

When a joint is in its close-packed position (i.e., joint surfaces are close together), the joint surfaces are fully congruent and held tightly together by maximal tension in the joint capsule and ligaments.[26] The position makes the ligaments and capsule taut and twisted, cinching the joint surfaces together and compressing the articular cartilage (Fig. 2-14a). This is the final limiting position of a joint. At the knee, the close-packed position is full extension with lateral rotation of the tibia. This combination locks the knee and is referred to as the screw-home mechanism.[26] In the foot, locking is achieved by the combined actions of subtalar supination and midtarsal pronation.

In the hand, the MCPs are close-packed when in full flexion and the IPs are close-packed when in full extension[27] (Fig. 2-15a). It is important to incorporate this positioning into an orthosis for the adult hand so as to preserve the length of the collateral ligaments and to maintain a full range of motion of the MCPs and IPs. Children are less susceptible to collateral ligament shortening than adults are; as a result, this type of range-preserving positioning is not required in children.

At the other extreme is a joint's loose-packed, or resting, position in which joint surfaces are minimally congruent and the joint capsule and ligaments are completely lax (Fig. 2-14b). The position is usually midrange, there is maximal joint play, and the joint surfaces can be distracted by moderate tensile forces.[26] The joint capsule has its greatest capacity when the joint is loose-packed. An effused joint will spontaneously assume the loose-packed position to minimize the tension in the capsule and ligaments and to minimize intra-articular pressure.[28] If an orthosis is applied when there is effusion, the joints should be supported in their loose-packed position because inflamed tissues should not be stretched.[29] In the hand, the MCPs are loose-packed when fully extended[27] (Fig. 2-15b).

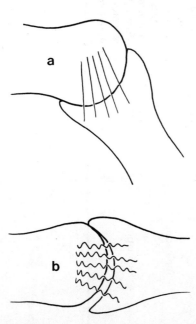

**FIGURE 2-14.** *(a)* Close-packed position of a joint, demonstrating fully congruent joint surfaces that are held tightly together by maximal tension in the joint ligaments. *(b)* Loose-packed position of a joint, demonstrating poor congruence between the joint surfaces and lax joint ligaments.

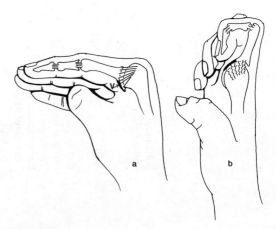

**FIGURE 2-15.** *(a)* Close-packed joints: MCPs in full flexion and IPs in full extension. The collateral ligaments are maximally taut. V = volar plate. *(b)* Loose-packed joints: MCPs extended joints. The collateral ligaments are slack.

These fundamental joint mechanics are important considerations when determining how to position a joint. When the objective is to maintain tissue length in the joint capsule and ligament, the close-packed position is appropriate because it creates the necessary tension to preserve the length of the articular soft tissues. When a joint is unstable and tending to sublux because of lax ligaments and joint capsule, the loose-packed position removes tension and promotes resorption of the articular soft tissues to restabilize the joint. Similarly, when tissues are inflamed, tension is contraindicated and loose-packed positioning is desirable.

## INTRA-ARTICULAR PRESSURE AND EFFUSED JOINTS

In 1964 Eyring and Murray[28] reported a landmark investigation of intra-articular pressure using a water manometer connected to a needle inserted into normal, effused, and cadaveric joints of human subjects. Their findings are contained in Table 2-1. They found that effused joints spontaneously assume a position of least pressure, which corresponds closely to a loose-packed position, to minimize discomfort.

The implication of these findings to orthotic intervention is that, when providing an orthosis for an effused joint, the objective should be to rest the joint in a position of least intra-articular pressure to minimize pain caused by the excess synovial fluid stretching the joint capsule (see Table 2-1). Attempts to position an effused joint otherwise will cause undue pain and a contraindicated stretch of the inflamed tissues.

## IMPACT OF JOINT POSITION ON TISSUE TENSION IN THE HAND

### Intrinsic Muscles

Passive MCP flexion and IP extension create length-preserving tension in the collateral ligaments of these joints. At the same time, this positioning produces slack in the intrinsic muscles, specifically the lumbricals and in-

terossei (Fig. 2-16*a*). It seems to be a paradox that the same position is achieved by the active contraction of the lumbricals and interossei. When there is effusion at the MCPs, the intrinsic muscles (i.e., the lumbricals and interossei) go into spasm, which is the body's natural defense mechanism to "splint" the inflamed joints. As a result, this position is referred to as the **intrinsic plus position.** Prolonged maintenance of the intrinsic plus position, either by muscle spasm or an orthosis, can cause intrinsic muscle shortening (also called **intrinsic tightness**). Consequently, orthoses for the vulnerable adult rheumatoid hand should position the MCPs in extension (or slight flexion) to exert length-preserving tension on the intrinsic muscles. In addition, the client should be instructed how to passively stretch the intrinsic muscles—gently flexing the IPs while extending the MCPs—when the joints are not inflamed (Fig. 2-16*b*). In this position, the intrinsics are maximally stretched.[25]

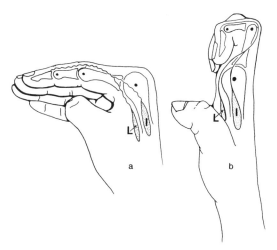

**FIGURE 2-16**. (*a*) The intrinsic muscles (L = lumbrical and I = interosseous) are fully slack when the MCPs are passively, fully flexed and the IPs are passively, fully extended. This position is called intrinsic plus. Note the course of the intrinsic tendons, passing to the volar side of the MCP axis (dot) and the dorsal side of the IP axes (dots). (*b*) The intrinsic muscles are maximally taut when the MCPs are passively, fully extended and the IPs are passively, fully flexed. In addition, the skin creases over the IP joints are fully unfolded, creating length-preserving tension in the dorsal skin over the fingers. This position is called intrinsic minus.

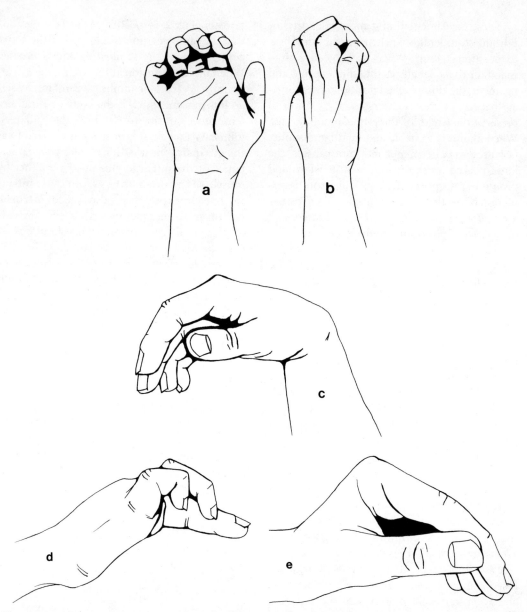

**FIGURE 2-17.**   Hand deformities due to muscle paralysis from peripheral nerve lesions. (*a*) and (*b*) Claw-hand deformity caused by loss of median and ulnar nerve innervation to the intrinsic muscles. The thenar and hypothenar eminences are atrophied and the first web space is contracted. (*c*) Wrist drop deformity resulting from midhumeral lesion of radial nerve. Active wrist extension, MCP extension, IP extension, and abduction of thumb are absent. (*d*) Partial clawhand deformity resulting from ulnar nerve lesion at the wrist. Ring and little fingers are hyperextended at MCPs and flexed at IPs. The hypothenar eminence is atrophied. (*e*) Ape-hand deformity resulting from a median nerve lesion at the wrist. When opposition is attempted, as shown here, the thumb cannot fully abduct and rotate to create a tip or tripod pinch because of paralysis of thenar muscles. Lateral pinch is substituted.

When a peripheral nerve injury paralyzes the intrinsic muscles, the MCPs spontaneously hyperextend and the IPs flex, creating a claw-hand deformity, called the **intrinsic minus position** (Fig. 2-17a and b). To preserve the length of the MCP collateral ligaments, provide an orthosis that positions the MCPs in about 60° of flexion.

## Dorsal Skin

In addition to preserving the length of intrinsic muscles, IP flexion maintains the folds in the dorsal skin over the IP joints. These wrinkles unfold during IP flexion and are essential to permit the full range of flexion. In the absence of length-preserving tension due to prolonged positioning in IP extension, the body will resorb the redundant skin and IP flexion will be restricted (see Fig. 2-8c and d).[11] If the IPs require immobilization in extension to maintain collateral ligament length, frequent active or passive IP flexion should be carried out, unless contraindicated, to prevent dorsal skin contracture.

## Extrinsic Muscles

Passive positioning to achieve composite flexion of the wrist, MCPs, and IPs creates tension in the extrinsic finger extensors and wrist extensors while the extrinsic finger flexors and wrist flexors are left slack (Fig. 2-18a). Conversely, composite extension of the wrist, MCPs, and IPs creates tension through the extrinsic finger flexors and wrist flexors while the extrinsic finger extensors and wrist extensors are left slack (Fig. 2-18b). The concern is that prolonged positioning that creates tension through a muscle group causes it to elongate to the point that it may be unable to generate enough tension to move the joints through their full active range. Conversely, the slack muscle group could shorten in the absence of length-preserving tension.

This situation can develop after a peripheral nerve injury. For example, when a midhumeral radial nerve injury results in **wrist drop** as seen in Figure 2-17c, the extrinsic extensors may elongate, while the extrinsic flexors may become contracted.[30] Orthotic intervention can position the joints to correct the forces through the muscles and prevent these changes in muscle length. For example, a wrist orthosis will

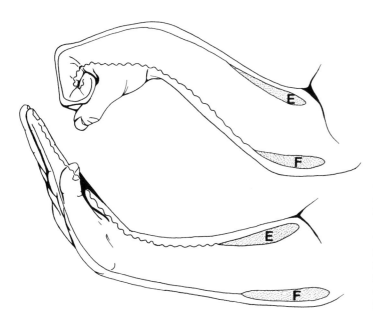

**FIGURE 2-18.** *(a)* Composite flexion of the wrist, MCPs and IPs creating tension through the wrist extensors and the extrinsic finger extensors (E) and leaving the wrist flexors and extrinsic finger flexors (F) fully slack. *(b)* Composite extension of the wrist, MCPs and IPs creating tension through the wrist flexors and the extrinsic finger flexors (F) and leaving the wrist extensors and extrinsic finger extensors (E) fully slack.

position the wrist to prevent contracture of the wrist flexors and enhance hand function (see Fig. 1-3*a*).

Sometimes the treatment protocol requires joint positioning that disrupts the balance of tension through the extrinsic muscles. For example, after surgical repair for a flexor tendon injury, an orthosis is applied to position the wrist, MCPs, and IPs in composite flexion to prevent injurious tension through the healing tendon (see Fig. 1-12). The therapist must always be cognizant of the forces that an orthosis is applying or neutralizing and the consequences of this force manipulation.

## Tenodesis

Tenodesis refers to the synergistic coupling of wrist extension with finger flexion and, conversely, the coupling of wrist flexion with finger extension (Fig. 2-19). This function occurs because wrist extension takes up the slack in the extrinsic finger flexors, creating sufficient tension in the tendons to passively pull the fingers into flexion. Conversely, wrist flexion absorbs the slack in the extrinsic finger extensors and creates sufficient tension to passively pull the fingers into extension.

Tenodesis occurs naturally during hand activities. When the hand is approaching an object to pick it up, the fingers extend and the wrist flexes. As the hand closes around the object, the fingers flex and the wrist extends.

In the case of wrist drop described earlier, the flexed wrist is accompanied by MCP extension that slackens the collateral ligaments (Fig. 2-17*c*). This posture should not be allowed to persist because the collateral ligaments will resorb, causing loss of MCP flexion range. Orthotic intervention is directed to preventing contracture of the collateral ligaments and wrist flexors, as well as enhancing hand function.

Individuals with a spinal cord injury between the fifth and sixth cervical (C6) vertebrae have innervation to the level of C6. As a result, the C6 myotome serving the wrist extensors is intact, whereas the C7 myotome to the finger extensors and the C8 myotome to the finger flexors are nonfunctional. A person with C6 **quadriplegia** learns to use wrist extension to achieve finger flexion to grasp objects, using the natural tenodesis function.[31] To release objects, the individual relaxes the wrist extensors, allowing the wrist to flex; this creates tension in the finger extensors, which in turn promotes finger extension. Orthotic intervention can help the individual learn tenodesis grasp and promote functional contractures of the finger flexors to strengthen the grasp (see Fig. 1-14).

## POWER GRASP AND WRIST POSITIONING

Whenever one attempts to grasp an object with a strong **power grip,** the wrist spontaneously extends, demonstrating the synergy between the wrist extensors and the finger flexors (Fig. 2-20). Wrist extension is essential to optimize the power of the finger flexors. The radial nerve innervates the wrist extensors. If this nerve is injured, wrist extension will be weakened, impairing the power grasp. If the muscles are completely paralyzed as in a radial nerve injury, active wrist extension is lost and the hand assumes a drop wrist posture (Fig. 2-17*c*). Similarly, if the muscles innervated by the ulnar nerve are paralyzed, power grasp is disrupted because the individual will be unable to adequately flex all the MCPs to achieve a strong

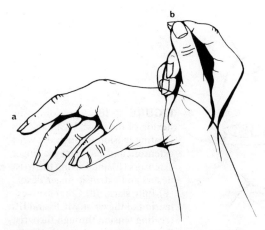

**FIGURE 2-19.**   Tenodesis. *(a)* Synergistic coupling of wrist flexion with finger extension. *(b)* Synergist coupling of wrist extension with finger flexion.

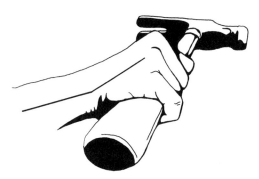

**FIGURE 2-20.**  Power grasp demonstrating pronounced wrist extension to create tension in the extrinsic finger flexors to grip the hammer tightly.

grip. The hand assumes the partial **clawhand deformity** characterized by MCP hyperextension and IP flexion of the ring and little fingers (Fig. 2-17*d*). Orthotic intervention can counteract the drop wrist posture and the partial clawhand. Specific orthoses are described in Chapters 10 and 11.

When a wrist orthosis is provided for the individual who needs gross grasp or a power grip, the wrist should be positioned in functional extension, ranging from 15° to 30°, depending on the task. The therapist should observe the amount of wrist extension that naturally occurs for each client during a power grasp and replicate it during the molding process.

In addition to the flexion-extension sagittal plane, the coronal plane should also be considered. While the forearm is positioned midway between pronation and supination, observe how the wrist deviates during a power grasp. Some wrists radially deviate, some ulnarly deviate, and some remain neutral (Fig. 2-21). When molding an orthosis to promote a power grasp, the naturally occurring deviation should be incorporated into the wrist positioning, along with the appropriate degree of wrist extension. An exception is when the deviation actually represents subluxation at the radiocarpal joint. A radial deviation deformity at the wrist often develops in the adult hand with **rheumatoid arthritis,** whereas the child with rheumatoid arthritis is more likely to develop an ulnar deviation wrist deformity.[25] In either circumstance, a wrist orthosis is designed to position the wrist in a neutral position in the coronal plane.

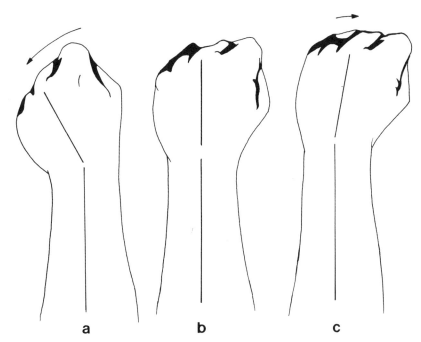

**FIGURE 2-21.**  Differing degrees of wrist deviation that can occur concomitantly with wrist extension. (*a*) Ulnar deviation. (*b*) Neutral. (*c*) Radial deviation.

## THE MOBILE DISTAL TRANSVERSE ARCH

As demonstrated in Figure 2-22a, during a relaxed grip, the metacarpal heads are aligned to form a gentle convex curve. This curve represents the distal transverse arch (DTA). However, when the fist is strongly clenched, the arch deepens because of the volar movement of the fourth and fifth MC heads (Fig. 2-21b). Mobility of the ulnar side of the hand is essential to a strong power grasp. Similarly, when the thumb opposes the tip of the little finger, the fifth MC head moves volarly.

These observations have implications in orthotic fabrication. To enable full MCP flexion, preserve the mobility of the fourth and fifth metacarpals, and allow the DTA to deepen, it is important to correctly position the distal edge of a wrist orthosis as discussed in Chapter 3. When molding an orthosis into the palm of the hand, conform the material to the contour of the transverse arch, with the apex at the third MC head (Fig. 2-21c). The client should feel the support in the palm of the hand.

## FINGER FLEXION TOWARD THE SCAPHOID

Individually each finger flexes toward the scaphoid bone. Pure sagittal flexion occurs only in the long finger. During flexion, the MCP of the index rotates slightly ulnarly, while the MCP of the ring finger rotates slightly radially (Fig. 2-23a). The little finger exhibits the great-

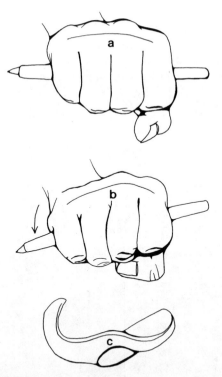

**FIGURE 2-22.** The distal transverse arch depicted by the curve of the metacarpal heads. (a) When the pen is loosely held in the hand, the curve is gently convex. (b) When the pen is firmly grasped in the hand, the convex curve deepens as the fourth and fifth metacarpal heads move volarly. (c) Palmar contour of a thumb-hole wrist orthosis conforming to the contour of the distal transverse arch.

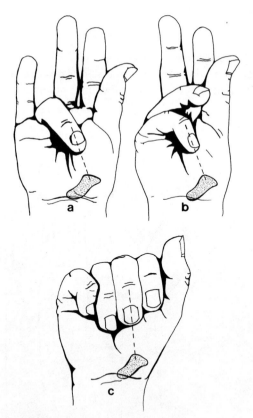

**FIGURE 2-23.** Flexion of the fingers toward the scaphoid (shaded). (a) Moderate radial orientation of the ring finger toward the scaphoid. (b) Pronounced radial orientation of the little finger toward the scaphoid. (c) Flexion of all fingers generally toward the scaphoid.

est amount of rotation as it flexes with a pronounced radial orientation at the MCP (Fig. 2-23*b*). When all four fingers flex together, the scaphoid orientation is less pronounced, but still apparent (Fig. 2-23*c*). This phenomenon has implications when making a dynamic or static-progressive orthosis that pulls the fingers into flexion (e.g., for a flexor tendon injury or to correct MCP and IP contractures). As discussed in Chapter 3, the therapist must position the pulleys so that the flexion force pulls the fingers toward the scaphoid.

## PRECISION FUNCTION AND THUMB POSITIONING

Whereas the mobility of the two ulnar **rays** is important to generate force during power grasp, the three radial rays endow the hand with dexterous fine prehension. The thumb abducts and rotates to oppose the index in the **tip pinch,** which is commonly used to pick up and hold small objects (Fig. 2-24*a*). In the **tripod pinch** (also called three-jaw chuck), the thumb opposes the index and long finger and is used, for example, to grip a pen when writing (Fig. 2-24*b*).

Thumb opposition, which occurs in both the tip pinch and tripod pinch, requires median nerve innervation to the thenar muscles. If the motor branch of the median nerve is lacerated, the resulting paralysis to the thenar muscles will mean the loss of thumb abduction and rotation. Consequently, thumb opposition is lost, resulting in the **ape-hand deformity** depicted in Figure 2-17*e*. Orthotic intervention can counteract the deforming posture and prevent a web space contracture. If the median nerve is not completely disrupted, but rather compromised by excess pressure in the carpal tunnel, active thumb opposition may be weakened, depending on the extent of the nerve damage.

When an object is gripped between the thumb and side of the index in the **lateral (or key) pinch** (Fig. 2-24*c*), the first dorsal interosseous muscle counteracts the force applied by adductor pollicus. The ulnar nerve innervates both of these muscles. As a result, when an injury to this nerve

impairs the innervation of these muscles, the lateral pinch is weakened or lost.

In the rheumatoid hand, intrinsic muscle weakness leaves the first dorsal interosseous

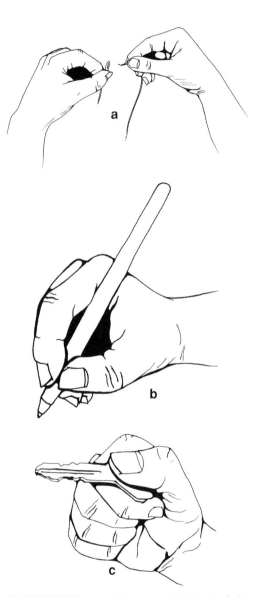

**FIGURE 2-24.** Precision grips. (*a*) Tip pinch, between the tip of the thumb and the index, demonstrated in both hands when threading a needle. Note the slightly flexed position of the wrists for this precision activity. (*b*) Tripod pinch (three-jaw chuck) between the tip of the thumb and the tips of the index and long fingers, commonly used to grasp a pen. (*c*) Lateral (or key) pinch between the pad of the thumb and the lateral side of the index, commonly used to grasp a key.

muscle unable to counteract the ulnar force of the thumb. As a result, lateral pinch, in addition to other pathomechanics, can contribute to the development of **ulnar drift.** The susceptible client should be educated to avoid lateral pinch and to use adapted keys with long levers to avoid unnecessary ulnar stress. Specific orthoses, designed to protect against ulnar drift and compensate for weak intrinsic muscles, are described in Chapters 10 and 11.

## ORTHOTIC INTERVENTION TO ENABLE PRECISION FUNCTION

To enable precision function of the hand, the thumb must be able to position itself to easily contact the index and long fingers. If an orthosis is designed to leave the thumb free, it is important to permit full range of motion. This is achieved by ensuring that the thenar eminence is fully exposed. For this purpose, the thenar crease serves as a suitable reference as described in Chapter 7.

If the orthosis is designed to restrict thumb motion, as required to rest inflamed tendons in **de Quervain's tenosynovitis,** it is important to immobilize the thumb in a position that will enable easy opposition. If the thumb is poorly positioned, the index and long fingers will need to radially deviate to make contact and the hand must work unnaturally in attempting a precision grip. During orthotic molding, position the thumb so that it can readily oppose the index and long fingers (Fig. 2-25). Having the client grip a pen in a tripod pinch while the thermoplastic cools can facilitate positioning.

When a nerve lesion paralyzes the thenar muscles, the thumb assumes an adducted position (Fig. 2-17a and e). If the first web space is not preserved with an orthosis, when the thenar muscles are reinnervated they will be unable to overcome the contracture to oppose the thumb. Therefore, thumb mobility requires preservation of the first web space to be able to achieve a tip or tripod pinch (Fig. 2-26).

Unlike gross grasp, which requires wrist extension to generate sufficient power in the finger flexors, precision function often requires neutral alignment or flexion of the wrist to position the fingers to pick up and manipulate objects (Fig. 2-27a). If an orthosis has positioned the wrist in

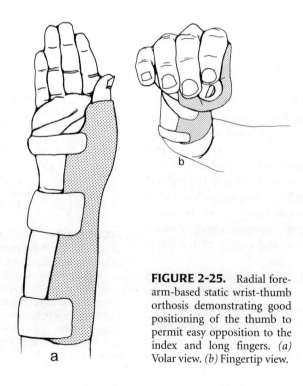

**FIGURE 2-25.** Radial forearm-based static wrist-thumb orthosis demonstrating good positioning of the thumb to permit easy opposition to the index and long fingers. *(a)* Volar view. *(b)* Fingertip view.

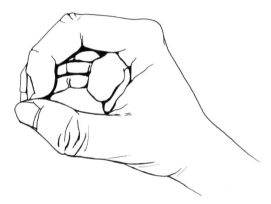

**FIGURE 2-26.** Position of thumb to preserve the C-shaped first web space.

extension, the individual must compensate with shoulder abduction to position the fingers for fine prehensive activities (Fig. 2-27*b*). As a result, the therapist must consider the best compromise position in which to immobilize the wrist—extension to promote a power grasp or neutral to slight flexion to promote precision function. This consideration requires the client's input and an analysis of the type of activities the individual performs. An ideal orthosis might have a wrist positioner that the client can easily adjust to change the angle of the wrist flexion-extension, in much the same way that hand prostheses have wrist flexion units.

If an orthosis is designed to enable handwriting, it is important to analyze the client's wrist position while doing this task. Although most right-handed individuals extend their wrist when writing (Fig. 2-28*a*), the left-handed writer may flex the wrist to prevent smearing the text that has been written (Fig. 2-28*b*). Each client deserves individual consideration concerning the wrist position that will best promote function. In addition, not everyone uses a tripod pinch to grip a pen. Again, observation of the individual's writing approach is necessary to ensure that the orthosis will enable the client's individual prehensive style.

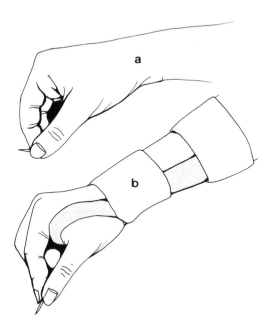

**FIGURE 2-27.** (*a*) To pick up an object, the wrist naturally flexes slightly. (*b*) An orthosis that positions the wrist in extension interferes with the ease of picking up small objects. To compensate, the shoulder must abduct to orient the fingertips to reach the tabletop.

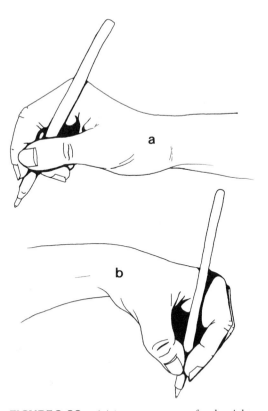

**FIGURE 2-28.** (*a*) A common grasp for the right-handed writer, positioning the wrist in extension. (*b*) A common grasp for the left-handed writer, positioning the wrist in flexion.

## ASSESSMENT OF OPTIMAL WRIST POSITION BEFORE WRIST FUSION

If surgical fusion of the wrist is warranted, presurgical considerations should include an evaluation of the optimal position in which to fuse the wrist to promote functional use of the hand. A therapist can fabricate a series of wrist orthoses, immobilizing the wrist in various degrees of extension/flexion and deviation to determine the position that is the best compromise. For this purpose, a low-temperature thermoplastic with memory facilitates multiple reheatings and remoldings. In addition, a circumferential wrist orthosis provides more rigid immobilization than a half-shell design and better replicates the rigidity of a wrist fusion.

## ● Selected Applications of Orthotic Intervention

### CARPAL TUNNEL SYNDROME

Figure 2-29 shows a cross-sectional view through the wrist revealing the complex arrangement of flexor and extensor tendons, intrinsic muscles, restraining retinacula, nerves and blood vessels, and the arched configuration of the carpal bones forming the immobile proximal transverse arch. The flexor retinaculum bridges across from the hamate to the trapezium, forming the roof of the carpal tunnel, which contains the tendons of flexor carpi radialis, flexor pollicus longus, flexor digitorum superficialis, and flexor digitorum profundus. Synovial sheaths, which contain a minus-

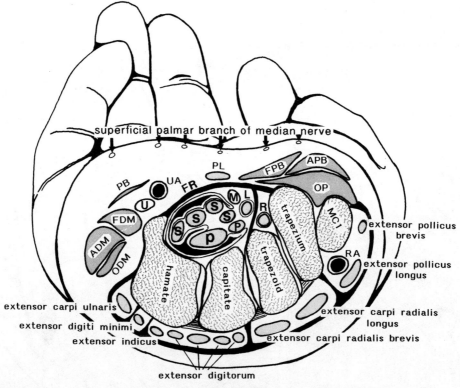

**FIGURE 2-29.**   Cross section through distal row of carpal bones. ADM = abductor digiti minimi; APB = abductor pollicus brevis; FDM = flexor digiti minimi; FPB = flexor pollicus brevis; FR = flexor retinaculum; L = flexor pollicus longus; M = median nerve; MC1 = first metacarpal; ODM = opponens digiti minimi; P = flexor digitorum profundus; PB = palmaris brevis; PCM = palmar cutaneous branches of the median nerve; PL = palmaris longus; R = flexor carpi radialis; RA = radial artery; S = flexor digitorum superficialis; U = ulnar nerve; UA = ulnar artery. (Redrawn with permission from Snell,[83] p 231.)

cule amount of synovial fluid to lubricate the inner walls, surround the tendons.

Also contained in the carpal tunnel is the vulnerable median nerve, which contains motor fibers destined for the thenar muscles and sensory fibers traveling from the radial three and one-half fingers. The superficial palmar branch (sensory) of the median nerve courses over the flexor retinaculum. As a result, when pressure within the carpal tunnel rises because of synovial sheath synovitis, local tissue swelling, or wrist flexion, sensory disturbance is felt in the radial fingers, but not in the palm. This paresthesia is typical of **carpal tunnel syndrome.** If the median nerve compression persists, the motor fibers are secondarily affected, causing the later symptom of thenar muscle weakness. Some studies have shown that orthotic positioning of the wrist in neutral to a few degrees of flexion minimizes the pressure in the carpal tunnel, thereby relieving the compression on the median nerve.[32–34]

Carpal tunnel syndrome is often attributed to poor wrist posture associated with using a standard computer keyboard. To position the fingers over the home row, the wrist is forced to ulnarly deviate. A keyboard that is too low will promote wrist flexion, whereas a keyboard that is too high will promote wrist extension. Intracarpal pressure increases as the wrist position moves further from neutral.[28] To correct the wrist posture and relieve the symptoms of carpal tunnel syndrome, a wrist orthosis is commonly prescribed. Unfortunately, most wrist orthoses are likely to interfere with keyboarding because they are designed to block the offending wrist postures that are required to position the fingers over the keys. Because complete wrist immobilization is usually unnecessary, consider a semiflexible design, especially for daytime use. In addition, orthotic intervention for carpal tunnel syndrome attributed to keyboarding should be preceded by an ergonomic assessment of the computer workstation to enhance the setup of the keyboard, mouse, monitor, document holder, and chair. Ergonomic keyboards that tilt the keyboard down at the back and orient the keys to neutralize the wrist position should be considered as an alternative or adjunct to orthotic intervention.

# INFLAMMATION

As previously discussed, the therapist should avoid causing inflammation by excessive stress while attempting to correct contractures. Furthermore, the presence of inflammation is a contraindication for even very gentle stretching. Efforts to resolve a soft tissue contracture with concomitant inflammation should wait until the inflammation has subsided. This guideline is particularly important for clients with rheumatoid arthritis, autonomic dysreflexias, and hemophilia, when the tissues are already chronically or acutely inflamed.[18]

However, the use of a static orthosis to promote local rest is known to reduce inflammation.[35] In addition, the orthosis protects the inflamed tissues from stressful forces and movements that would further aggravate the condition and promote deformity.[36] As the inflammatory process subsides, so does the pain. The body part is then more comfortable to use in functional activity.

Inflamed joints should be supported in a loose-packed position to minimize stressful forces on the joint capsule and ligaments. This is a form of joint protection. Inflamed tendons should also be rested in a slack position to minimize aggravating tensile forces.

The therapist should be aware that immobilizing one joint, for example the wrist, causes increased stress on adjacent joints, which could become inflamed or subluxed.[36]

# RHEUMATOID ARTHRITIS

The preceding discussion of inflammation also applies to rheumatoid arthritis, as well as other inflammatory joint conditions. Orthoses should be designed to support inflamed joints in their loose-packed position or position of least intra-articular pressure (see earlier discussion) to minimize pain and prevent or correct deformity such as the following:

- Volar subluxation and radial drift at the wrist
- Volar subluxation and ulnar drift at the MCPs

- Swan-neck or boutonnière deformity through the IPs
- Intrinsic muscle tightness
- Knee flexion contracture
- Carpal tunnel syndrome

## TENDON INJURIES

Immediately after surgical repair of a tendon injury in the hand, early protected joint movement and tendon excursion are promoted with a dynamic orthosis to maintain nourishment of the injured tendons and uninjured cartilage[37] (see Fig. 1-12). In addition, gentle stress favorably influences the scar tissue, guiding the newly synthesized collagen fibers to orient themselves along the lines of stress and to elongate the inevitable **peritendinous** adhesions.[37] As a result, injured tendons that are mobilized early show progressively greater tensile strength and maintain their glide. In contrast, tendons that are immobilized develop restrictive adhesions and are slow to regain tensile strength.[5]

## SPASTICITY

Individuals with upper motor neuron lesions, such as closed-head injury, stroke (cerebral vascular accident), or cerebral palsy, often exhibit spasticity, which is a state of increased muscular tone. The spastic upper extremity has a pattern of flexion, internal rotation, and thumb adduction. Orthotic intervention for spasticity is directed toward reducing muscle tone, preventing or reducing contractures, and preventing breakdown of skin in the hand.[38–48] When muscles are allowed to remain in a state of prolonged contraction, they adapt and shorten, causing contractures. Early orthotic intervention, before contractures are established, is recommended.

Orthotic intervention for spasticity is controversial and lacks consensus. The literature documents various orthotic approaches and rationales for managing spasticity. Some of the theories recommend molding a hand orthosis to the volar surface of the forearm and hand to block sensory input that might stimulate the spastic flexor muscles. In contrast, other theories recommend a dorsal forearm base, arguing that the material over the dorsal surface stimulates the weak, antagonistic, extensor muscles. A study by Aalderks et al.[44] found no difference in effectiveness between volar and dorsal placement of the forearm base.

Some therapists advocate positioning the hand joints in maximal extension to keep the spastic flexors on a full stretch.[42] Others contend that this actually increases muscle tone and instead advocate submaximal extension (5° to 10° less than maximal).[47]

Another controversy is static versus dynamic. A static orthosis is used to maintain the hand in a reflex-inhibiting posture for extended periods of time to facilitate muscle relaxation.[46] Advocates of dynamic orthoses claim that dynamic extension forces provide a more uniform stretch to spastic muscles.[44,47]

Abduction of the thumb often helps break the flexor pattern of spasticity. This can be achieved with a thumb abduction strap, as shown in Chapter 11. Some hand orthoses keep the thumb and fingers in full abduction, again to inhibit flexor spasticity.[45,50] A volar hand-based finger-abduction orthosis can be worn while performing weight-bearing exercises through the upper extremity.[49]

Another approach is to place a hard cone in the hand. The rationale is that the spastic fingers will firmly grip the cone, creating deep pressure on the tendon insertions in the fingers and palm, inhibiting the flexor muscle tone.[50] In contrast, some therapists prefer soft, circumferential orthoses that provide neutral warmth, which is thought to affect the temperature receptors in the hypothalamus and stimulate the parasympathetic nervous system to promote relaxation.[41,51,52] Soft orthoses are particularly well suited to long-term care facilities in which active rehabilitation may be lacking or orthoses may be poorly monitored for adverse effects.

Regardless of the orthotic design, orthoses should be regarded as an adjunct to therapy, to help maintain the range and relaxation gained by tone-reducing techniques. Often a trial and error approach is required to determine the orthotic design that will yield the best outcome for each individual. Unfortunately, muscle relaxation does not usually persist long after the orthosis is removed, and while the tone-inhibiting orthosis is worn, hand function is blocked.[48] Orthoses have the greatest benefit by preventing contractures for individuals in whom high muscle tone will eventually subside.

## INTRA-ARTICULAR INTERPHALANGEAL JOINT FRACTURES

Following from the articular cartilage research by Salter and others that led to the development of CPM,[8] dynamic traction orthoses have evolved for the management of **intra-articular** joint fractures.[53–56] These devices maintain gentle, constant traction on a fractured interphalangeal joint, while permitting a full active arc of motion (see Fig. 1-13). Radiographic monitoring during the orthotic intervention has demonstrated gradual remodeling of the articular surface, improved alignment of the fracture fragments, and resolution of subluxation or dislocation. Joint movement has been credited with enhancing cartilage nutrition and preventing intra-articular adhesions.[54]

## FRACTURES OF LONG BONES

In 1791 John Hunter[60] of Great Britain was the first to report successful treatment of a proximal fracture of the femur with weight bearing. In 1855 H. H. Smith[57] of Philadelphia reported its success in treating fractures of the femur. He saw it as a means to avoid surgery or prolonged bed rest. At about the same time, the Germans developed "walking therapy" as a tool for fracture rehabilitation, and this was applied all over Europe. However, with the rising cost of equipment and the development of skeletal traction, mobilization therapy fell out of favor, and for many years thereafter, treatment centered on immobilization. Until recently, the standard treatment for fractured limbs has been to reduce and maintain the fracture in a plaster cast, immobilizing it and the adjacent joints above and below it for as long as 16 weeks.

Mobilization therapy was revived in 1963, when Sarmiento and others[61,62] reported the positive outcome of functional fracture bracing for tibial fractures. The prototype was a circumferential plaster of Paris cast that permitted free motion of the knee joint with early weight-bearing ambulation. This device evolved into a circumferential plastic orthosis that left both the knee and ankle free to move. The approach of stabilizing a fracture without joint immobilization has expanded to include fractures of the femoral shaft, humerus and forearm, metacarpals, and phalanges.[59–64]

The rationale for this treatment of fractures is that rigid immobilization is neither necessary nor desirable. Some motion at the fracture site enhances osteogenesis, and the maintenance of joint mobility prevents joint stiffness and fracture disease, caused by immobilization. Instead, fracture stabilization is achieved by circumferential compression of the soft tissues to maintain the alignment of the fracture site.[56]

In contrast to plaster casts, plastic circumferential orthoses are lightweight, durable, easy to apply, and adjustable to accommodate changes in limb girth due to atrophy and changes in edema. Velcro straps enable adjustability, ensuring optimal compression of the soft tissues to maintain fracture alignment. The joints adjacent to the fracture site are left free to move, and early graded weight-bearing is standard[65] (see Fig. 1-1*a*).

A fracture orthosis is generally applied 7 days to 6 weeks postinjury, when acute swelling and pain have subsided and the fracture has stabilized. For example, a fracture of the tibia may be casted in a long-leg cast, which immobilizes the knee and ankle for the first 1 to 3 weeks. After that time, a plastic fracture-stabilizing orthosis is applied, leaving the knee and ankle free. The client is encouraged to walk with crutches, beginning with partial weight bearing and progressing to full weight bearing without external support by about the sixth week postinjury. The orthosis is used until the fracture is completely healed, at which time the client is gradually weaned from it. In general, no physical therapy is required to restore joint mobility because the joints were not immobilized after initial casting.[65] However, physical therapy may be required to teach the client partial weight-bearing techniques when a fracture orthosis is first implemented.

Fractures of the humerus also lend themselves to fracture orthoses, which are usually applied 5 to 10 days postinjury. They should permit full elbow flexion and extension and full shoulder abduction. Sarmiento[65] recommended that gravity pendulum exercises for the shoulder be instituted as soon as acute symptoms had subsided to prevent adhesive capsulitis. In addition, activity of the forearm and hand musculature should be encouraged to reduce distal swelling.

Fractures of the ulna can also be managed with fracture orthoses, provided there is no associated injury of the radius or the joints adjacent to the fracture site. As with a tibial fracture, initial treatment is a full-length cast that immobilizes the elbow and wrist. When the pain and swelling have reduced, in about 1 week, the cast is replaced by a fracture orthosis. Early protocols recommended limiting pronation and supination during the healing process. However, this restriction is no longer seen as necessary. The ulnar fracture orthosis should permit full range of motion of the elbow and wrist, with minimal limitation of pronation and supination. In addition, full active range of motion of all upper limb joints should be encouraged.[60]

Since 1991 Sarmiento[65] has used orthoses for fractures of the radius and ulna after an initial 2 weeks of cast immobilization to establish fracture stability. Unlike other orthoses, the design for radial-ulnar fracture has a supracondylar extension block to prevent elbow extension past 60°. In addition, supination and pronation are restricted.

Orthoses can also be applied to fractures of the femur in the middle or proximal third of the bone shaft.[60] Generally, the orthosis is applied after the fracture alignment has been maintained by traction for 4 to 6 weeks, when callus formation is evident, the fracture has stabilized, and pain has subsided.

Fracture orthoses can be either removable, with an adjustable opening, or sealed shut and nonremovable. A removable orthosis permits cleaning and aeration of skin. Furthermore, it is adjustable with Velcro straps to accommodate changes in limb circumference due to fluctuations in edema or atrophy. However, when an orthosis is removable, it is important to educate the client well about when it can be removed. The client who is unlikely to adhere to the recommended protocol is not a good candidate for a removable fracture orthosis.

## SCAR MANAGEMENT

After a layer of new epithelium has closed a skin wound caused by burns or other trauma, the subsequent remodeling phase of the healing process is characterized by shrinkage of the scar tissue. During this phase, it is important to maintain the extensibility of the skin. Scar tissue shrinkage has been attributed to the action of the myofibroblast. This distinctive cell, found in healing connective tissues, contains contractile myofilaments similar to a smooth muscle cell.[66] Myofibroblasts pull the edge of the scar tissue together like a drawstring, often causing contracture of the skin and loss of joint mobility.

Another contributing factor during the remodeling phase is the hypervascularity of the new skin, causing an overproduction of oxygen-rich tissue fluid, which fuels the proliferating fibroblasts to produce excess collagen in the dermis.[67] The resulting **hypertrophic scar tissue** is raised, firm, and red. The normal balance between collagen synthesis and collagen lysis is disturbed because synthesis is oxygen dependent, whereas lysis is not.[68] However, this balance can be restored through the application of surface pressure that compresses the capillaries in the dermis, creating an ischemic environment that now favors collagen lysis.[70] Continuous pressure—applied with elastic bandages, Lycra garments (e.g., Jobst), cohesive tape, or elastomer—is most effective in controlling collagen formation if it is applied prophylactically, before the tissue has begun to hypertrophy. If the tissue has already hypertrophied, pressure can help soften and flatten the scars as long as it is still remodeling, which is indicated by its rosy appearance. As the remodeling phase draws to a close, up to 2 years postinjury, the redness fades and the vascularity and oxygen levels return to normal. The resulting mature scar is less responsive to pressure techniques to flatten any residual hypertrophic scar.

Orthotic intervention for the client with burns should strive to maintain or restore joint range of motion and optimize the appearance of the new skin. The remodeling scar tissue is favorably influenced by compression to suppress the overproduction of collagen and tension to oppose the skin-contracting action of the myofibroblasts. If contractures have developed, an orthosis can be used to exert prolonged, gentle tensile force that will direct the fibroblasts to create longer fibers of collagen, oriented in the direction of the tension. In this situation, the oxygen-rich environment is advantageous because the accelerated production of collagen helps the contracted tissue to grow rapidly under the influence of the tension. Therefore, the therapist must consider the factors influencing the physiology of scar control and adjust compression and tension mediated by an orthosis, according to the stage of healing and the condition of the scar tissue.

Compression therapy to control hypertrophic scarring was developed in the mid-1960s, using orthoses, bandages, or compression garments.[70] However, the latter tend to bridge over concave areas of the body, such as above the clavicles, thus lacking sufficient control of scar tissue in these areas.[71] Silicone elastomer was introduced in the early 1970s as an adjunct to orthoses or compression garments, to form highly conforming, rubberlike inserts that conform precisely to the contours of the scar tissue.[72,73]

In the early 1980s, silicone gel sheeting was found to control scar tissue in the absence of compression.[74] Although the mechanism of action is unclear, silicone gel hydrates, softens, and flattens scars; shortens scar maturation time; prevents scar shrinkage; and maintains joint range of motion.[74–79] Silicone gel sheeting is flexible and clings to the skin; therefore it is a stand-alone medium for scar management. Alternatively, it can be adhered to the inner surface of an orthosis if a device is molded to an area with scar tissue.

Another medium to soften scar tissue is plaster of Paris. It is used to form circumferential serial-static finger orthoses to correct IP flexion contractures.[80,81] Alternatively ¹⁄₁₆ or ³⁄₃₂ in. (1.6 or 2.4 mm) thick thermoplastics can be used.[81]

## ● Summary

Mobility and nutrition of dense connective tissues require joint movement, either active or passive, and control of edema (see Chapter 3).

Nutrition of the cartilage requires joint movement, either active or passive, and cyclical loading and unloading.

The length and tensile strength of dense connective tissues change in response to the requirements of their pattern of use: they atrophy when habitual forces are reduced, and they grow when held constantly in a slightly stretched position, within the elastic range of the tissue. The cells sense the tension and the collagen fibers grow longer (i.e., remodel), causing elongation, because gentle, prolonged stretch promotes soft tissue growth.

Corrective forces must be very low. The client should sense tension in the tissues but feel no pain.

Connective tissues need to be optimally stressed to either maintain their status or promote growth and strengthening. They respond adversely to both stress deprivation and stress overload.

Stress deprivation has the following effects within various tissues:

- Bone loses compressive and tensile strength and becomes osteoporotic (less dense).
- Tendons and ligaments lose their tensile strength.
- Cartilage becomes malnourished and friable.

Prolonged joint immobilization is generally undesirable because of the rapid loss of tissue strength; therefore, do not unnecessarily restrict joint motion. When immobilization is warranted to promote healing, reintroduce movement as soon as possible.

Position a joint in its loose-packed position to promote resorption of redundant soft tissues and thereby restabilize the joint.

Position a joint in its close-packed position to preserve the length of the articular soft tissues and thereby maintain joint mobility.

Rest an effused joint in a position of least intra-articular pressure to relieve pain and reduce inflammation.

To promote a power grasp, position the wrist in extension. To promote precision function, position the wrist in neutral or slight flexion. To promote handwriting, check each client's wrist position, and replicate that position when molding the orthosis.

Correctly position the distal edge of a wrist orthosis to enable full MCP flexion and preserve the mobility of the fourth and fifth metacarpals.

Finger flexion forces should pull each finger toward the scaphoid.

Ensure that the thumb can readily oppose the index and long fingers.

For carpal tunnel syndrome, position the wrist in neutral to a few degrees of flexion.

Inflammation is a contraindication for even very gentle stretching.

For tendon injuries, orthoses provide early, protected joint motion and tendon excursion to maintain nourishment of tendons and cartilage, guide the synthesis of collagen fibers, and elongate peritendinous adhesions.

For spasticity, orthotic intervention may reduce muscle tone, prevent or reduce contractures, and prevent skin breakdown in the hand.

## ● References

1. Carlstedt, CA, and Nordin, M: Biomechanics of tendons and ligaments. In Nordin, M, and Frankel, VH (eds): Basic Biomechanics of the Musculoskeletal System, ed 2. Lea & Febiger, Philadelphia, 1989.
2. Snell, RS: Clinical and Functional Histology for Medical Students. Little, Brown, Boston, 1984.
3. Salter, RB: History of rest and motion and the scientific basis for early continuous passive motion. Hand Clinics 12:8, 1996.
4. Fess, EE, and Philips, CA: Hand Splinting Principles and Methods. Mosby, St. Louis, 1987.
5. Gelberman, RH, and Woo, SL: The physiological basis for application of controlled stress in the rehabilitation of flexor tendon injuries. J Hand Ther 2:66, 1989.
6. Mow, VC, Proctor, CS, and Kelly, MA: Biomechanics of articular cartilage. In Nordin, M, and Frankel, VH (eds): Basic Biomechanics of the Musculoskeletal System, ed 2. Lea & Febiger, Philadelphia, 1989.
7. Jobe, C, Jobe, FW, and Pink, M: The sports medicine rehabilitation center. In Nickel, VL, and Botte, MJ (eds): Orthopaedic Rehabilitation, ed 2. Churchill Livingstone, New York, 1992.
8. Coutts, RD, et al: The use of continuous passive motion in the rehabilitation of orthopaedic problems. Cont Orthop 16:75, 1988.
9. Prosser, M: The value of continuous passive motion in hand therapy. Presentation at the 10th World Congress of Physical Therapists, Sydney, Australia, 1987.
10. Nordin, M, and Frankel, V: Biomechanics of bone. In Nordin, M, and Frankel, VH (eds): Basic Biomechanics of the Musculoskeletal System, ed 2. Lea & Febiger, Philadelphia, 1989.
11. Brand, PW, and Hollister, A: Clinical Mechanics of the Hand, ed 2. Mosby, St. Louis, 1993.
12. Brand, PW: Mechanical factors in joint stiffness and tissue growth. J Hand Ther 8:91, 1995.
13. Tillman, LJ, and Cummings, GS: Biologic mechanisms of connective tissue. In Currier, DP, and Nelson, RM (eds): Dynamics of Human Biologic Tissues. FA Davis, Philadelphia, 1992, p 1.
14. Johnson, RD, et al: Tissue expansion as an alternative to skin grafting for closure of skin deficits. J Am Podiatr Med Assoc 82:249, 1992.
15. Spence, RJ: Experience with novel uses of tissue expanders in burn reconstruction of the face and neck. Ann Plast Surg 28:453, 1992.
16. Malata, CM, et al: Tissue expansion: an overview. J Wound Care 4:37, 1995.
17. Hudson, DA, and Grobbelaar, AO: The use of tissue expansion in children with burns of the head and neck. Burns 21:209, 1995.
18. Cummings, GS, and Tillman, LJ: Remodeling of dense connective tissue in normal adult tissues. In Currier, DP, and Nelson, RM (eds): Dynamics of Human Biologic Tissues. FA Davis, Philadelphia, 1992, p 45.
19. Chow, J, and Schenck, RR: Early continuous passive movement in hand surgery. Curr Surg 46:97, 1989.
20. Strickland, JW: Biological rationale, clinical application, and results of early motion following flexor tendon repair. J Hand Ther 2:71, 1989.
21. Flowers, KR, and LaStayo, P: Effect of total end range time. J Hand Ther 7:42, 1994.
22. Thompson, DE: Dynamic properties of soft tissues and their interface with materials. J Hand Ther 8:85, 1995.
23. Fess, EE: Force magnitude of commercial spring-coil and spring-wire splints designed to extend the proximal interphalangeal joint. J Hand Ther 1:86, 1988.
24. Hepburn, GR: Case studies: Contracture and stiff joint management with Dynasplint. J Orthop Sports Phys Ther 8:498, 1987.
25. Melvin, JL: Rheumatic Disease in the Adult and Child, Occupational Therapy and Rehabilitation, ed 3. FA Davis, Philadelphia, 1989.
26. Norkin, CC, and Levangie, PK: Joint Structure and Function: A Comprehensive Analysis. FA Davis, Philadelphia, 1983.
27. Magee, DJ: Orthopedic Physical Assessment, ed 2. WB Saunders, Philadelphia, 1992.
28. Eyring, EJ, and Murray, WR: The effect of joint position on the pressure of intra-articular effusion. J Bone Joint Surg 46A:1235, 1964.
29. MacBain, KP, Galbraith, M, and Brady, F: Non-operative Management of Adult-Onset Rheumatoid Arthritis. The Arthritis Society, BC Division, Vancouver, 1981.
30. Skirven, T: Nerve injuries. In Stanley, BG, and Tribuzi, SM (eds): Concepts in Hand Rehabilitation. FA Davis, Philadelphia, 1992.

31. Hollar, LD: Spinal cord injury. In Trombly, CA (ed): Occupational Therapy for Physical Dysfunction, ed. 4 Williams & Wilkins, Baltimore, 1995.

32. Dolhanty, D: Effectiveness of splinting for carpal tunnel syndrome. Can J Occup Ther 53:275, 1986.

33. Burke, DT, et al: Splinting for carpal tunnel syndrome: In search of the optimal angle. Arch Phys Med Rehabil 75:1241, 1994.

34. Weiss, ND, et al: Position of the wrist associated with the lowest carpal tunnel pressure: implications for splint design. J Bone Joint Surg 77a:1695, 1995.

35. Hanes, B: Orthotics, splinting, and lifestyle factors. In Walker, JM, and Helewa, A (eds): Physical Therapy in Arthritis. WB Saunders, Philadelphia, 1996.

36. Marx, H: Rheumatoid arthritis. In Stanley, BG, and Tribuzi, SM (eds): Concepts in Hand Rehabilitation. FA Davis, Philadelphia, 1992.

37. Thomes, LJ, and Thomes, BJ: Early mobilization for surgically repaired zone III extensor tendons. J Hand Ther 8:195, 1995.

38. McPherson, JJ, et al: A comparison of dorsal and volar resting hand splints in the reduction of hypertonus. Am J Occup Ther 36:664, 1982.

39. Mills, V: Electromyographic results of inhibitory splinting. Phys Ther 64:190, 1984.

40. Johnstone, M: Restoration of Motor Function in the Stroke Patient: A Physiotherapist's Approach. Churchill Livingstone, New York, 1983.

41. Eggers, O: Occupational Therapy in the Treatment of Adult Hemiplegia. William Heineman Medical, London, 1983.

42. Snook, JH: Spasticity reduction splint. Am J Occup Ther 33:648, 1979.

43. Bobath, B: Adult hemiplegia: Evaluation and treatment. Heineman Medical Books Limited, London, 1978.

44. Aalderks, M, et al: A comparison of dorsal and volar resting hand splints in the reduction of hypertonus. Am J Occup Ther 36:664, 1982.

45. Rose, V, and Shah, S: A comparative study on the immediate effects of hand orthosis on reduction of hypertonus. Aust Occup Ther J 34(2):59, 1987.

46. Scherling, E, and Johnson, H: A tone reducing wrist hand orthosis. Am J Occup Ther 43(9):609, 1989.

47. McPherson, J, Becker, A, et al: Dynamic splint to reduce the passive component of hypertonicity. Arch Phys Med Rehabil 66:249, 1985.

48. McPherson, JJ: Objective evaluation of a splint designed to reduce hypertonicity. Am J Occup Ther 35:189, 1981.

49. Kinghorn, J, and Roberts, G: The effect of an inhibitive weight-bearing splint on tone and function: A single-case study. Am J Occup Ther 50:807, 1996.

50. Farber, S: Neurorehabilitation: A Multidisciplinary Approach. WB Saunders, Toronto, 1982.

51. Johnstone, M: The Stroke Patient: Principles of Rehabilitation. Churchill Livingstone, New York, 1982.

52. Schmidt, R: Fundamentals of Sensory Physiology. Springer Verlag, New York, 1978.

53. Schenck, R: Dynamic traction and early passive movement for fracture of the proximal interphalangeal joint. J Hand Surg 11A:851, 1986.

54. Dennys, LJ, Hurst, LN, and Cox, J: Management of proximal interphalangeal joint fractures using a new dynamic traction splint and early active movement. J Hand Ther 4:16, 1992.

55. Byrne, A, et al: A modified dynamic traction splint for unstable intra-articular fractures of the proximal interphalangeal joint. J Hand Ther 8:216, 1995.

56. Smith & Nephew: Functional Bracing: Principles and Progress Reviewed. Smith & Nephew, Hull, England, 1988.

57. Sarmiento, A, et al: Prefabricated functional braces for the treatment of fractures of the tibial diaphysis. J Bone Joint Surg 66A:1328, 1984.

58. Sarmiento, A: A functional below-the-knee cast for tibial fractures. J Bone Joint Surg 52A:855, 1967.

59. Sarmiento, A, and Sinclair, WR: Application of prosthetic-orthotic principles to orthopaedics. Artif Limbs 2:2, 1967.

60. Sarmiento, A: Functional bracing of tibial and femoral shaft fractures. Clin Orthop Res 82:1, 1972.

61. Sarmiento, A, Cooper, JS, and Sinclair, WF: Forearm fractures: early functional bracing—a preliminary report. J Bone Joint Surg 57A:297, 1975.

62. Sarmiento, A, and Latta, LL: Closed Functional Treatment of Fractures. Springer-Verlag, New York, 1981.

63. Schultz, KH: Hand-based metacarpal fracture brace and forearm ulnar or radius fracture brace. J Hand Ther 5:158, 1992.

64. Oxford, K, and Hildreth, D: Fracture bracing for proximal phalanx fractures. J Hand Ther 9:404, 1996.

65. Sarmiento, A, Ross, SDK, and Racette, WL: Functional fracture bracing. In American Academy of Orthopedic Surgeons: Atlas of Orthotics: Biomechanical Principles and Applications, ed 2. Mosby, St. Louis, 1985. (Also available at www.orthoamerica.com:80/500lit 4a.html.)

66. Hardy, MA: The biology of scar formation. Phys Ther 69:1014, 1989.

67. Dockery, GL: Hypertrophic and keloid scars. J Am Podiatr Med Assoc 85:57, 1995.

68. Leveridge, A: The use of silicone gel in the control of hypertrophic scarring after burn surgery and hand surgery. J Hand Rehab 21:73, 1990.

69. Nicholson, B: Evaluation of the hand. In Stanley, BG, and Tribuzi, SM (eds): Concepts in Hand Rehabilitation. FA Davis, Philadelphia, 1992.

70. Gibbons, M, et al: Experience with silastic gel sheeting in pediatric scarring. J Burn Care Rehab 15:69, 1992.

71. Gollop, R: The use of silicone gel sheets in the control of hypertrophic scar tissue. Br J Occup Ther 51:248, 1988.

72. Feldman, AE, Thompson, JT, and MacMillan, BT: The moulded silicone shoe in the prevention of contractures involving the burn-injured foot. Burns 1:83, 1974.

73. Malick, MH, and Carr, JA: Flexible Elastomer molds in burn scar control. Am J Occup Ther 34:603, 1980.

74. Perkins, K, Davey, RB, and Wallis, KA: Silicone gel: A new treatment for burn scars and contractures. Burns 9:201, 1983.

75. Wessling, N, et al: Evidence that use of a silicone gel sheet increases range of motion over burn wound contractures. J Burn Care Rehabil 6:503, 1985.

76. Katz, B: Silicone gel sheeting in scar therapy. Cutis 56:65, 1995.

77. McNee, J: The use of silicone gel in the control of hypertrophic scarring. Physiotherapy 76:194, 1990.

78. Carney, SA, et al: Cica-care gel sheeting in the management of hypertrophic scarring. Burns 10:163, 1994.

79. Farquhar, K: Silicone gel and hypertrophic scar formation: A literature review. Can J Occup Ther 59:78, 1992.

80. Bell, J: Plaster casting for the remodeling of soft tissue. In Fess, EE, and Philips, CA (eds): Hand Splinting Principles and Methods. Mosby, St. Louis, 1987.

81. Bell-Krotoski, JA, and Figarola, JH: Biomechanics of soft-tissue growth and remodeling with plaster casting. J Hand Ther 8:131, 1995.

82. Kapandji, IA: The Physiology of Joints: Volume 1: Upper Limb. Churchill Livingstone, New York, 1982.

83. Snell, RS: Atlas of Clinical Anatomy. Little, Brown, Boston, 1978.

# Design and Fabrication Principles

## ● Biomechanical Principles

### JOINT POSITIONING

When positioning one or more joints with an orthosis, consider the following factors, in this order:

1. Pathology
2. Joint biomechanics and tissue tension
3. Function

Refer to Chapter 2 for rationale.

### Pathology

The first consideration is whether pathology dictates the position. Examples include the following:

- Carpal tunnel syndrome—the wrist should be positioned in neutral or a few degrees of flexion, to minimize the pressure in the carpal tunnel.[1-3]
- Rheumatoid arthritis—inflamed joints should be positioned in their loose-packed position to minimize tensile forces in the joint capsule and ligaments.[4]
- Flexor tendon lacerations (surgically repaired)—the wrist and MCPs should be positioned in flexion to prevent injury to sutured tendons from tensile forces.[5]
- Burns to the dorsum of the fingers—interphalangeal joints should be kept in complete extension to prevent flexion that could rupture the extensor mechanism.[6]

- Tissue contractures—joint(s) should be positioned to apply gentle, prolonged stretch, promoting tissue growth.[7,8]

Consider also the possibility that certain joint positions could actually promote pathology. For example, positioning the wrist in flexion could irritate the median nerve in the carpal tunnel. The therapist should be aware that immobilizing one joint, for example the wrist, increases stress on adjacent joints, which could become inflamed or subluxed.[9]

### Joint Biomechanics and Tissue Tension

If pathology does not dictate joint positioning, the next factor is joint biomechanics and tissue tension, as discussed in Chapter 2. For example, a forearm-based wrist-hand orthosis for an adult should position the metacarpophalangeals (MCPs) in full flexion to keep the MCP collateral ligaments taut to preserve their length.[10] However, this position causes the long finger flexors to be slack and puts the long finger extensors in tension. Therefore, to balance the tension in the flexors and extensors, the wrist should be positioned in extension to counterbalance the MCP flexion (see Fig. 2-9).

### Function

If neither pathology nor joint biomechanics is an influencing factor for a particular situation, joint positioning should enable function. This is the case, for example, with **de Quervain's tenosynovitis**—inflammation of abductor pollicus longus and extensor pollicus brevis at the wrist. The objective of the orthosis is to rest the inflamed tendon sheaths by immobilizing the joints that the tendons cross—wrist, thumb, carpometacarpal (CMC), and MCP. If, for example, the client needs to write while wearing the orthosis, the therapist should position the wrist and thumb to facilitate the precision grip that the client uses to grasp a pen (see Fig. 2-28). If the orthosis restricts thumb opposition, function will be unnecessarily limited and compliance will be jeopardized.

Consider the position of the wrist in an orthosis that is designed to enable function. De-

termine the type of activities that the client will be performing with the orthosis. Do they involve primarily gross power grasp or fine prehension grip? The former is facilitated by positioning the wrist in extension (see Fig. 2-20); the latter, in neutral or slight flexion (see Fig. 2-24a). Personal hygiene and precision activities are restricted by an orthosis that positions the wrist in extension. As a result, it may be appropriate to provide an orthosis with an adjustable wrist positioner or to provide two orthoses—one with wrist extension, the other with wrist neutral or slightly flexed.

Even if pathology or joint biomechanics is the primary factor influencing joint position, efforts to optimize function should still be considered. For the client with MCP volar subluxation caused by rheumatoid arthritis, consideration of pathology and joint biomechanics leads the therapist to position the MCPs in their loose-packed position (i.e., slight flexion) to promote resorption of the lax ligaments. However, consideration of function leads the therapist to position the MCPs in slightly more flexion (e.g., 20°) to facilitate opposition. To facilitate compliance, the positioning may be a compromise between the dictates of pathology or joint biomechanics and the considerations for function.

## SURFACE AREA

The trough of the orthosis needs to be sufficiently deep so that the limb is well seated and the orthosis fits securely (Fig. 3-1). If the trough is too shallow, the limb will "overflow" the sides of the trough, and the straps will need to be applied tighter to secure the orthosis in

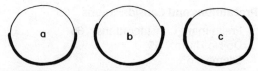

**FIGURE 3-1.**   Schematic cross section through a limb showing different trough depths. *(a)* Too low: The limb overflows the sides of the trough. *(b)* Just right: Slightly more than halfway up the sides of the limb. *(c)* Too deep: Too difficult to apply to a forearm if the thermoplastic is inflexible.

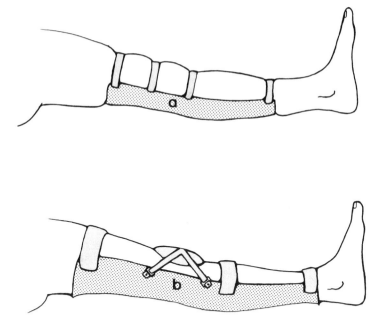

**FIGURE 3-2.** Static posterior knee orthoses. *(a)* Poor design: The limb "overflows" the orthosis because the trough is too shallow and the lever arms above and below the knee are too short; the straps are too narrow and inadequately secure the knee. *(b)* Good design: The limb is well seated because the trough extends a little over halfway up the sides; the straps are adequately wide, and the conforming knee pad is well positioned to keep the knee extended.

place (Figs. 3-1*a* and 3-2*a*). As a general rule, the trough should extend slightly more than halfway up the sides of the limb, as shown in Figures 3-1*b* and 3-2*b*. The greater the surface area of the trough, the less the pressure, because pressure (*P*) equals force (*F*) divided by surface area (*SA*) (*P* = *F/SA*). However, if the trough is too deep, as shown in Figure 3-1*c*, and the material is inflexible, the orthosis will be difficult to apply and remove.

An exception is the **circumferential orthosis,** which encircles the body part. When fabricating hand- or forearm-based circumferential orthoses, it is best to use ¹⁄₁₆ or ³⁄₃₂ in. (1.6 or 2.4 mm) low-temperature thermoplastics (LTTs) rather than the standard ⅛ in. (3.2 mm) thickness. The thinner materials are more flexible, making it easier to apply and remove the orthosis. However, ⅛ in. (3.2 mm) thick LTTs are suitable for large circumferential orthoses (e.g., for the humerus or tibia).

If the area of force application is too small, high pressure results, causing discomfort and possibly skin irritation. To reduce discomfort and improve the force distribution, increase the surface area. For example, if a strap is too narrow, as in Figure 3-2*a*, it may cut into the client's skin. Replace it with a wider, more con-

forming strap, as in Figure 3-2*b*, especially if the client is obese or the part is edematous. A diagonal orientation also increases the contact area of a strap.

## CONFORMITY TO CONTOUR

The thermoplastic should conform to the contours of the body, without any gapping. Material that does not contact the body serves no purpose and should be removed. Conformity is enhanced by using the more conforming Category C or D materials (see Chapter 4).

Straps should also conform to the body contours, to enhance comfort and to increase the distribution area of the securing force. Using padded or stretchy strap materials such as Velfoam, CushionStrap, Beta Pile, Vel-Stretch, or neoprene enhances strap conformity. This is particularly important for the dorsal wrist strap when it lies over a prominent ulnar head.

Thermoplastic that is molded over bony prominences must conform to the contours to prevent pressure points over these sensitive areas. Alternatively, pad bony prominences before molding the orthosis (see Chapter 7).

## ROUND ALL CORNERS

All corners should be rounded to improve the aesthetics of the orthosis and to eliminate sharp corners that could injure the skin.

## FLARE THE PROXIMAL WEIGHT-BEARING EDGE

Many functional activities are performed with the forearm pronated. As a result, it is common to bear weight on the forearm trough of an orthosis when seated at a table. To prevent the proximal edge from causing a pressure point, it

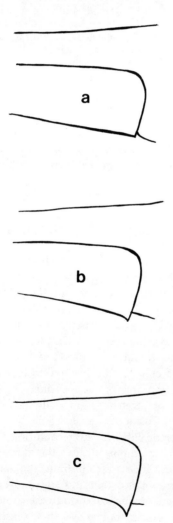

**FIGURE 3-3.** The proximal edge. *(a)* Unflared. *(b)* Just the right amount of flare. *(c)* Too much flare.

should be slightly flared (Fig. 3-3). Similarly, orthoses molded to the posterior aspect of the thigh or calf should have their proximal edge slightly flared to prevent a pressure point when the client lies in bed or sits in a chair (Fig. 3-2*b*).

## LEVER ARM

Orthoses, even static ones, apply torque to each joint on which they act. **Torque (moment of force)** is the extent to which a force tends to cause rotation of an object (body part) about an axis. Torque ($T$) is the product of force ($F$) multiplied by the lever arm ($LA$) ($T = F \times LA$) (Fig. 3-4). **Lever arm** is the perpendicular distance from the axis of rotation to the line of application of the force. When the lever arm is lengthened, less force is required to generate sufficient torque to produce rotation (Fig. 3-4*b*). In orthotics, the axis of rotation is the joint axis. The magnitude of the torque exerted by an orthosis on a joint depends on the amount of force applied by the orthosis and the length of the lever arm through which it is applied. As a general rule, to optimize the mechanical advan-

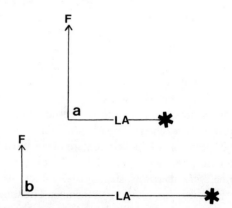

**FIGURE 3-4.**    Torque = force × lever arm.
* = axis of rotation.
F = force (the length of the arrow represents the magnitude of the force)
LA = lever arm (the perpendicular distance from the axis of rotation to the line of application of a force)
The torque generated in *(a)* is equivalent to the torque in *(b)*, but the lever arms and forces are different. In *(a)* the lever arm is shorter and, to compensate, the force must be larger. In *(b)* less force is required to generate sufficient torque to cause rotation at the axis because the lever arm is longer.

tage of an orthosis, use the longest lever arm possible without restricting the motion of other joints.

To understand this concept, consider the technique used to bend a piece of wire. A torque is applied to each side of the bending site while a counterforce is applied at the bending site (Fig. 3-5a). The bending site corresponds to the axis of joint rotation. Torque is determined by the magnitude of each force ($F^1$ and $F^2$) and the lengths of the respective lever arms ($LA^1$ and $LA^2$). To bend the wire, the torque on each side of the bending site must be sufficient to overcome the stiffness of the wire (Fig. 3-5b).

Now, consider the application of forces required to extend the wrist. As in bending the wire, torque is applied to each side of the bending site (i.e., wrist axis) while a counterforce is applied over the bending site (Fig. 3-5c). Biomechanically, these torques are equal and balanced on each side of the joint axis; that is, $F^1 \times LA^1 = F^2 \times LA^2$. The lever arm distal to the wrist ends in the palm of the hand. If this force were applied more distally, it would no longer focus on the target joint; instead, the force would be distributed among all the joints it crosses, which would not be appropriate for a wrist orthosis. The correct lever arm is short because of the anatomy of the hand; as a result, a relatively high force must be applied to generate sufficient torque to position the wrist. In contrast, the lever arm proximal to the wrist can take advantage of the full length of the forearm; the longer the lever arm, the less the force required to generate the required amount of torque.

To apply these concepts to orthotic design, consider the static volar forearm-based wrist orthosis, which counteracts the force of gravity that pulls the wrist into flexion when the forearm is pronated (Fig. 3-5d). One torque is distal to the wrist, with the lever arm beginning at the wrist joint axis and ending at the distal edge of the orthosis in the palm. The proximal torque, equal in magnitude to the distal one, begins at the wrist joint axis and ends at the proximal edge of the orthosis. Once again, the longer the lever arm, the less force required to generate the required amount of torque. How-

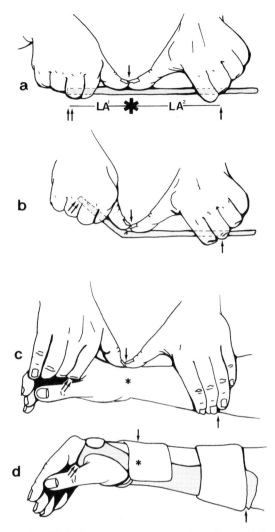

**FIGURE 3-5.** Generating torque in orthotics. *(a)* Position of the hands preparing to bend a piece of wire. Forces (arrows) are applied at the end of each lever arm (LA$^1$ and LA$^2$). The thumbs are positioned to apply a counter force at the bending site, that is, the axis of rotation (*), creating a system of three forces. *(b)* Sufficient torque has been generated to bend the wire. *(c)* Position of the hands to apply torque to extend the wrist. Again, a system of three forces is applied—one at each end of the lever arm and a counterforce over the axis of rotation. *(d)* A volar forearm-based static wrist orthosis designed to resist wrist flexion, showing the system of three forces and the lever arms. Note the location of the key strap over the axis of rotation (i.e., wrist joint axis). Notice also that the key strap is wide to distribute its force over a large area to reduce pressure.

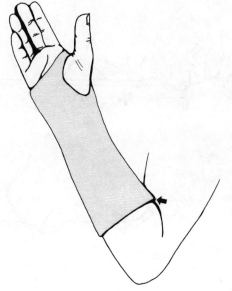

**FIGURE 3-6.** Poor orthotic design. The forearm base is too long, extending more than two thirds up the forearm from the wrist, restricting elbow flexion and irritating the tissues above the elbow (arrow).

ever, if the proximal lever arm extends beyond two thirds up the length of the forearm, elbow flexion becomes restricted and the proximal edge irritates the soft tissues above the elbow (Fig. 3-6). The wrist strap applies the counterforce. Therefore, to control each joint, a system of three forces and two lever arms is required.

## FIXATION

To be optimally effective, a volar forearm-based orthosis needs a counterforce centered directly over the target joint axis (i.e., wrist). Thus, the wrist strap applies the key force to keep the wrist positioned in the orthosis (Fig. 3-5*d*). To maximize the distribution of this force and thereby enhance comfort, use a 2 in. (5 cm) wide strap. In contrast, Figure 3-7 demonstrates an ineffective wrist strap.

To reiterate, when an orthosis that resists flexion (i.e., applies extension force) is molded to the flexor surface of the limb, the key force, applied by the key strap, crosses the extensor surface. Ideally, the key strap is centered over the target joint axis and its force is distributed over a large area to enhance comfort. To opti-

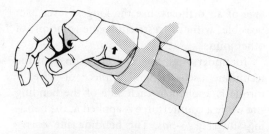

**FIGURE 3-7.** Ineffective wrist strap. The strap over the wrist is too narrow and positioned too proximally, providing inadequate joint control and allowing the wrist to flex out of the orthosis (arrow).

mize conformity, use padded or stretchy strap materials such as Velfoam, Beta Pile, Cushion-Strap, Vel-Stretch, or neoprene.

Consider the posterior knee orthosis designed to resist flexion by applying extension force to the knee (Fig. 3-2*b*). Like the wrist orthosis described previously, it is molded to the flexor (posterior) surface and its key force crosses the extensor surface of the target joint. To be optimally effective, this force should be distributed over a large area and centered over the knee joint axis, using a contoured kneepad. The biomechanics of the controlling force is superior when using the centered knee pad, rather than a pair of straps above and below the knee, as shown in Figure 3-2*a*. Even a painful, inflamed knee is usually able to tolerate the extension force if the surface area is large and the pad conforms to the knee contours. In addition, apply the principle of lever arm to optimize control of the knee—maximize the lever arm above and below the knee, extending them as close as possible to the hip and ankle joints, without restricting their motion or irritating tissues.

Different mechanics are involved when an orthosis that is resisting flexion has a **dorsal** base, with the proximal lever arm over the extensor surface (Fig. 3-8*a*). The key force is not over the target joint but instead at the proximal edge of the orthosis. The leverage of this design is more obvious than the volar- or posterior-based orthoses. It is easier to appreciate that the longer the lever arm, the lower the force required to extend the joint. With this orthotic design, the proximal lever arm can be used to "lever" the joint into extension, using the same

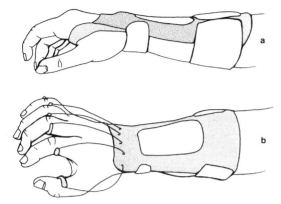

**FIGURE 3-8.** Orthoses for radial nerve injury presenting with paralysis of wrist, finger metacarpophalangeal (MCP), and thumb extensors. *(a)* Dorsal forearm-based static wrist orthosis. *(b)* Dorsal forearm-based dynamic arching spring-wire wrist and D2-5 MCP assistive-extension orthosis.

mechanics as a crowbar (see Fig. 1-16). To increase the extension torque, lengthen the proximal lever arm. This orthotic design is easy to apply to spastic limbs. As with the volar- or posterior-based orthoses, optimize the pressure distribution of the key force by using a wide (2 in./5 cm) strap.

Two common strap designs are overlap and D-ring (Fig. 3-9). An overlap strap is easy to make by cutting a length of strap material and attaching it to hook Velcro. D-ring straps require a D-ring to be sewn to one end of the strap; alternatively, prefabricated D-ring straps can be purchased. It is often easier for the client to secure an orthosis with a D-ring strap. See Chapter 7 for strap fabrication techniques.

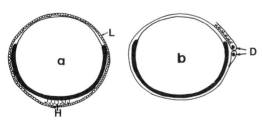

**FIGURE 3-9.** Cross-sectional view through half-shell orthoses on a limb, demonstrating two styles of straps. L = loop Velcro; H = hook Velcro; D = D-ring. *(a)* Overlap. *(b)* D-ring closure.

## TISSUE-SPECIFIC FORCES

When an orthosis is designed to apply tensile forces to reduce a soft tissue contracture, the **magnitude** of the force should be low (i.e., in the elastic range) and prolonged to stimulate growth and subsequent lengthening of the contracted tissues. If the magnitude of the corrective force exceeds the elastic limit of the tissues, the resulting microtrauma may elicit pain and a counterproductive inflammatory response.[7,8]

If limited range of motion is the problem requiring orthotic intervention, it is essential to identify the specific structures responsible for the limited mobility—joint capsule, ligaments, intrinsic muscles, extrinsic muscles or tendons, or bony block. Once the range-limiting tissues or structures have been identified, the orthosis can then be designed to be joint or tissue specific in directing its corrective forces. However, if a bony block has been identified, corrective forces are in vain and nothing short of surgery will enhance the range of motion.

The orthotic design must take into account the direction of static or dynamic forces. For example, when the objective is to shorten lax radial collateral ligaments of the MCP joints in rheumatoid arthritis, the orthosis should apply force to pull the MCPs in a radial direction to unload the lax radial MCP collateral ligaments and promote their resorption (see Fig. 2-13).

## OUTRIGGERS

Dynamic extension orthoses are commonly fabricated for the client with radial nerve injury or post-MCP **arthroplasty**. Many incorporate an outrigger that serves as the anchor or pulley for the traction mechanism. Before the 1980s most extension dynamic orthoses were **high profile** (Figs. 3-10*a* and 3-11*a*). In this design, elastic bands are anchored to the end of the outrigger, which is positioned some distance above the limb (therefore "high profile") to ensure adequate excursion of the elastic. In the early 1980s **low profile** extension outriggers became popular, to lower the profile of the outrigger closer to the hand.[11] The outrigger changed from being the traction anchor to be-

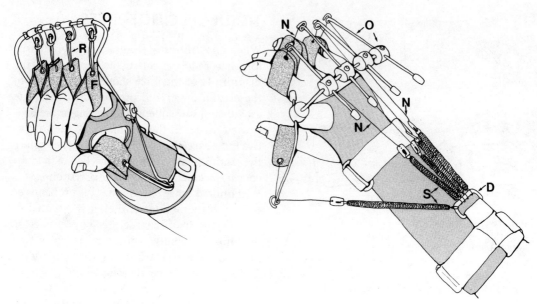

**FIGURE 3-10** *(Left)* Volar forearm-based dynamic high-profile D1-5 MCP assistive-extension orthosis (prefabricated Rolyan® High-Profile Outrigger Splint[12]). Rubber bands (R), attached to finger loops (F), are anchored to the metal outrigger (O). *(Right)* Dorsal forearm-based dynamic low-profile D1-5 MCP assistive-extension orthosis. (Rolyan® Adjustable Outrigger Kit for Extension). Nylon lines (N), attached to finger loops, are connected to springs that provide the dynamic extension force. The springs (S) are anchored to the orthosis by a D-ring (D).

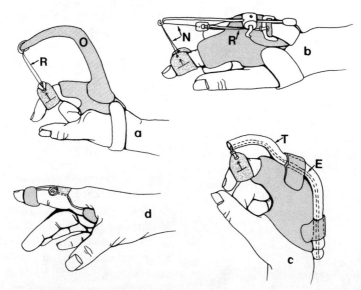

**FIGURE 3-11.** Various outrigger designs for dynamic proximal interphalangeal joint (PIP) corrective extension. *(a)* Circumferential hand-based dynamic high-profile D2 PIP corrective extension orthosis. The outrigger acts as the anchor site for the elastic band. *(b)* Circumferential hand-based dynamic low-profile D2 PIP-corrective extension orthosis (Rolyan® Adjustable Outrigger Kit (Patent No 4,765,320). The outrigger acts as a pulley to redirect the traction force. This Rolyan® extension outrigger has unique adjustability, allowing the pulley wire to be angled higher or lower and moved proximally or distally. This allows the direction of the traction force to be easily adjusted to accommodate changes in the condition. *(c)* Circumferential hand-based dynamic tube outrigger D2 PIP corrective extension orthosis. The tube (T) transmits the elastic cord (E) to the finger loop. *(d)* Three-point finger-based dynamic joint-aligned coil-spring D2 PIP corrective extension orthosis; joint-aligned coil springs keep the orthosis close to the body, creating no profile.

ing a pulley to redirect the traction force (Figs. 3-10*b* and 3-11*b*). In the 1990s tube outriggers were introduced in which the full length of the tube acts as a pulley to transmit the elastic cord to the finger loop (Fig. 3-11*c*).

The spring wire design shown in Figure 3-8*b* also has a low profile. The wires arch over the hand; when the fingers are fully flexed, the wires come closer to the hand, allowing the hand to slip into a pocket. Arching spring wire is effective for applying assistive forces; however, it cannot exert sufficient corrective force to reduce a tissue contracture. The most compact dynamic orthoses have no profile; the extension force is exerted through joint-aligned coil springs (Fig. 3-11*d*).[13] As a general rule, design the outrigger to be as close to the hand as possible. This creates a more compact, less conspicuous orthosis, which has a positive impact on compliance.[14] In addition, the force should always pull 90° to the long axis of the bone to prevent stress to the collateral ligaments (Fig. 3-11*a, b,* and *c*).

Orthoses designed to promote composite MCP and IP flexion, either to protect healing flexor tendons or to reduce extension contractures, should flex each finger toward the scaphoid, which is the natural direction in which the fingers point during flexion (see Fig. 2-23).

# ● Optimizing Compliance–Design and Psychosocial Considerations

*Compliance* refers to the client's adherence to the prescribed orthotic program. The client who is noncompliant is often viewed as uncooperative; however, many factors influencing compliance are the responsibility of the therapist. For example, knowledge of orthotic principles and fabrication skills affect the quality of the finished product. The therapist's interpersonal skills also influence compliance.

## OFFER OPTIONS

Ensure that the entire process is client centered, and encourage client participation in the deci-

sion-making process. Begin by offering options to the client before the definitive orthosis is dispensed. Options include prefabricated or custom fabricated, dorsal or volar, static or dynamic, color of thermoplastic and Velcro, degree of perforation and thickness of thermoplastic, and method of fixation.

## EXERCISE IN EMPATHY

When students are learning orthotic skills, a useful exercise is for them to wear a wrist orthosis fabricated by a fellow student for a 24-hour period. They will experience firsthand how having the wrist immobilized in a fixed position can affect function. Also apparent is discomfort from pressure points; attention that the orthosis attracts in public; and the heat and sweat retained by the plastic material. This experience reinforces the importance of optimal joint positioning, no unnecessary restriction of function, optimal cosmesis, and discrete design.

## NO UNNECESSARY RESTRICTION OF FUNCTION

Determine which joints (if any) are to be incorporated into the orthosis, taking into consideration the targeted tissues or structures. *Do not incorporate more joints than necessary.* Any joints excluded from the orthosis should be permitted full mobility. For example, an orthosis designed to immobilize the wrist should not interfere with finger MCP or thumb or elbow mobility (Figs. 3-5*d*, 3-6, 3-12, 3-13, and 3-14). A forearm-based orthosis should extend no more than two thirds up the forearm from the wrist. Similarly, an orthosis designed to immobilize the thumb CMC and MCP joints should not restrict wrist, finger MCP, or thumb IP movements. Needless restriction of joint motion will interfere with function and adversely affect compliance.

However, when designing a corrective or assistive orthosis, it may be necessary to stabilize one or more joints immediately proximal to the targeted joint(s) (Fig. 3-11). Another exception is that it is sometimes beneficial to block the movement of one of more flexible joints proximal to a stiff joint to encourage an active force

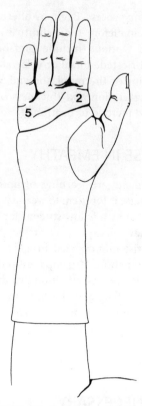

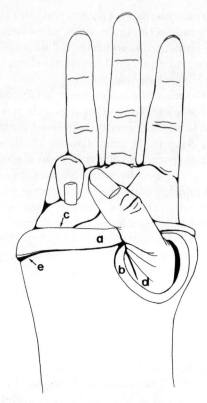

**FIGURE 3-12.**   Volar forearm-based thumb-hole wrist orthosis: good design. The distal edge permits full flexion of the MCPs and allows the distal transverse arch to deepen during a power grasp. It ends at the proximal edge of the second MC head (2) and ¼ in. (½ cm) proximal to the fifth MC head (5). The thenar eminence is completely exposed to permit full mobility of the thumb to enable precision function of the hand.

**FIGURE 3-13.**   Volar forearm-based thumb-hole wrist orthosis: poor design. (a) The thermoplastic has been folded back at the distal edge, creating unnecessary bulk. (b) Similarly, the material around the thumb has been rolled, creating a thick ridge that interferes with grasp. (c) The distal edge is too long, restricting full MCP flexion. Because of the folded material, the resulting double thickness would be difficult to cut through even if it were heated. (d) The thenar eminence has not been well cleared. As a result, thumb mobility is severely restricted and the thumb is unable to oppose the little finger. (e) The distal folded edge is poorly sealed. The resulting crevice is difficult to clean and is a breeding ground for bacteria.

to be directed to the target joint. For example, in Figure 3-15 the more flexible MCP and PIP are stabilized with a static orthosis, to enable the flexor digitorum profundus to direct its force to the stiff DIP.

When deciding whether a wrist orthosis should be volar (Fig. 3-5*d*) or dorsal based (Fig. 3-8), bear in mind that the volar surface of the hand is used for important sensory input. As a general rule, design the orthosis to block the volar surface area as little as possible.

## OPTIMIZE COSMESIS

The physical appearance of the orthosis deserves careful attention. The device becomes a part of the client's microenvironment and, like any item of clothing, is often seen by others, especially one for the hand or face. To optimize compliance, it should be aesthetically acceptable to the client. Furthermore, the orthosis is a product of your therapeutic intervention that will be on display, representing you and your profession, and as such should meet basic standards. Common cosmetic defects include pen marks, rough edges, and surface impressions. Efforts to optimize cosmesis should not be viewed as time-consuming and unimportant.

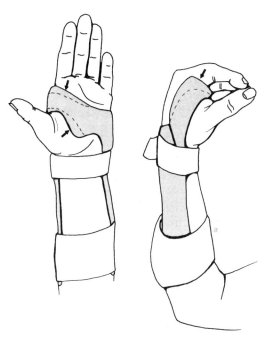

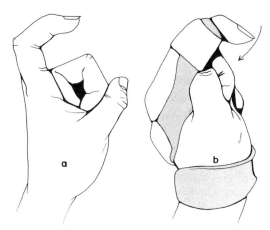

**FIGURE 3-15.** Restriction of joints proximal to the target joint. *(a)* Active DIP flexion of the index is limited by capsular tightness. *(b)* Circumferential hand-based D2 MCP-PIP flexion-blocking orthosis. This orthosis blocks the two joints proximal to the stiff joint so that flexor digitorum profundus can direct all its force to the distal interphalangeal (DIP) joint.

**FIGURE 3-14.** Dorsal forearm-based static wrist orthosis demonstrating unnecessary joint restriction (arrows). The distal edge is too long, restricting full MCP flexion. The palmar support partly covers the thenar eminence, restricting full mobility of the thumb. Broken lines show recommended trim lines.

To ensure optimal orthotic cosmesis in the minimal amount of time, begin the fabrication process by cutting off pattern lines with long, even strokes to create a clean, smooth edge.

Applying a strip of flannel-like, self-adhesive moleskin immediately disguises any ragged edges with a soft cover. However, this short-sighted solution is generally inappropriate because the moleskin cannot be cleaned and it becomes dirty, smelly, and shabby, especially on a hand orthosis. Generally, it is preferable in the long run to provide an orthosis with smooth, finished, thermoplastic edges.

Edge covering is appropriate and necessary with maxi-perforated materials, primarily to ensure comfort. Rather than using moleskin, use a strip of a durable, washable covering such as ⅟₁₆ in. (1.6 mm) self-adhesive Plastazote, Aquaplast Ultra-Thin Edging Material, or a thin version of the same LTT.

Consider the color of the thermoplastic and Velcro strapping. What is pleasing to one client may be unacceptable to another.

Most clients prefer the orthosis to be inconspicuous and not to draw attention. Exceptions sometimes include young or athletic clients. It is especially important to create a compact design for a dynamic orthosis using a low-profile outrigger that uses pulleys to bring the apparatus as close to the hand as possible.

## LIGHTWEIGHT

As a general rule, create an orthosis that is as lightweight as possible for the application and the client. The weight of the orthosis is determined primarily by the thickness and degree of perforation of the thermoplastic. A common but inappropriate practice in orthotic fabrication is the routine use of ⅛ in. (3.2 mm) thick materials for forearm- or hand-based orthoses, when ³⁄₃₂ or ⅟₁₆ in. (2.4 or 1.6 mm) thickness would provide adequate support and be more comfortable and lighter for the client. Once the material has been contoured to conform to the body, it is stronger than it was before molding. As a general rule, use the thinnest LTT that will provide adequate support. This is particularly important for children or clients with muscle weakness or fatigue.

Another common but sometimes inappropriate practice is rolling or folding back ⅛ in. (3.2 mm) thick material at the MCP heads and around the thenar eminence (Fig. 3-13). This technique is used to deal quickly with redundant material rather than cutting it off when a precise, **custom** pattern is not made. Although folding creates a smooth edge that requires no further finishing, the folded material creates additional bulk and interferes with the easy grasp of items in the palm of the hand. If the therapist chooses to fold the edges when using ⅛ in. (3.2 mm) thick LTTs, we advise against folding more than once to avoid creating a bulky edge. To ensure full thumb opposition, stretch the warm thermoplastic to expose the thenar eminence during molding. Fold carefully, because if insufficient material is folded back to permit full MCP flexion and thumb opposition, it is difficult to cut through two (or more) layers of ⅛ in. (3.2 mm) thick material. When a precise custom pattern is made, trimming is minimized. If trimming is required, do so before the material has completely cooled. In contrast, when using ¹⁄₁₆ or ³⁄₃₂ in. (1.6 or 2.4 mm) thick LTTs, folding back the edges proximally, at the MCP heads, and around the thenar eminence may be desirable to enhance the rigidity of the orthosis.

## DURABILITY

Consider the durability of the thermoplastic, straps, spring wires, and outrigger attachment. Begin by selecting a thermoplastic that can withstand the stresses that will be imposed by the client during activities. For example, circumferential orthoses must withstand bending forces every time they are applied and removed; some LTTs are too rigid and will develop fatigue cracks.

Low-temperature thermoplastics become malleable in hot water or dry heat, ranging from 135° to 180°F (57° to 82°C), depending on the material. As a result, it is important to advise the client or caregiver that the molded orthosis may lose its shape if washed in very hot tap water, left in a car on a sunny day, or placed near a heat source.

Velcro loop straps are usually secured to the orthosis with a patch of self-adhesive hook Velcro. Ensure that the patch is well secured to prevent it from peeling off with repeated detachment of the loop strap. If the hook Velcro patch becomes detached, the orthosis cannot be secured to the client and it becomes useless. The same problem develops if the loop Velcro strap becomes detached and is lost. See "Methods of Fixation" in Chapter 7 for solutions. With extended use, some padded straps lose their sensitivity to hook Velcro; standard loop Velcro is more durable.

Spring wire, used in some dynamic orthoses, is easily deformable. Consider the client and the type of activities for which the orthosis will be used. For example, a spring-wire assistive-extension orthosis for radial nerve injury may not be suitable for a child (Fig. 3-8*b*). If the orthosis is dropped, the wires may become deformed. For this situation, consider a more durable type of outrigger or perhaps provide only a static orthosis (Fig. 3-8*a*).

Outriggers are secured to the base of the orthosis, usually by embedding the wire and then reinforcing the attachment with a bonded layer of thermoplastic. Ensure that the outrigger has been securely attached without the possibility of its breaking away. Outrigger attachment techniques are described in Chapter 7.

## EASY TO APPLY AND REMOVE

Unless removal of an orthosis is contraindicated, it is important to ensure that the client understands how to apply and remove the orthosis and is physically able to do so. For clients with poor prehension caused by weak or painful hands, consider the mode of fixation. To facilitate manipulation of Velcro straps, one technique is to cut a hole in the end of the loop Velcro strap (Fig. 3-16). D-ring closure makes it easier to cinch an orthosis snugly in place. If a zipper closure is used, attach a loop to the end of the runner to eliminate the need for fingertip prehension.

If the thermoplastic is too high on the sides of the trough and the material is fairly rigid, it will be difficult to place the limb into the or-

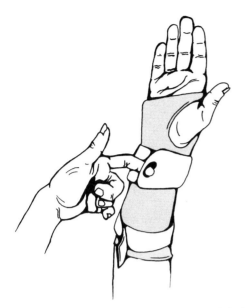

**FIGURE 3-16.** Volar forearm-based thumb-hole wrist orthosis with a long proximal strap and a hole in the wrist strap to make it easier for a client with poor prehension to grasp the strap.

thosis (Fig. 3-1*c*). To correct this problem, trim the sides of the trough. If the orthosis is circumferential, ensure that the client can easily apply it with minimal stress and effort. This is facilitated by using thinner materials, 1/16 or 3/32 in. (1.6 or 2.4 mm) thick, which are more flexible than the standard 1/8 in. (3.2 mm) thermoplastics.

An easily removable orthosis is not always appropriate. If removal of the orthosis puts injured tissues at risk (e.g., ruptured tendon in mallet finger, healing lacerated tendon, or unstable fracture) and the client will not keep the orthosis on, it should not be removable.

Ensure that the client or caregiver knows how to apply and remove the orthosis and when it is to be worn.

## SIMPLE IN DESIGN

Design the orthosis to be as simple as possible. This is particularly important when creating a dynamic orthosis. The more complex the design, the more confusing it is for the client to apply and maintain and the more likely it will

become damaged or inappropriately applied. It might be better to provide two or more different orthoses rather than one complex orthosis.

For example, after a peripheral nerve injury, a dynamic orthosis may provide a client with more natural prehension than a static one; however, the complexity of the dynamic orthosis may be unsuitable for some clients or situations. As a result, the therapist could provide the client with various options to consider before fabrication, including a simple static orthosis. The client with a radial nerve injury could be provided with a dynamic orthosis that would apply passive extension forces to the wrist and MCPs to enable natural prehension (Fig. 3-8*b*). However, some clients might prefer a static wrist orthosis that simply supports the wrist in a fixed degree of functional extension, to counteract the wrist drop, without addressing the lack of MCP extension (Fig. 3-8*a*). Other clients might appreciate the function that is enabled by a dynamic orthosis for self-care, work activities, and leisure activities but prefer to use a less conspicuous static wrist orthosis in certain social situations. For these individuals, more than one orthosis may be required to meet their emotional and functional needs.

## EASY TO ADJUST

Orthoses intended for correction of contractures require frequent adjustment to accommodate the soft tissue growth that is stimulated by gentle, prolonged tensile forces. As a result, these orthoses should be designed for easy adjustability. If the orthosis is serial static, the use of a thermoplastic with memory facilitates the required frequent remolding. If the orthosis is static progressive or dynamic corrective, ensure that the outrigger used to apply the corrective forces can be easily adjusted. Some prefabricated outriggers are specifically designed for easy adjustability (Figs. 3-10*b*, 3-11*b*).

## EASY TO CLEAN AND SOIL RESISTANT

Thermoplastics with a smooth surface coating, designed to prevent accidental self-bonding during fabrication, have the highest degree of soil resistance. In contrast, although Turbocast is easy to mold, it soils easily and is difficult to clean because of its fuzzy surface. Orfilined, Kushionsplint, QuickCast, and Dynacast Rapide incorporate a terry lining. These linings help pad the orthosis and absorb perspiration; however, they are difficult to clean.

To wick away perspiration and reduce soiling on the inside of the orthosis, the client can apply a tubular, cotton or polypropylene bandage (e.g., Stockinette or Tubigrip) over the limb before donning the orthosis (Fig. 3-17). Alternatively, a presewn splint liner provides an absorbent interface with prefinished edges that will not fray (Fig. 3-18).

If the thermoplastic is folded over or bonded together, the seams must be well sealed because crevices are hard to clean and become a breeding ground for bacteria (Fig. 3-13).

## CLIENT EDUCATION

In some circumstances, the client will have less pain and be more functional while wearing an orthosis. Relief from pain and enhanced function have positive effects on compliance. In contrast, compliance may be adversely affected if

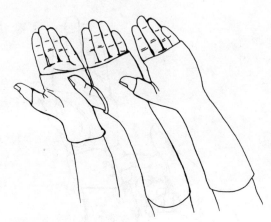

**FIGURE 3-18.** Prefabricated splint liners with prefinished, sewn edges that will not fray.

benefits of orthotic intervention are long term or the orthosis limits function to prevent deformity or injury to optimize future function.

The therapist should consider how the orthosis will affect the client's ability to perform activities pertaining to self-care (e.g., eating, dressing, personal hygiene), productivity (e.g., writing, computer keyboarding, operating machinery, driving), and leisure (e.g., skiing, swimming, art activities). Client education about the purpose of orthotic intervention is an integral component of the process. When function is temporarily compromised, it is particularly important that the client or caregiver clearly understand the merits of orthotic intervention.

Educate the client about the following:

- Objectives of the orthotic regimen and consequences of noncompliance
- Correct application and removal of the orthosis
- Wearing schedule and circumstances when it can be removed
- Care of the orthosis—how to clean it, precautions against leaving it in a hot environment, and how to make minor adjustments if necessary
- Indications of poor fit (such as pressure points) that need prompt attention

Whenever possible, provide this information in a written format. Use everyday language and avoid jargon or anatomic terms. If there is a language barrier, a translator should be en-

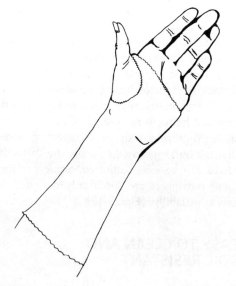

**FIGURE 3-17.** Tubular cotton bandage to be worn under an orthosis to absorb the perspiration.

listed. Consider the client's level of education, literacy, and comprehension. Ensure that the client knows how to and is physically able to apply and remove the orthosis and manage the straps or other mode of fixation.

A few days after dispensing the orthosis, follow up with an appointment or a telephone call to ensure that any problems are identified and resolved.

## PSYCHOSOCIAL ADJUSTMENT

A client with a long-term, progressive condition may become used to ongoing medical intervention and thus accept an orthosis more readily than a client confronted with sudden trauma. However, some clients requiring long-term intervention develop "gadget intolerance" and may resist additional devices. In addition, an orthosis for short-term use is usually easier to accept than one prescribed for an indefinite period or with delayed benefits.

Another important factor in acceptance is the reaction of family, friends, peers, and strangers to the orthosis. If adverse reaction by others is likely to occur, provide education about the objectives of orthotic intervention to significant individuals in the client's social network. It is important to enlist their support to optimize compliance.

## ● Precautions and Considerations

### PRELIMINARY CONSIDERATIONS

Although a client may have been referred for an orthosis, the therapist must apply professional judgment and seek input from the client, caregiver (if appropriate), and other team members to determine whether an orthosis is warranted.

If the preliminary assessment supports the need for an orthosis, it is important to estimate likely compliance and determine whether the orthosis will be adequately and correctly used. For example, a circumferential orthosis may be more comfortable and functional than a plaster of Paris or fiberglass cast to promote fracture healing. However, the orthosis is removable, and the client must accept the responsibility to keep it on except when following the well-defined guidelines for removal, cleaning, and therapeutic activities. Fracture healing will be seriously compromised if the client does not follow these guidelines and misuses the ability to remove the orthosis.

## DO NO HARM

The provision of an orthosis should not be taken lightly. It is important for the therapist to appreciate that the orthosis has a great influence on soft tissues, joints and bone, and function—either promoting or temporarily restricting it. If the orthosis fails to achieve its intended outcome, the least it should do is no harm. Avoidable harmful consequences include the following:

- Injury to skin or compression of nerves caused by pressure points
- Burns caused by molding overheated LTTs to the skin
- Failure to protect injured structures during the healing process
- Undue stress to tendons or joints caused by poor design or joint positioning
- Inflammation of and injury to shortened soft tissues caused by excessive tensile forces intended to reduce contractures[13]
- Disuse atrophy
- Edema

To prevent pressure points, note the location of bony prominences over which the thermoplastic is to be formed. Before the molding process, pad the bony prominences with a thin layer of self-stick foam or gel padding, or flare the material away (see Chapter 7). After the orthosis has been molded, check the skin for the presence of red areas that indicate pressure points; ensure that corrections have been made before giving the orthosis to the client. Be especially vigilant if sensation is impaired by nerve injury, stroke, head injury, or spinal cord injury. Similarly, check the temperature of the heated LTT on an area of sensitive skin before molding to prevent burns.

As previously stated, immobilizing one joint, for example the wrist, increases stress on adjacent joints, which could become inflamed or subluxed, especially if those joints are arthritic.[10] The therapist must also clearly understand the natural plane of motion of every joint the orthosis acts on. For example, when attempting to improve thumb abduction, the orthosis must apply its corrective force to the CMC joint, where the motion occurs. In this situation, it is easy to inadvertently and inappropriately apply radial deviation stress to the first MCP.

Although it is important to minimize the potential for secondary pathology as a result of orthotic intervention, in some circumstances it may be necessary to accept some negative consequences to achieve the desired outcomes. For example, while positioning the wrist and MCPs in flexion during the healing of lacerated finger flexor tendons, some loss of extension range may occur. This is viewed as an acceptable risk, and contractures can be corrected after the tendons are fully healed.

Occasionally the client's skin will respond adversely to contact with the thermoplastic. If the client develops a rash, provide a tubular bandage or splint liner as an interface between the skin and the LTT (Figs. 3-17 and 3-18). If this fails to relieve the problem, remold the orthosis with a different LTT.

# EDEMA

Consider the presence of, or potential for, edema. It poses a serious threat to joint mobility and tendon excursion, and efforts to control it are a fundamental component of rehabilitation, especially when it involves the hand. Unlike the volar skin of the hand, which is naturally adherent and unyielding, the dorsal skin is loose and mobile. Consequently, when the hand becomes edematous, excess tissue fluid accumulates in the dorsum, creating tension in the dorsal skin that pulls the MCPs into hyperextension, the IPs into flexion, and the thumb into adduction.[15] The resulting clawhand posture shown in Figure 2-10*a* must not be allowed to persist because MCP extension and IP flexion are the loose-packed positions for these joints; their collateral ligaments are left slack and the body will resorb what it perceives as redundant tissue.[16,17] In the absence of length-preserving tension that is generated by MCP flexion, the MCP collateral ligaments will shorten and the joints will stiffen in extension. To prevent this sequela, the clawhand posture must be opposed by a hand orthosis that positions the MCPs in 50° to 70° of flexion, the IPs in extension (or slight flexion), and the thumb well abducted with a well-rounded first web space[15] (see Fig. 2-10*b*)

## Strategies to Control Edema[17,18]

- Elevate the edematous limb above the level of the heart so that gravity can assist venous and lymphatic return.
- Avoid slings because they position the hand below the heart and promote immobility of the entire limb and iatrogenic stiffness.
- Encourage active movement because muscle contraction enlists the skeletal muscle pump to promote the return of lymphatic fluid and venous blood from the extremities. For example, if the wrist is injured and immobilized by an orthosis, the client should be encouraged to frequently move all the MCPs and IPs through a full range of motion. This creates a favorable muscle pumping action on the blood vessels and preserves the extensibility of the uninvolved tissues.
- Apply compression to create a pressure gradient, promoting distal-to-proximal return of lymphatic fluid and venous blood via
  - Continuous compression
    - Figure-eight wrapping of fingers and limbs with Cohesive tape (e.g., Coban) or elastic bandage
    - Elasticized finger sleeves for individual finger compression
    - Elastic tubular bandage (e.g., Tubigrip)
    - Prefabricated or custom-fabricated pressure gradient Lycra garments (e.g., Jobst)
    - Air cast splints

- ▪ String wrapping
  - ○ Intermittent compression pumps
- Continuous passive motion orthoses help decrease wound edema by milking fluid out of the extremity.[19]
- **Cryotherapy.** Apply cooling agents to acutely edematous tissue, especially during the initial period after injury or whenever the tissues are inflamed, to promote vasoconstriction and suppress capillary leakage. In contrast, superficial heating is contraindicated because it causes vasodilation and greater capillary permeability, aggravating the inflammatory response, which in turn causes increased edema.
- Contrast baths.
- Retrograde (distal to proximal) massage.

Because edema tends to fluctuate, mold the orthosis when edema is most pronounced because it is better to have an orthosis that is a little too loose (after edema subsides) than one that is too tight (if edema increases).

Use a thinner thermoplastic (³⁄₃₂ in./2.4 mm for wrist-hand orthoses; ¹⁄₁₆ in./1.6 mm for wrist orthoses) or use a thermoplastic that is more flexible when cool. This allows easy "cold adjustment" to spread apart the sides of the orthosis to accommodate increased edema or squeeze in the sides of the orthosis to accommodate decreased edema. The therapist can teach these techniques to the client or caregiver.

If the completed orthosis is not readily cold-adjustable, it may be necessary to reheat and remold the orthosis to accommodate the change in limb girth resulting from fluctuating edema. Furthermore, straps may be unsuitable when edema is severe (Fig. 3-19) and should be replaced with bandage fixation.

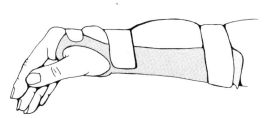

**FIGURE 3-19.** The consequence of strap fixation when the limb has marked *edema*. Tissue fluid has accumulated between the straps.

To minimize edema while the orthosis is worn, encourage the client to elevate the limb whenever possible and move unrestricted joints to actively contract the muscles; this enlists the skeletal muscle pump to assist venous blood return from the limb.

## ● Summary

1. When positioning one or more joints with an orthosis, take into consideration the pathology, joint biomechanics and tissue tension, and function.
2. As a general rule, the trough should extend slightly more than halfway up the sides of the limb.
3. To reduce discomfort and improve the force distribution, increase the surface area.
4. Mold the orthosis to conform to the body contours.
5. Pad bony prominences before molding.
6. Round all corners.
7. Flare the proximal weight-bearing edge.
8. Use the longest lever arm possible without restricting the motion of other joints.
9. Straps apply securing forces to keep the orthosis in place. Ensure that their location optimizes the lever arm and joint-controlling forces. Adequate width and conformity to body contour maximizes surface area so that the securing force is distributed over a large area.
10. Design corrective forces to be tissue specific.
11. Design the orthosis to be inconspicuous and outriggers to be as close to the hand as possible.
12. Dynamic finger extension forces should pull 90° to the long axis of the bone.
13. Dynamic finger flexion forces should direct each finger toward the scaphoid.
14. Do not incorporate more joints than necessary.
15. Do not restrict joint motion unnecessarily.
16. Design the orthosis to block the volar surface of the hand as little as possible.
17. Optimize cosmesis by eliminating pen marks, rough edges, and surface impressions.
18. Use the thinnest LTT that will provide adequate support.

19. Ensure that the orthosis is easy to apply and remove, unless removal is contraindicated.
20. Keep the design simple.
21. Design the orthosis for easy adjustability.
22. Consider soil resistance and ease of cleaning when selecting materials.
23. Provide client and caregiver complete wearing and care instructions.
24. Consider psychosocial factors that will influence compliance.
25. Minimize harmful consequences of orthotic intervention.
26. Consider the presence of, or potential for, edema.

● **References**

1. Dolhanty, D: Effectiveness of splinting for carpal tunnel syndrome. Can J Occup Ther 53:275, 1986.
2. Burke, DT, et al: Splinting for carpal tunnel syndrome: in search of the optimal angle. Arch Phys Med Rehabil 75:1241, 1994.
3. Weiss, ND, et al: Position of the wrist associated with the lowest carpal-tunnel pressure: implications for splint design. J Bone Joint Surg 77a:1695, 1995.
4. Hanes, B: Orthotics, splinting, and lifestyle factors. In Walker, JM, and Helewa, A (eds): Physical Therapy in Arthritis. WB Saunders, Philadelphia, 1996.
5. Strickland, JW: Biologic rationale, clinical application, and results of early motion following flexor tendon repair. J Hand Ther 2:71 1989.
6. Malick, MH, and Carr, JA: Manual on Management of the Burn Patient. Harmarville Rehabilitation Center, Pittsburgh, 1982.
7. Brand, PW, and Hollister, A: Clinical Mechanics of the Hand, ed 2. Mosby, St. Louis, 1993.
8. Brand, PW: Mechanical factors in joint stiffness and tissue growth. J Hand Ther 8:91, 1995.
9. Magee, DJ: Orthopedic Physical Assessment, ed 2. WB Saunders, Philadelphia, 1992.
10. Marx H: Rheumatoid arthritis. In Stanley, BG, and Tribuzi, SM (eds): Concepts in Hand Rehabilitation. FA Davis, Philadelphia, 1992.
11. Colditz, JC: Low profile dynamic splint of the injured hand. Am J Occup Ther 37:182, 1983.
12. Smith & Nephew, Inc.: Rehabilitation Catalog, 1997. Rolyan® is a trademark of Smith & Nephew, Inc.
13. Prosser, R: Splinting in the management of proximal IP joint flexion contracture. J Hand Ther 9:378, 1996.
14. Fess, EE: Force magnitude of commercial spring-coil and spring-wire splints designed to extend the proximal interphalangeal joint. J Hand Ther 1:86, 1988.
15. Malick, MH, and Carr, JA: Manual on Management of the Burn Patient. Health South Harmarville Rehabilitation Center, Pittsburgh, 1982.
16. Brand, PW, and Hollister, A: Clinical Mechanics of the Hand, ed 2. Mosby, St. Louis, 1993.
17. Brand, PW: Mechanical factors in joint stiffness and tissue growth. J Hand Ther 8:91, 1995.
18. Hardy, MA: The biology of scar formation. Phys Ther 69:1014, 1989.
19. Coutts, RD, et al: Symposium: The use of continuous passive motion in the rehabilitation of orthopaedic problems. Contemporary Orthopaedics 16:75, 1988.

# Orthotic Materials

## ● Thermoplastic Categories

Until the late 1960s leather, metal, and plaster of Paris bandage were the predominant materials in orthotic fabrication. Today, most therapists use thermoplastics to fabricate orthoses. Thermoplastics are plastics that become malleable when heated and are divided into two broad categories: high-temperature and low-temperature thermoplastics.

# HIGH-TEMPERATURE THERMOPLASTICS

The term *high-temperature thermoplastic* indicates that when the plastic is malleable for contouring, its temperature is too high to be molded directly on the client's skin without causing severe burns. High-temperature thermoplastics, such as polyethylene, are usually molded to a positive plaster replica of the body part, which is generated from a negative plaster of Paris bandage cast. The process of positive-negative casting is messy and time-consuming and is more commonly undertaken by orthotists than therapists.

# LOW-TEMPERATURE THERMOPLASTICS

In contrast, when low-temperature thermoplastics (LTTs) are malleable for molding, the temperature of the material is low enough to be molded directly to the client's skin. The fabrication procedure is shorter and less complicated than for high-temperature thermoplastics. In therapy departments and clinics, most orthoses are fabricated using LTTs.

In addition to their application in orthotics, LTTs are used in radiation therapy and theater. The mask worn in the musical "The Phantom of the Opera" was originally created out of Polyform, a highly conforming thermoplastic from Smith & Nephew Inc.[1] Thermoplastics are also used to adapt handles of utensils, pens, and tools to promote independent function. This Chapter focuses on low-temperature thermoplastics— their characteristics, applications, and equivalent materials that can be used interchangeably.

Low-temperature thermoplastics are available as flat sheets—12 × 18 in., 18 × 24 in., and 24 × 36 in. (30 × 46 cm, 46 × 61 cm, and 61 × 91 cm)—ranging in thickness from ⅟₃₂ to ⁶⁄₃₂ in. (0.8 to 4.8 mm) and in a wide range of colors. They are also available as **precuts** or **preformed** orthoses.

Each year, new materials are introduced, creating a competitive, dynamic industry. Therapists have at least 40 LTTs to select from, with the choices increasing each year. That is not to say that there are 40 *different* materials, only that there are 40 differently *named* materials made by a small number of manufacturers (see Appendix A). Many of the materials are almost replicas of each other. Two or more different suppliers may distribute a material made by one manufacturer, each supplier applying a different trade name. For example, in the late 1980s and early 1990s, Polymed manufactured a material that was marketed as NCM Preferred by North Coast Medical and Custom Splint by Remington Medical and Polymed itself.[2] A supplier may specifically request that the named material be manufactured with specific colors or slightly different properties to distinguish its brand of materials from those of the other suppliers made by the same manufacturer.

Not only are there numerous materials on the market, but the names rarely identify the handling characteristics of the thermoplastic. An effort to reduce this confusion was made by Smith & Nephew Inc. They renamed Greenstripe Aquaplast T as Aquaplast Resilient T and renamed Bluestripe Aquaplast T as Aquaplast Prodrape T. As the names suggest, the latter is more conforming than the former.

With the exception of Smith & Nephew Inc., most suppliers do not make their own thermoplastics and most manufacturers do not sell the thermoplastics that they make. This company is unusual in that it both manufactures and sells its own materials (see Appendix D). Many suppliers are reluctant to reveal the manufacturer of their plastics. In fact, over the years, many materials made by an individual manufacturer have been marketed and named differently by various suppliers.

The principal ingredient of many thermoplastics is polycaprolactone. Exceptions are San-Splint, Orthoplast, Orthoform, and Kay-Prene, which are equivalent materials composed of isoprene, a synthetic rubber from Japan. San-Splint and Orthoplast were the first successful LTTs introduced to the rehabilitation field.[3] The name "San-Splint" was derived from Smith and Nephew.

The LTTs can be subdivided into two categories: those that turn translucent when heated, referred to as translucent materials; and those that remain opaque when heated, referred to as opaque materials (see Appendix A).

## Conformability Categories

Tables 1 and 2 in Appendix A categorize the LTTs according to their handling characteristics, in particular, the degree of **conformability** when heated. We devised these categories by comparing 1/8 in. (3.2 mm) thick unperforated materials. Translucent materials demonstrate four degrees of conformability—A, B, C, and D—in which category A is the least conforming and category D is the most conforming. In contrast, the opaque materials demonstrate a range of eight conformabilities, from low to high—A1, A2, B1, B2, C1, C2, D1, and D2.

Materials in the same column demonstrate similar performance when warm and can be used interchangeably. For example, if a therapist is familiar with the handling properties of NCM Preferred, any other material from category C2 could be substituted. The next closest substitute would be a material from category C1 or D1.

### TRANSLUCENT-WHEN-HEATED THERMOPLASTICS

Materials that turn **translucent** when heated (e.g., Aquaplast, Kay-Plast, Orfit, Prism, and Turbocast) enable the therapist to view bony prominences and skin creases during molding. In addition, the translucency of the warm thermoplastic indicates that the material is fully heated. Translucent LTTs have 100% memory, which means that they will return to their original shape when reheated.

### OPAQUE-WHEN-HEATED THERMOPLASTICS

**Opaque** A1 materials (San-Splint, Orthoplast, Orthoform, and Kay-Prene) are the only LTTs with isoprene rubber, which imparts the distinctive, low-conforming quality when warm and rubbery flexibility when cool. Opaque B1 materials are distinguished by their 100 percent memory, which is unusual for an opaque material. Ezeform, the only B2 material, has a uniquely granular texture when pulled, and although it is fairly resistant to stretch, it has ab-

solutely no elastic rebound; it stays where it is put like thin, soft metal. Opaque C1 and C2 materials demonstrate a distinctive rebound when stretched because of partial memory. Opaque D materials, the most conforming of all, have absolutely no rebound properties and drape like soft pastry dough when warm.

Variables that influence the therapist's choice of materials include handling properties when warm, appearance, durability, and cost, as well as service of suppliers and rapport with sales representatives.

## ● Characteristics of Low-Temperature Thermoplastics

- Molding characteristics
  - Translucency
  - Memory
  - Conformability
  - Stretch
  - Ease of finishing the edges
  - Surface impressionability
  - Surface stickiness and self-adherence
  - Working temperature
  - Working time
  - Shrinkage
- Appearance
  - Size of sheet
  - Thickness
  - Perforations
  - Color
  - Surface texture/sheen
- Durability
  - Resistance to fatigue cracks (particularly relevant to circumferential and weight-bearing orthoses)
  - Resistance to deformation
- Resistance to soiling and ease of cleaning
- Cost
  - Material costs—thermoplastic, Velcro, dynamic components
  - Labor costs
- Supplier
  - Service
  - Rapport established with sales representatives

# MOLDING CHARACTERISTICS

## Translucency

Translucent materials that have no pigment are white when cold and turn completely transparent when warm. Translucent materials are also available in a wide range of colors. However, the color pigment reduces the translucency of the material—the darker the pigment, the less translucent the material and the more difficult it is to view the skin features through the warm material.

## Memory

One hundred percent memory is a feature common to translucent materials. In contrast, only a few opaque materials have 100% memory.

One hundred percent memory means that the material will recover its original shape, size, and flatness when reheated. This property is created when polycaprolactone is exposed to electron beam radiation, which creates cross-linking between molecules.[4] This quality is useful to correct errors and for serial-static orthoses when it is necessary to repeatedly remold an orthosis to gradually increase the range of motion of a stiff joint. This property is also useful for the therapist unskilled in orthotic fabrication, allowing a poorly molded orthosis to be remolded as many times as necessary.

Opaque category C materials have a moderate degree of memory and are characterized by a tendency to rebound when warm. That is, when a category C material is stretched, then released, the elasticity of the material will cause it to partially recoil. In addition, these materials are relatively flexible when cold so they are suitable for circumferential stabilizing orthoses. This flexibility makes it easier to apply and remove a circumferential orthosis.

However, memory is not always helpful. Spot heating materials with memory for local adjustment can be a frustrating experience because it can leave a ridge (hot-cold line) between the heated spot and the remainder of the orthosis left unheated. Often it is easier to completely reheat and remold the orthosis. In addition, it is difficult to embed wire into category B translucent materials with 100 percent memory (e.g., Resilient Aquaplast T, Orfit Stiff, and Prism). The technique of heating outrigger wire and embedding it into the orthotic base is often unsuccessful because as the material cools, it "rejects" the embedded wire, causing the wire to become loose.

## Conformability

Conformability, or drape, is the degree to which the heated material readily conforms to the contours of the body part over which it is being molded. As previously discussed, the translucent materials have been categorized according to four degrees of conformability (see Table 1 in Appendix A) and the opaque materials according to eight degrees of conformability (see Table 2 in Appendix A). The degree of conformability when warm does not correspond to the degree of flexibility when cool.

Category A is the least conforming and is well suited for large orthoses. Its low conformability is appropriate when gross contour is adequate or when the therapist needs to maintain the highest degree of control over the material or needs to apply strong forces during fabrication to position the joints. Common applications include circumferential orthoses for the tibia or humerus, knee orthoses, tone-reducing orthoses for spasticity, and shoulder orthoses.

Category A materials have the lowest degree of surface impressionability and can be handled aggressively without leaving impressions from finger or bandages on the surface. An elastic bandage can be used during the molding process to help achieve the contouring, leaving minimal impressions of the bandage in the surface. This category is suitable for gravity-resisted molding described in Chapter 7 under "Positioning the Client."

Category A materials require firm pressure or stretch to achieve even gross contours. As a result, this category is not suitable for molding on clients with painful joints or soft tissues as seen in arthritis.

At the other end of the scale, warm category D materials are the most conforming and readily drape over the body contours like soft pastry dough. They are best suited for small orthoses when precise, detailed contouring is desirable.

When warm, category D materials are limp and inclined to drape and must be handled carefully. The client should be positioned so that all or most of the thermoplastic is on the top surface of the body part. Gravity, as well as gentle stroking motions, can assist the material to flow into the contours of the body part. This technique is called gravity-assisted molding and is described in Chapter 7.

Category C materials have the broadest applications. Their conformability is sufficient for the smallest hand or finger orthoses, especially if thinner versions are used. Yet its controlled stretch allows it to be used in large-area circumferential orthoses for the forearm, arm, or leg (e.g., tibia/fibula) using the vertical molding technique described in Chapter 7.

Category B materials are used in similar applications as category A, but they are slightly more conforming and require relatively less force to create contours.

Thinner or perforated versions of any material are more conforming than the corresponding unperforated ⅛ in. (3.2 mm) thickness.

## Stretch

Generally speaking, the degree of stretch correlates to the degree of conformity or drape—the less conforming the material, the greater its resistance to stretch. Materials with memory are more resistant to stretch than those without memory. Opaque category C materials have a distinctive rebound when stretched caused by their partial memory.

## Ease of Finishing

For client comfort and orthotic cosmesis, the edges should be smooth. Strategies to ensure a smooth edge begin when the orthotic pattern is cut from the thermoplastic sheet. Heating the thermoplastic before cutting it helps achieve a smoother edge.

Edges of an orthosis made from any category C or D material can be heat smoothed. That is, they can be smoothed by heating the edges with a heat gun or by submerging the edges in warm water; any irregularities can be blended in using the thenar eminence or thumb. To smooth the rough edges of category A or B materials, either heat and recut the edges or use a power hand grinder (see Chapter 5). Edge grinding is more time-consuming than edge smoothing and requires a special tool. As a result, some therapists prefer materials from categories C or D because of the greater ease of edge finishing. Generally speaking, opaque C or D materials smooth more readily with heat than translucent C or D materials. However, Turbocast, a translucent material, has exceptional heat smoothing capabilities.

*Covering a rough edge with self-adhesive moleskin is usually a poor solution. Although this method masks and softens the uneven edges, moleskin cannot be cleaned and after a few days becomes dirty, shabby, and smelly.*

Edge finishing is complicated by the presence of perforations. If the material is lightly perforated with well-spaced holes, try to cut between the holes when cutting out the pattern. Maxi- or superperforated materials require an edge covering. Select Aquaplast Ultra-Thin Edging Material, Microfoam tape from Smith & Nephew, Inc., or a washable, self-adhesive foam material such as ¹⁄₁₆ in. (1.6 mm) Plastazote.

## Surface Impressionability

This undesirable quality refers to the susceptibility of the surface to become marked by fingerprints or other textures while it is soft. In general, the more conforming the material, the more susceptible it is to impressions. Another generalization is that translucent materials are relatively less impressionable than opaque materials because of their 100 percent memory. When handling a warm, impressionable material, the therapist should avoid a static grip and should mold it gently, stroking it with extended fingers and the palm (see Chapter 7, *"Molding the Material"*).

## Surface Stickiness

Surface stickiness can pose a problem during molding because it makes the material self-adherent and it can accidentally bond to itself. However, a moderate degree of surface tackiness is useful because it helps the material cling to the client's skin to achieve more precise contouring during molding.

Some LTTs can be softened with either dry or wet heat. Dry heating, for example in an oven, often enhances the stickiness of the surface.

Some LTTs have surface coating to prevent accidental self-adherence during molding. Unfortunately, this surface treatment makes it more challenging to adhere two pieces of thermoplastic together such as when applying outriggers to orthoses. To help ensure a permanent bond, scrape off the coating on the surfaces to be bonded or use a solvent or bonding agent to dissolve the coating. However, solvents are harsh chemicals with strong fumes, and many thermoplastics now have coatings that can be dissolved with 100 percent isopropyl alcohol. Another strategy is to use dry heat (i.e., a heat gun), rather than moist heat, to soften the material to be bonded because this enhances surface stickiness. Other strategies for thermoplastic bonding are discussed in Chapter 7.

Uncoated materials include most opaque category A and B materials, as well as Orfit Classic and Aquaplast Original. Their nonsticky equivalents are Orfit NS, in which "NS" means "nonstick," and Aquaplast T where "T" means "treated." The newest nonstick coatings include the fuzzy finish on Turbocast and the terry cloth lining on one side of Orfit creating a material called Orfilined.

## Working Temperature

Thermoplastics absorb heat to soften. Although LTTs are designed for molding directly to the client's skin, the plastic can absorb enough heat to burn the skin. Therapists should always check the temperature of the LTT on their own skin first, and then on the client's forearm be-fore proceeding with molding. Some clients are more sensitive to heat than others.

It should be noted that Synergy absorbs more heat than other thermoplastics and should not be molded directly on the skin of children or other heat-sensitive clients. To reduce discomfort and risk of skin injury, one or two layers of tubular bandage could be applied to the limb before molding Synergy. Alternatively, a prefabricated splint liner can be used to protect the skin (see Figs. 3-17 and 3-18).

Perforated LTTs should be thoroughly dried before molding because the perforations hold water that could burn the skin.

## Working Time

This refers to the cooling time or length of time the therapist has to work with the material while it is still malleable. For 1/8 in. (3.2 mm) thick materials, the working time is generally 3 to 5 minutes. Aquaplast and isoprene-based LTTs have the longest working time of 4 to 6 minutes. The working time is increased if the warm plastic is wrapped in place with an elastic bandage, which retains heat and slows the cooling process.

Working time is greatly affected by the thickness of the material and the degree of perforation. The thinner the material, or the greater number of the perforations, the shorter the working time.

Pigment may reduce the working time—the darker the color, the shorter the working time.[1] As a result, the Watercolors version of Aquaplast, colored Prism, and the ColorFit version of Orfit set faster than their respective counterparts, Aquaplast T (white), Prism (white), and Orfit (peach). In addition, pigment makes the plastic more resistant to stretch.[1]

The therapist needs an adequate amount of time to position all the incorporated joints and shape the material. Therefore, the length of the working time should be considered for each application. Complex orthoses and low-conforming materials require a longer working time for precise molding. However, if the client has **spasticity** or is not fully cooperative, a shorter working time may be desirable. To use the working time to its best advantage, position the client near the heating appliance.

*To hasten the cooling of the thermoplastic:*
- *Apply a cold pack.*
- *Wrap low-conforming material with an elastic bandage that has been soaked in ice water.*
- *Wrap LTTs with Thera-Band that has been stored in a freezer.*
- *Remove orthosis when partially set and run under cold water.*
- *Use an environmentally friendly cold spray that will not degrade the ozone layer. Surprisingly, some cold sprays for orthotic fabrication are "not for use on skin." Read the label or catalog description before using.*

## Shrinkage

When materials with memory have been stretched during the fabrication process, they will "shrink back" toward their original size as they cool. Indeed, they continue to contract over the first few hours after molding as they finish hardening. As a result, an orthosis that seems to fit well after it has been molded will "shrink" further after the client leaves the clinic. The client should be shown how to stretch the sides of the trough if the orthosis becomes too small (see Fig. 6-3).

Shrinkage of materials with memory is particularly problematic when the orthosis has a circumferential component. For example, when molding circumferentially around the thumb, the material will contract around the proximal phalanx as it cools, and it may become difficult to slide it off over the more bulbous distal phalanx. Similarly, when molding an anti–swan-neck orthosis around the finger, the component around the proximal phalanx may not slide over the larger PIP joint. If this should happen, apply a lubricant to the skin and allow the client to pull the orthosis off.

Precautions should be taken to ensure a safety margin for shrinkage by molding the orthosis slightly larger. This technique is described in Chapter 7.

Landec Corporation makes a distinctive, heat-shrink material called QuickCast (by North Coast Medical and Sammons Preston) or Dynacast Rapide (by supplier Smith & Nephew Inc.). It is a fiberglass fabric coated with a lightweight, temperature-sensitive polymer, which is activated by the heat of a hair dryer and shrinks about 50 percent to fit the contours of the body. Although it is available in sheet form, it is principally marketed as pre-sized, circumferential precuts for the thumb, wrist, wrist-thumb (Fig. 4-1*a*), wrist-hand, elbow, knee, and ankle. It has a plush terry liner and requires little skill to produce a bulky but soft orthosis that is unlikely to cause pressure points.

# APPEARANCE

## Sheet Size

The standard sheet size is 18 × 24 in. (46 × 61 cm). Some materials are also available in double-size sheets of 24 × 36 in. (61 × 91 cm) or half-size sheets of 12 × 18 in. (30 × 46 cm). The double-size sheets are more difficult to handle and store and are required only for very large orthoses.

## Thickness

Thermoplastics are available in thicknesses ranging from ⅟₃₂ in. (0.8 mm) to ³⁄₁₆ in. (4.8 mm), with the most popular being ⅛ in. (3.2 mm) (Fig. 4-2*a*). Other commonly used thicknesses are ⅟₁₆ in. (1.6 mm), sometimes referred to as "light," and ³⁄₃₂ in. (2.4 mm). Turbocast is the only material available in the thinnest version of ⅟₃₂ in. (0.8 mm). However, this thickness has limited applications although it is useful for finishing the edges of orthoses made from highly perforated materials. Smith & Nephew Inc. markets Aquaplast Ultra-Thin Edging material designed specifically for this purpose.

A common flaw in orthotic fabrication is the use of ⅛ in. (3.2 mm) thick material when ³⁄₃₂ in. (2.4 mm) or ⅟₁₆ in. (1.6 mm) would be adequate. As a general rule, use the thinnest material that will provide adequate support and en-

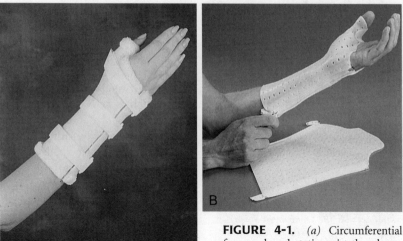

**FIGURE 4-1.** *(a)* Circumferential forearm-based static wrist-thumb orthosis fabricated from QuickCast (also called Dynacast Rapide) thumb spica forearm precut. *(b)* Circumferential forearm-based static wrist-thumb orthosis with zipper closure fabricated from a Rolyan® Aquaform wrist-thumb zipper precut. (Rolyan® is a trademark of Smith & Nephew, Inc.)

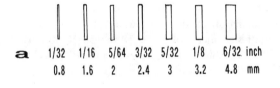

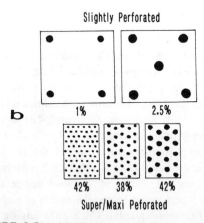

**FIGURE 4-2.** *(a)* Thicknesses of thermoplastics (drawn half scale). 5/64 and 5/32 in. (2 and 3 mm) are less common than the other thicknesses. *(b)* Degrees of perforation. Super/maxi perforated versions are available only in translucent materials, whereas slightly perforated version is available in opaque and translucent materials.

sure enough working time for the application. However, students and therapists unskilled in orthotic fabrication could begin with ⅛ in. (3.2 mm) thickness to ensure sufficient working time while developing molding skills.

Thinner materials are suitable for smaller orthoses. They also shorten the working time, are more conforming when warm, and flexible when cold. An important advantage of using thinner materials is that they produce a lighter orthosis, which is desirable for clients with muscle weakness and arthritis. Another benefit is that thinner materials can be cut cold without stress to the therapist's hands, reducing the risk of cumulative trauma to the joints and soft tissues. Further discussion of ergonomic considerations can be found in Chapter 6. Recommended applications for the different material thicknesses are shown in Table 3 in Appendix A.

## Perforations

Thermoplastic sheets are available in solid form (i.e., unperforated) and with varying degrees of perforations (Fig. 4-2b). Perforations provide ventilation, decrease the weight of the orthosis, increase the conformability during molding, reduce the working time, complicate the finishing process, and increase the flexibility of the orthosis.

Ventilation is desirable because the contact of plastic against the skin promotes perspiration. However, when a perforated material is worn directly against the limb, only the skin adjacent to each perforation is exposed to air; at least 35 percent perforation is recommended to achieve adequate ventilation. This degree of perforation is available only in translucent materials.

When using materials that are minimally perforated, a thin air space between the plastic and the skin can be achieved by a sleeve of cotton or polypropylene tubular bandage (Stockinette or Tubigrip) or splint liner worn underneath the finished orthosis (see Figs. 3-17 and 3-18). Lines made of cotton absorbs perspiration and can be readily washed. Client comfort and compliance may be higher when an interface is worn under the orthosis.

The more perforated the material, the lighter the weight of the orthosis. For clients with muscular weakness or arthritis, as well as infants, it is especially desirable to minimize the weight. To reduce the weight of an orthosis, choose a thinner material or a material that is at least 35 percent perforated (called maxi- or superperforated). The greater the perforation, the more conforming the material will be during molding.

However, perforations have the disadvantage of shortening the working time and requiring more effort to finish the edges. They are also contraindicated over wounds with exudate. Another consideration is the more perforated the material, the more flexible the orthosis and the more likely it will be deformed by force.

The most ventilated thermoplastic is Hexcelite, which is a resin-impregnated open-weave material and is discussed in more detail later in this chapter.

## Color

Low-temperature thermoplastics are available in a wide range of colors. Color influences the appeal of the orthosis for the client. However, the pigment added to the formula may shorten the working time.

Opaque materials are generally available in subdued tones of white, buff, oyster, beige, soft pink, and light blue. In contrast, translucent materials are available in white, peach, pastels, and vibrant colors (see Table 4 in Appendix A).

Common applications of brightly colored materials are for children, inpatients, or **unilateral neglect.** The wide range of bright colors available in translucent materials is popular in pediatric settings because of their appeal to children. Sammons Preston sells permanent, nontoxic splint markers, which can used to decorate an orthosis before heating. They may improve compliance and help identify orthoses belonging to different clients.

In addition to the cosmetic appeal of bright colors, colored LTT helps distinguish the orthosis from the bed linens of the inpatient and thus prevent inadvertent laundering or loss of the orthosis. Bright colors also serve as a visual attraction to help counteract the tendency toward unilateral neglect when used on the hand of a client who has experienced a stroke or head injury.

However, for the most part, adults tend to prefer colors that are "skin-colored." The peach color of Orfit or Turbocast is particularly appealing to pale-skinned clients. Kay-Splint Basics II and III from Sammons Preston are available in a wide range of beige/brown flesh tones. Consider also the wide variety of colors available in Velcro strapping material. Colored Velcro can either coordinate or contrast with the color of the thermoplastic.

## Surface Texture/Sheen

The smooth surface coating applied to reduce the surface stickiness of warm thermoplastic makes the surface smoother, with a higher sheen than uncoated materials. The coating enhances the resistance to soiling.

Heating can change the surface texture of some thermoplastics. For example, before heating, Ezeform is shiny; after heating it has a distinctive, slightly granular surface that becomes more noticeable as the material is stretched. Similarly, Polyform develops a distinctive surface texture after heating that resembles human skin.

The unique, nonstick fuzzy coating of Turbocast is initially soft like velvet but becomes harder and less comfortable for the client after heating. Despite this factor, many therapists enjoy the lack of self-adherence provided by the fuzzy coating during molding and find the material to be aesthetically pleasing. Turbocast is especially easy for the unskilled orthotic fabricator to use. In contrast, Prism and ColorFit have a distinctively high sheen that remains unchanged by heat.

### Resistance to Soiling and Ease of Cleaning

The smooth surface coating applied to reduce the surface stickiness of warm thermoplastic makes the surface more soil resistant. Materials with a coating include all opaque C and D materials, as well as Aquaplast and Orfit materials. Some opaque category A or B materials lack a surface coating and thus soil more readily and are less easily cleaned. Although Turbocast is coated to eliminate surface stickiness, the fuzzy coating is textured and prone to soiling.

## DURABILITY

The durability of a thermoplastic can be measured by its resistance to fatigue cracks and deformation. Resistance to fatigue cracks is generally an issue only with weight-bearing foot orthoses and circumferential orthoses. Many LTTs cannot withstand dynamic weight-bearing stresses and begin to show fatigue cracks within a few weeks. The most durable thermoplastic foot orthoses are $\frac{1}{12}$ in. (2 mm) San-Splint, $\frac{1}{16}$ in. (1.6 mm) Aquaplast or Orfit.

Exposing an orthosis to heat from stoves, radiators, heat registers, direct sunlight (e.g., window ledge or car dashboard), very hot water, or clothes dryer can cause it to lose its shape because the LTT is heat sensitive. Caution the client and caregiver about this inherent susceptibility.

## ● Suggested Materials to Stock

Many clinics and organizations do not like to stock a wide variety of materials and may restrict their stock to one material for all applications. Generally speaking, category C materials in either opaque or translucent categories are the most versatile. They are suitable for small, detailed orthoses yet have enough control in their stretch to allow them to be used for large, circumferential orthoses. In the opaque materials, Sammons Preston, North Coast Medical, and Remington Medical have two category C thermoplastics—C1 and C2. North Coast Medical applies the name "Preferred" to their most popular material, which is a category C2. The student or inexperienced therapist may prefer to use a C1 material, which is slightly more resistant to stretch and easier to control.

If many of the applications involve medium (wrist-hand) or small (wrist or hand only) orthoses, it is better to use $\frac{3}{32}$ or $\frac{1}{16}$ in. (2.4 or 1.6 mm) rather than the standard $\frac{1}{8}$ in. (3.2 mm) thickness. Thinner thermoplastics require less force to cut when cold and mold more readily to body contours. In addition, they are lighter for the client.

If memory is a requirement to serially reduce contractures, select either a translucent material or one of the opaque B1 materials (see Appendix A).

If detailed, highly conforming medium or small orthoses are required and the therapist has well-developed orthotic skills, a category D material is appropriate.

## ● Identifying Features

Many opaque materials are available in white or a pale, neutral color with no distinguishing characteristics, and if the identifying labels have been cut off it is difficult to tell them apart when cold. However, many materials have distinctive handling properties when warm.

- Category A materials have a high resistance to stretch because of their isoprene rubber content.
- Category B1 materials have 100 percent memory when reheated, like most of the translucent materials.
- Ezeform (category B2), which is shiny before heating, can be distinguished by its unique granular texture, which becomes apparent when stretched.
- Category C materials have a distinctive rebound when stretched, whereas category D materials have none.

## ● Other Thermoplastics

Beyond the commonly used LTTs already described, there are four other types of thermoplastics:

- Heat-moldable foam thermoplastics—Plastazote, AliPlast, NickelPlast, PE LITE
- Kushionsplint
- Hexcelite (also called X-Lite)
- Heat-shrink thermoplastics—QuickCast and Dynacast Rapide

### FOAM THERMOPLASTICS

Materials such as Plastazote, AliPlast, NickelPlast, and PE LITE are closed-cell foam thermoplastics, made from a high-temperature thermoplastic called polyethylene. The process of expanding and cross-linking the polyethylene converts it to a thermoplastic that can be safely molded directly to the client's skin. Foam thermoplastics require dry oven heating at 240°F (140°C) in a well-ventilated area.

Closed-cell foam materials will not absorb perspiration, bacteria, or odors. They have a smooth surface and are easy to clean. In contrast, open-cell foam materials tend to absorb moisture, bacteria, and odors.

Foam thermoplastics come in a wide range of thicknesses and degrees of firmness (see Table 5 in Appendix A). According to the Shore

A Firmness Scale, the lower the rating, the softer, more conforming, more cushioning, and more compressible the material. "Shore" is a classification of firmness of materials. For example, human soft tissue has a Shore A Firmness Scale of 20 to 30. The higher the rating, the greater the resistance to compression and "bottoming out." Bottoming out refers to permanent compression that occurs over time when the material is used in a weight-bearing application such as a resilient foot orthosis. To prevent this problem from occurring, select a medium-firm material ranging from Shore A 35 to 42. Although a low-density Plastazote or AliPlast seems more desirable because it will be more cushioning under the foot of an individual with arthritis, it will soon compress and lose its cushioning under the metatarsal heads and heel because of body weight. Therefore, low-density materials are best used in non–weight-bearing applications such as cervical collars or for cushioning. The firmest foam thermoplastics will not compress under body weight and are stiff enough to be used as outersoles of shoes. NickelPlast, an alloy of ethylene vinyl acetate and polyethylene, is more resistant to bottoming out than the simpler expanded polyethylenes such as AliPlast and Plastazote.

Plastazote is particularly well suited as a shoe liner or an insole for the delicate skin of the diabetic foot. We have found this material to promote reepithelialization of pressure sores. With the exception of cervical collars and insoles, Plastazote and AliPlast are not generally suitable to fabricate a full orthosis because of their bulk and lack of rigidity and conformability. AliPlast has a smoother surface than Plastazote and is less irritating to the skin. Common applications for the foam thermoplastics are identified in Table 5 in Appendix A. Foam thermoplastics are also useful to line an orthosis or pad specific parts of the orthosis (e.g., over bony prominences). For this purpose, use thinner versions that are self-adhesive.

Plastazote also comes laminated to PPT (from *Professional Protective Technology*, the name of the manufacturer) in a product called Diab-A-Sheet (from AliMed) so named because of its application in foot orthoses for individuals with diabetes.

## KUSHIONSPLINT

This distinctive ¼ in. (6.4 mm) thick material is a laminate of two foam layers plus terry cloth. Like other foam thermoplastics, it becomes moldable with dry heat and produces a semi-rigid, low-conforming, lightweight orthosis. Sammons Preston markets a prefabricated Freedom Thumb Spica Splint (radial forearm-based, wrist-thumb orthosis) for de Quervain's tenosynovitis made out of Kushionsplint.

## HEXCELITE (ALSO CALLED X-LITE)

Hexcelite is a resin-impregnated open-weave material that is sold in 72 in. (180 cm) long rolls in widths of 2, 3, 4, 5, or 6 in. (5, 7.5, 10, 12.5, or 15 cm). It is also sold in sheets of various widths and lengths. It is a flimsy material that requires two or more layers bonded together to achieve adequate rigidity. It can be used to make low-conforming orthoses. Its greatest advantage is its high degree of perforation that permits good ventilation and light weight, which is desirable for arthritic clients. Hexcelite is useful to create "hoods" to protect replants or skeletal traction hardware (see Fig. 10-18g).

## HEAT-SHRINK THERMOPLASTICS

Landec Corporation makes a distinctive, heat-shrink material called QuickCast (by suppliers North Coast Medical and Sammons Preston) or Dynacast Rapide (by supplier Smith & Nephew Inc.). It is a fiberglass fabric coated with a lightweight, temperature-sensitive polymer, which is activated by the heat of a hair dryer causing it to shrink about 50 percent to fit the contours of the body. Although it is available in sheet form, it is principally marketed as presized, circumferential precuts with a plush terrylike liner for the thumb, wrist,

wrist-thumb (Fig. 4-1a), wrist-hand, elbow, and knee.

## ● Thermoplastic Precuts

A large variety of precut designs in a wide range of materials are available from various suppliers. These are intended to eliminate the time (and associated labor cost) required to create a pattern, transfer it to the thermoplastic, heat, and cut it out. The time saved should more than compensate for increased material cost. However, many precuts are large and require a lot of trimming to fit the client. This trimming offsets the advantage of using a precut. Furthermore, there are no standards for sizing the precuts; as a result a small thumbhole wrist precut from one supplier may not be the same size as one from a different supplier. Therapists are urged to try precuts from different suppliers to find the sizes that best suit their client populations. If a certain minimum number are ordered, many suppliers will prepare custom precuts of any design to meet the therapist's specific needs.

## ● Circumferential Zipper Precuts

Zipper orthoses were first developed by Orfit Industries of Belgium in 1989. At this time there are two manufacturers of precut circumferential orthoses with a zipper sewn into the sides (see Table 6 in Appendix A). The zipper provides the method of fixation and makes it easy to mold the orthosis, applying uniform compression around the enclosed limb (Fig. 4-1b).

Orfizip precuts have a core of Orfit Classic covered on both sides with a thin cloth material; the zipper is sewn to the material along its length. Similarly, the Aquaform precuts have a longitudinal zipper, but it is sewn directly to the Aquaplast without a covering. Although the covering of the Orfizip precuts provides a perspiration-absorbent interface between the skin and the plastic, it soils easily and is difficult to clean.

Whether using an Orfizip or Aquaform pre-cut, it is important to realize that these are made from translucent materials with memory. As a result, they contract during cooling, and because of their circumferential nature, the orthosis can become too tight and constricting. To prevent excessive shrinking as the material cools and hardens, mold the orthosis over one or two layers of tubular bandage or a splint liner. For thumb orthoses, a layer of ¹⁄₁₆ in. (1.6 mm) self-adhesive Plastazote can be applied around the thumb before molding.

## ● Plaster of Paris

Plaster of Paris was commonly used to fabricate half-shell splints (in this circumstance *splint* is a more appropriate term than *orthosis*) before the introduction of LTTs in the mid-1960s. Currently, this material has two common applications in orthotics. Plaster of Paris bandage is used to generate a negative cast of a body part. Plaster of Paris powder is then mixed with water and poured into the negative cast to create a positive plaster mold over which a high-temperature thermoplastic can be molded to make a durable orthosis. The second application is to fabricate circumferential static progressive orthoses to soften scar tissue and reduce interphalangeal (IP) joint contractures.

## ● Soft Materials

Occasionally, soft materials such as webbing, elastic, and Stockinette are used to fabricate an orthosis as seen in Figures 9-16, 9-17, and 12-17.

## ● Interface Materials

Interface materials are used for lining, for padding, for absorbing perspiration, and for managing scars. Lining refers to the application of a layer of self-adhesive material over the entire inner surface of an orthosis. Padding refers to the application of a patch of self-adhesive, cushioning, or gel material over an isolated spot on the inner surface of an orthosis, usually to pad and protect a bony prominence, prevent a dynamic orthosis from "migrating," or to soften scar tissue. A full range of materials for lining or padding is found in Tables 7, 8, and 9 in Appendix A.

## LINING

A principle of orthotic design is to create an orthosis that is as thin and lightweight as possible. Therefore, unless the skin is especially fragile or cushioning is required, lining the entire inner surface is generally not recommended because it makes the orthosis bulkier, adding to its weight and thickness. Furthermore, lining is usually more difficult to clean than the smooth surface of a thermoplastic. Follow these guidelines when considering a lining for an orthosis:

- Lining should not be added to absorb perspiration—instead apply a washable tubular cotton bandage (e.g., Stockinette or Tubigrip) or splint liner over the limb.
- Do not line the orthosis to compensate for poor contouring—reheat the material and remold.
- Lining an orthosis with moleskin is generally not desirable because it cannot be washed.
- If lining is warranted, select a ¹⁄₁₆ in. (1.6 mm) thick, closed-cell (therefore washable) material and mold the orthosis with the lining in place.
- If the limb is large and more cushioning is required, choose ⅛ in. (3.2 mm) thick lining.
- To prevent migration, apply a strip of ¹⁄₃₂ in. (0.8 mm) thick self-adhesive gel sheeting (e.g., Krystal Gel) or Dycem.

## PADDING

On the other hand, padding over bony prominences is often appropriate as long as the padding is incorporated during the original molding of the thermoplastic. Another reason to pad part of the inner surface is to soften burn or surgical scar tissue using silicone, polymer gel (also called hydro gel), or elastomer.

Padding techniques are described under "Protecting the Bony Prominences" in Chapter 7. Padding should not be added *after* the molding because the space required for the padding was not accounted for, thus creating poor contour and potential pressure points.

### Lining and Padding Materials

The preferred lining and padding materials do not absorb moisture or odors and are easily washable. Select a self-adhesive, closed-cell or gel material from Tables 7 and 9 in Appendix A. Prefabricated, self-adhesive gel disks are specially designed to pad the ulnar head.

## TUBULAR BANDAGE INTERFACE

Generally, it is desirable to provide the client with an interface between the thermoplastic and the skin to absorb perspiration. The preferred type of interface is a layer of tubular cotton or polypropylene bandage (e.g., Stockinette) worn over the limb, under the orthosis. This interface is removable and easily washable. Risk of skin maceration is reduced because the cotton absorbs perspiration and allows for air circulation.

Elasticized tubular bandage (e.g., Tubigrip) is a popular alternative to Stockinette. Its elastic quality ensures that it will fit the contours of the limb without wrinkling. Also, it provides circumferential compression to help support the circulation. A variation is cushioned tubular bandage, with or without elastic reinforcement, which is lined with foam. Yet another variation is gel-lined tubular bandage, for example Thero-Gel Body Sleeve/Liner from Sammons Preston, Silopad sleeving from North Coast Medical, or Ped-A-Ligne.

One of the problems with tubular bandages is that the required length is cut from a roll and the cut edges fray, detracting from the cosmesis of the orthosis. Prefinished, nonfray, two-ply Stockinette splint liners are now available to wear under thumb, wrist-thumb, and wrist-hand orthoses.

## PRELINED THERMOPLASTICS AND PRECUTS

As previously mentioned, some thermoplastic sheets are available with an absorbent lining bonded to one side. These include Orfilined (Orfit with a terry lining on one side) and Kushionsplint (a foam thermoplastic with a terry lining on one side). Some precuts, discussed earlier, also come prelined. These include Orfizip, QuickCast, and Dynacast Rapide. When considering prelined thermoplastics and precuts, bear in mind that the lining will soil and is not easily washable.

## MATERIALS FOR SCAR MANAGEMENT

The theories regarding the mechanism by which pressure helps prevent or soften hypertrophic scar tissue are discussed in Chapter 2. Materials used to control scar tissue fall into four categories: elastic compression garments, elastomer products, prosthetic foam, and gel sheets. The last three are compared in Table 9 in Appendix A.

### Elastic Compression Garments

These custom-made or prefabricated garments, introduced about 30 years ago by Jobst (now Beiersdorf Jobst) of Toledo, Ohio, are widely used for both the prevention and correction of hypertrophic scars. However, uniform pressure is often difficult to obtain because the Lycra material bridges over concave areas of the body.

### Elastomer Products

These silicone products were introduced in the 1970s and are used to create highly conforming inserts that are worn under compression garments or orthoses to fill in the concave areas to provide uniform pressure. Elastomer is sold as a liquid or putty base to which a catalyst is added, causing the base to harden.

### Prosthetic Foam

As the name suggests, this material was developed to use as a lightweight filler for prosthetic limbs. However, it can also be used alone or in combination with elastomer to create a conforming insert that is firmer than elastomer alone. The combination is ideal for large inserts.

### Gel Sheets

There are two types of gel sheets: silicone and polymer (or hydro). Their properties are compared in Table 9 in Appendix A. They are generally less durable than elastomer inserts, but they are skin adherent and thus can be used without compressive garments or orthoses to keep them in place.

Silicone gel sheets are flexible, washable, durable, and skin adherent to varying degrees, depending on the brand. Some of the manufacturers claim their products moisturize the scar. Gel sheets should be washed with a glycerin soap to ensure maximum durability and cleanliness. Silicone gel sheets can be used alone or under compression garments or orthoses. Several reports state that silicone gel sheets are a safe and effective treatment for hypertrophic and keloid scars.[5–8] However, silicone gel treatment may cause rash, itchiness, and skin maceration.[9,10]

Polymer gel (also called hydrogel) sheets are skin adherent, mineral oil based, and silicone free. They release mineral oil onto the skin to soften and help reduce keloid and hypertrophic scar formation. The gel lubricates the skin while reducing shear forces and conforms to the most contoured areas. Polymer gel is hypoallergenic and nonsupportive of bacterial growth. It is available as sheets, seamless elastic tubing or wrap, body sleeves, gloves, and digital caps. It can be used alone or under compressive garments or orthoses.

## ● Strapping Materials

### VELCRO STRAPS

Velcro straps using hook and loop are commonly used to secure an orthosis in place. The term *Velcro* was derived from *velv*et and *cro*chet hook. Typically, a length of loop Velcro is used for the strap, and patches of self-stick hook Velcro, adhered to the orthosis, are used for the attachments.

Velcro strapping materials are available in a variety of widths and colors, with or without self-stick backing. Strapping materials can be chosen to match the color of the thermoplastic or contrast it. Younger clients tend to prefer bright colors, whereas older clients prefer that their orthosis be as inconspicuous as possible. The therapist may recommend brightly colored straps to minimize the likelihood of a detachable strap from getting lost.

Velcro rolls are available in widths of ½ in. (1.3 cm), 1 in. (2.5 cm), 1½ in. (3.8 cm), and 2 in. (5 cm). Most therapists stock 1 in. (2.5 cm) and 2 in. (5 cm) widths. For finger orthoses, there is ½ in. (1.3 cm), low plush loop Velcro called R-Thin (from Smith & Nephew Inc.), or Extra-Thin (from North Coast Medical), or Narrow Strapping Material (from Sammons Preston). Refer to suppliers' catalogs for the full range of options.

### Precut Self-Stick Hook Tabs

Precut tabs of hook Velcro are available in a variety of sizes and shapes. They are approximately 70 percent more expensive than cutting Velcro pieces from a roll (based on a cost comparison of North Coast Medical catalog prices). However, they save time and eliminate the accumulation of adhesive residue on scissors.

### Loop Strap Alternatives

The most economical strap material is plain loop Velcro. Alternatives that are more conforming include the following:

- Elasticized loop Velcro (e.g., Vel-Stretch).
- Padded straps (e.g., Velfoam, Beta Pile, and CushionStrap), which have a foam core with hook-compatible fabric on the outer surface. Padded straps are highly desirable because they conform to the body contours and distribute the securing forces over a larger surface area. The edges of Al-

phaStrap and SoftStrap are self-sealing when they are cut, creating a more finished appearance. In general, padded straps are less durable than standard loop Velcro and require more frequent replacement.

- Neoprene straps, which have a hook-sensitive surface and a rubber core.

Nonpadded alternatives include the following:

- Back-to-back hook and loop
- Omni-Tape with hook and loop on the same side
- Poly-Lock or Dual Lock, made of two intermeshing grids, which is five times stronger than conventional hook and loop Velcro

Prefabricated overlap straps are strips of plain loop Velcro or padded material, available in varying lengths and widths, with a 3 in. (7.5 cm) length of self-stick hook Velcro attached at one end.

Prefabricated D-ring straps have a length of loop Velcro with a hook portion attached at one end. A D-ring is sewn to the other end. They are available in self-stick and nonstick versions.

Prefabricated strap pads slip over loop Velcro straps. Occasionally, straps are fabricated from webbing with or without foam padding, as seen in Figure 9-2.

## STRAP ACCESSORIES

To secure one end of the loop Velcro strap to the orthosis to prevent loss, various devices can be used:

- Metal rivet—also called rapid or speedy rivet (Fig. 4-3*a*)
- Pop rivet (metal)
- Finger rivets (plastic)
- Plastic screw (Fig. 4-3*b*)
- Aluminum, bookbinder, or Chicago screw (metal) (Fig. 4-3*b*)

Pop rivets require a pop rivet gun to apply. Metal rivets are secured by a rivet setter or by hammering together, creating a permanent attachment that can be removed only by drilling through the rivet. Similarly, plastic finger rivets

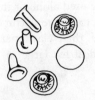

Metal rapid rivets · Chicago/Plastic screws

Various styles of D-Rings

**FIGURE 4-3.**   Accessories for straps.

create a secure attachment, but the interlocking pieces are snapped together by the fingers. In contrast, metal or plastic screws can be unfastened to detach the straps for washing or replacing. If spontaneous loosening of the screw is a problem, apply Loctite or Vibratite (available from hardware stores) to the screw before fastening.

A metal or plastic D-ring can be sewn to one end of the strap to easily cinch the orthosis closed. The size of the D-ring should match the width of the Velcro strap (Fig. 4-3*c*).

## ● Outrigger Components

The numbers in [square brackets] refer to the following suppliers of outrigger components:

1. Alimed
2. North Coast Medical
3. Orfit Industries
4. Physio E.R.P.
5. Sammons Preston
6. Smith & Nephew, Inc.
7. Vaillancourt (Canada only)

### OUTRIGGER WIRE

This is used to form the frame of a high- or low-profile outrigger. (see Figs. 1-11*f*, 10-15). Use pliers, a 90° wire bender, or a bending bar, which are described in Chapter 5. Select a light gauge wire that is easy to bend. Choices include:

- $\frac{1}{16}$ in. (1.6 mm), $\frac{3}{32}$ in. (2.4 mm), $\frac{1}{8}$ in. (3.2 mm) [1,2,4,5,6]
- Coat hanger wire

## PREFABRICATED ENERGY-STORING COMPONENTS

### Prefabricated Spiral Springs

- Universal springs—1 or $1\frac{3}{4}$ in. (2.5 or 4 cm) [2]
- Graded springs with color-coded tension [6]
- Gyovai finger springs—universal 1 in. (2.5 cm) spring with outrigger line attached at one end and Velcro tab attached at the other end [2]

### Prefabricated Spring Wire Coil Springs [3,7]

See Figure 4-4.

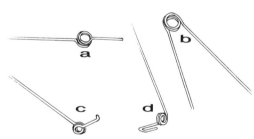

**FIGURE 4-4.** Prefabricated spring wire coil springs. *(a)* Joint jack coil spring (0.7 mm gauge). See Figure 1-11e. This spring aligns with the proximal interphalangeal (PIP) joint axis and is used in pairs to increase the extension range of the PIP joint. *(b)* Knuckle bender coil spring (0.9 mm gauge). See Figures 11-7 and 11-9. This spring aligns with the fifth metacarpophalangeal (MCP) joint axis and is used to correct MCP hyperextension in ulnar nerve palsy. *(c)* Wrist extension coiled spring (1.5 mm gauge). See Figure 10-8. This spring aligns with wrist joint axis and is used in pairs to counteract wrist drop in radial nerve palsy. *(d)* Finger extension assist (0.9 mm gauge). See Figures 3-8b and 10-13. This spring arches over the dorsum of the hand to extend the MCP joint and is used in a dynamic orthosis for radial nerve palsy.

### Rolyan® P.I.P.E. Splint (*Proximal Interphalangeal Extension*) [6]

This kit comes with five pairs of interchangeable dynamic coil springs that align with the PIP joint to apply a desired amount of force to increase the extension range of the PIP joint (see Fig. 11-21*a*).

## ENERGY-STORING MATERIALS

### Spring Wire

This is used to fabricate joint-aligned coil springs or arching spring wire outriggers using a wire bending jig or round-nosed pliers as described in Chapter 5.

- 0.9 mm gauge [3,7]
- 15 gauge [4]
- 16.5 gauge [6]

### Rubber/Elastic

- Rubber bands
- Elastic thread (wrapped elastic cord)—available in various strengths [2,6,7](see Fig. 3-11*c*)
- Thera-Band/Orfiband [1–7]
- Thera-Band strips [1,4]
- Thera-Band tubing [1,2,4,5,6]

## NONELASTIC NYLON/POLYESTER LINE AND CONNECTORS (FIG. 4-5)

- Nylon line is sold as outrigger line, fishing line, or monofilament [1–7]
- Outrigger line connectors [2,6]. Crimp the connector with pliers to attach outrigger line to finger loop or sling to eliminate the need to tie knots.
- Tension-adjustable connecting pieces [6] (see Fig. 3-11*b*).

## FINGER ATTACHMENTS

- Finger loops or slings (see Figs. 3-10 and 3-11) are used for orthoses that exert flexion or extension force [1,2,4,5,6]. They are

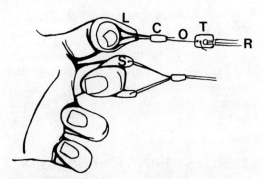

**FIGURE 4-5.** Attachment to fingers to apply extension force (as shown) or flexion force. L = finger loop; S = finger sling; O = outrigger line (monofilament); C = outrigger line connector; T = tension-adjustable connecting piece—the two small holes adjust the outrigger line tension while the larger hole is used for tying on a rubber band (R).

made from Velfoam, ultrasuede, vinyl, or loop Velcro. Prefabricated loops and slings are available with or without metal eyelets, or you can make your own.

- Glue-on finger hooks [1,2,4,5,6]. Metal dressmaker's hooks are adhered to the fingernail with an instant adhesive such as Krazy Glue and detached with nail polish remover (see Fig. 1-12).
- Contoured finger hooks [2,6]. This variation of the finger hook is contoured and covers a larger surface area of the nail.
- Rolyan® wrap-on finger hooks [6]. These have a Dycem nonslip lining that prevents distal migration. They are secured with Velcro.
- Silicone finger caps [3,7].
- Rolyan® Biodynamic Flexion/Extension System [6] promotes composite flexion or extension of finger MCP and IPs (see Fig. 10-24).

## LINE GUIDES

These are used to change the direction of the line.

- Plastic pulley [1,5]
- Super/maxi-perforated translucent material such as Aquaplast or Orfit (see Figs. 1-11*d* and 10-15)

- Metal eyelets—this is the "eye" of the dressmaker's "hook and eye" [2]
- Paper clip (see Fig. 10-24)
- Safety pin

## TUBES FOR TUBE OUTRIGGERS AND LINE GUIDES

Aquatubes and ThermoTubes require heating to be shaped, whereas Orfitubes are bendable with the hands without heating (see Figs. 3-11*c* and 11-12*b*).

- Aquatubes (made of white Aquaplast T) ³⁄₁₆, ¼, and ⅜ in. (4.8, 6.4, and 9.5 mm) diameters [6]
- ThermoTubes (made of white Prism) [2]
- Orfitubes (clear plastic)—use with metal Orfitube ends [3,7]

## HINGES

A variety of prefabricated metal hinges are available for the wrist, elbow, knee, and ankle [1,2,6,7].

## PREFABRICATED ADJUSTABLE OUTRIGGERS

These use a slotted pulley that is aligned using an Allen wrench. The pulley comes mounted on a preformed outrigger wire form, which is embedded into the thermoplastic base. They are designed for a single finger or all digits. Two common makes are Phoenix (see Fig. 1-11*f*) [1,2,4,5,6] and Rolyan® (see Figs. 3-10*b* and 3-11*b*) [6].

## MERIT STATIC PROGRESSIVE COMPONENT

This thumb screw resembles the nut on stringed instruments used to adjust the tension in the string (see Figs. 10-16 and 11-12*a*) [1,6].

# Liquids

Various liquids may be required for the molding or finishing process, including the following:

- Liquid disinfectant (e.g., Hibiclens from North Coast Medical) added to the heating pan water helps reduce the risk of cross-infection and helps prevent accidental adherence of thermoplastics when they are heating.
- Hand lotion applied to the client's skin prevents unwanted adherence of thermoplastics that are excessively surface sticky when warm. The therapist also finds it easier to manipulate sticky thermoplastics with lubricated hands.
- Solvent or 100 percent alcohol dissolves the surface coating to prime it for bonding.
- Cold spray hastens the cooling of the thermoplastic during the molding procedure. Select a spray that will not degrade the ozone layer and is safe for the skin.

- Contact cement is required to adhere LTT to Plastazote or AliPlast for some orthoses. Select a brand that is solvent free. Rubber cement does not work.
- Instant adhesive (e.g., Krazy Glue) adheres dressing hooks to fingernails for orthoses that pull the fingers into flexion.
- Nail polish remover dissolves the instant adhesive to remove fingernail hooks.

## References

1. Clark, J: Personal communication, June 1996.
2. Johnson, E: Personal communication, September 1996.
3. Durant, M: Personal communication, August 1996.
4. Kirk, J: Personal communication, June 1996.
5. Ahn, ST, et al: Topical silicone gel: A new treatment for hypertrophic scars. Surgery 106:781, 1989.
6. Katz, BE: Silicone gel sheeting in scar therapy. Curtis 56:65, 1995.
7. Quinn, KJ, et al: Non-pressure treatment of hypertrophic scars. Burns 12:102, 1985.
8. Mercer, NSG: Silicone gel in the treatment of keloid scar. Br J Plast Surg 42:83, 1989.
9. McNee, J: The use of silicone gel in the control of hypertrophic scarring. Physiotherapy 76:194, 1990.
10. Gibbons, M, et al: Experience with silastic gel sheeting in pediatric scarring. J Burn Care Rehabil 15:69, 1994.

CHAPTER **5**

# Equipment and Tools

Equipment is available from several rehabilitation suppliers. Many tools are also sold in hardware, department, and hobby stores, where they are often less expensive than comparable tools in rehabilitation catalogs. Suppliers for all equipment and tools are listed in Table 5-1. Addresses of suppliers can be found in Appendix D.

When purchasing power equipment, ensure that it meets safety standards. In North America, look for either the Underwriters Laboratories (UL) or the Canadian Standards Association (CSA) seal of approval. Check equipment and tools frequently to ensure that they are in optimal working condition.

Height-adjustable chairs, tables, and plinths are required to optimally position the therapist and client during the fabrication process. Ergonomic considerations are discussed in Chapter 6. Techniques for using various equipment and tools are described in Chapter 7.

## ● Creating and Transferring Patterns

Paper towels or flexible clear plastic sheets are useful for making patterns. A flexible tape measure is required for circumferential limb measurements to generate patterns for some orthoses.

To mark patterns or trim lines on thermoplastic, the therapist can use a light-colored grease pencil, scratch awl, ballpoint pen, or permanent marker. Avoid nonpermanent felt-tipped markers because the ink will run in wa-

**TABLE 5–1. Suppliers of Equipment and Tools**

| | AliMed | North Coast Medical | Physio E.R.P. | Sammons Preston | Smith & Nephew Inc. | Orfit or Vaillancourt | Various Nonrehabilitation Suppliers |
|---|---|---|---|---|---|---|---|
| **Creating the Pattern** | | | | | | | |
| Flexible tape measure | ✓ | ✓ | ✓ | ✓ | ✓ | | Housewares |
| White or yellow grease pencil | | ✓ | | | | | Office supplies |
| Scratch awl | | ✓ | | ✓ | | | Tool/department store |
| Ballpoint pen or permanent marker | | | | | | | Office supplies |
| Decorative splint markers | | | | ✓ | | | |
| **Moist Heating** | | | | | | | |
| Splinting pan | ✓ | ✓ | ✓ | ✓ | ✓ | ✓ | |
| Rolyan®Large Heat Pan | | | | | ✓ | | |
| Small heat pan (electric frying pan) | ✓ | ✓ | ✓ | | | | Department/appliance store |
| Splinting pan timer | | ✓ | | | ✓ | | |
| Heavy-duty cart | ✓ | | | ✓ | ✓ | | |
| Hydrocollator | | ✓ | ✓ | ✓ | ✓ | | |
| Cooking thermometer | ✓ | ✓ | ✓ | ✓ | ✓ | | Housewares/department store |
| Hibiclens | | ✓ | | | | | Substitute another from a pharmacy |
| Microwave oven | | | | | | | Department/appliance store |
| Towels/sheets/pillowcases | | | | | | | Housewares/department store |
| Spatula | | ✓ | ✓ | | ✓ | | Housewares/department store |
| Baster | | ✓ | ✓ | | | | Housewares/department store |
| Large syringe | | | | | | | From hospital supplies |
| **Dry Heating** | | | | | | | |
| Countertop convection oven | ✓ | | | | | | Department/appliance store |
| Kitchen oven | | | | | | | Department/appliance store |
| Splinting oven | | | ✓ | | | | Restaurant equipment |
| Heat gun | ✓ | ✓ | ✓ | ✓ | ✓ | ✓ | Substitute a paint stripper tool |
| Hair dryer | | ✓ | | ✓ | ✓ | | Department store |
| Metal baking sheets | | | | | | | Housewares/department store |
| Potholders or insulating work gloves | | | | | | | Department store |
| Cornstarch or talcum powder | | | | | | | Department store |
| **Cutting Thermoplastics** | | | | | | | |
| Scissors | ✓ | ✓ | ✓ | ✓ | ✓ | ✓ | Department/tool store |
| Utility knife | ✓ | ✓ | ✓ | ✓ | ✓ | | Department/tool/hobby store |
| Knife with retractable, break-off blades | | | | | | | Department/tool store |
| Metal straight edge | | | | | | | Department/tool store |
| Rolyan® Cutting Tool | | | | ✓ | | | |

*(continued)*

**TABLE 5-1.   Suppliers of Equipment and Tools (Continued)**

| | AliMed | North Coast Medical | Physio E.R.P. | Sammons Preston | Smith & Nephew Inc. | Orfit or Vaillancourt | Various Nonrehabilitation Suppliers |
|---|---|---|---|---|---|---|---|
| **Bandage Wrapping** | | | | | | | |
| Elastic bandage | ✓ | | | ✓ | ✓ | | Pharmacy or medical supplies |
| Thera-Band | ✓ | ✓ | ✓ | ✓ | ✓ | | |
| Orfiband | | | | | | ✓ | |
| **Edge Finishing/Safety Tools** | | | | | | | |
| Hand grinder | | | | | ✓ | | Department/tool/hobby store |
| Bench grinder with vacuum | ✓ | | | | | | Department/tool store |
| Face shield | ✓ | | | | | | Safety supply store |
| Goggles | ✓ | | | | | | Department/tool store |
| Filter mask | ✓ | | | | | | Department/tool store |
| **Strapping** | | | | | | | |
| Revolving hole punch | ✓ | ✓ | ✓ | ✓ | ✓ | ✓ | Department/tool store |
| Manual drill | ✓ | ✓ | ✓ | | ✓ | | Department/tool store |
| Power drill | | | | | | | Department/tool store |
| Rivet gun | | ✓ | ✓ | ✓ | | | Department/tool store |
| Hammer | | | | | | | Department/tool store |
| Anvil | | | | | | | Department/tool store |
| Sewing machine | | | | | | | Department store |
| **Wire Bending/Cutting** | | | | | | | |
| Flat-nose or needle-nose pliers | | | ✓ | ✓ | ✓ | | Department/tool store |
| Round-nose pliers | | | | | | ✓ | Department/tool store |
| Ergonomic pliers | | | | | ✓ | | Specialty tool store |
| Heavy-duty wire cutter | ✓ | | ✓ | ✓ | ✓ | | Department/tool store |
| 90° wire bender | | ✓ | | | ✓ | | |
| Wire bending bar | | ✓ | | ✓ | | | |
| Wire bending jig | | | | | ✓ | | |
| **Tool Organizers and Carriers** | | | | | | | |
| Tool tote | | | | | | | Tool store |
| Tool pouch | | | | ✓ | ✓ | | |
| Carrying cart with wheels | | | | | | | Luggage store |
| Rolyan® Port-a-Splint Kit | | | | | ✓ | | |
| **Spring Gauges** | ✓ | ✓ | ✓ | ✓ | | | |

ter. Every effort should be made to cut off the pen or pencil lines when cutting or trimming the orthosis. Pen or pencil markings detract from the cosmesis of the finished orthosis.

Sammons Preston sells permanent, nontoxic splint markers that can be used to decorate an orthosis before heating. They may improve compliance and help identify orthoses belonging to different clients.

# ● Moist Heating

Various appliances are designed to heat water. They differ in cost, size, and appearance.

Electric "splinting" pans are available in a wide variety of sizes, with or without lids. Most pans have variable heat settings to accommodate the heating temperatures of all thermoplastics. The Rolyan® Large Heat Pan has the largest surface area; however, it has only one heat setting of 160°F (70°C) (Fig. 5-1a). This temperature accommodates all thermoplastics except Orfit Classic, which is best heated at 140°F (60°C); when heated at a higher temperature, Orfit Classic becomes more sticky. A useful accessory is a timer that automatically turns the pan on and off.

A household electric frying pan provides a satisfactory, low-cost alternative; however, it has a much smaller surface area than a splinting pan (Fig. 5-1b). It is sold by rehabilitation suppliers as a small heat pan and is easily portable for the traveling therapist visiting clients in their homes. To heat a long piece of thermoplastic material in a small pan, fold the material back and forth on itself, inserting a paper towel between the layers to prevent material adhesion. If the ability to wheel a pan between different locations is desirable, consider a heavy-duty utility cart (Fig. 5-2a).

Another moist heat source is the hydrocollator, a deep container designed to heat hot packs (Fig. 5-2b). The hydrocollator can be used for category A or B materials, or if the hydrocollator has a horizontal shelf, category C or D materials can be heated without distortion. Alternatively, the material can be lowered into the water on a net liner to keep it horizontal. It is not recommended to heat category C or D materials by suspending them vertically in the hydrocollator because they will easily stretch in length, distorting their shape.

The therapist can heat water in a skillet on a stove or pour boiling water from a kettle into a deep-dish pan. The key to successful thermoplastic heating without the aid of a thermostat is to have the water steaming, not boiling. These heating techniques may be more commonly used by home care or traveling therapists. A cooking thermometer may be desirable to ensure the proper water temperature if thermostatically controlled appliances are not used. When fabricating orthoses for neonates in the

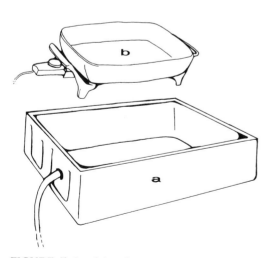

**FIGURE 5-1.** *(a)* Rolyan® Large Heat Pan. *(b)* Small heat pan (electric frying pan).

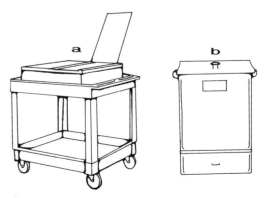

**FIGURE 5-2.** *(a)* Splinting pan with lid and heavy-duty cart. *(b)* Hydrocollator.

neonatal intensive care unit, use an insulated coffee mug to maintain the temperature of the water.

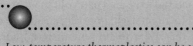

*Low-temperature thermoplastics can be soft-ened in a microwave oven. Place the material in a container of water and heat on high for 1 to 2 minutes, depending on the size and thick-ness of the material and output of the oven. For more information on this topic, see Afor, JD: Microwave proves effective for softening low temperature splinting materials. Advance for Occupational Therapists June 26, 1989.*

When using moist heat sources, especially large heating pans, consider adding an antimicrobial cleanser such as Hibiclens to the water to reduce the risk of cross infection and to prevent accidental adherence of thermoplastics when they are heating.

A plastic spatula is useful to lift LTTs out of hot water (Fig. 5-3a). Basters (Fig. 5-3b) or large syringes (Fig. 5-3c), available from hospital suppliers, can be used to spot heat with hot water withdrawn from a heating pan. Towels, sheets, or pillowcases are needed to dry moist-heated materials before molding. It is especially important to dry perforated materials because the perforations retain the hot water and could burn the skin.

Check the power requirement of any heating appliance before you purchase it. Some pans draw as much as 13 amps. Most North American electric circuits provide only 15 amps. Each circuit may have several receptacles. However, you may be able to use only one pan plus perhaps a power hand grinder on one circuit. If you want to use both a heating pan and heat gun simultaneously, you probably need two separate electrical circuits.

## ● Dry Heating

Dry heating is required for foam thermoplastics (e.g., Plastazote, AliPlast, and Kushion-Splint), which soften at 250° to 300°F (140° to 170°C) and high-temperature thermoplastics (e.g., polyethylene heated at 250°F/140°C). Choices include a countertop convection oven, a kitchen oven, and a splinting oven (Fig. 5-4). The latter looks like a pizza oven and has a large interior. Isoprene-based opaque materials (category A1) can be oven heated. This provides a useful alternative for softening pieces of thermoplastic that are too large for a heating pan. Splinting ovens and kitchen ovens usually require 220 volts. Install a ventilation unit or fan above the oven to remove hazardous fumes from the area.

An electric heat gun is used to spot heat thermoplastic materials. Two popular models are the heavy-duty model and the lightweight, silent heat gun (Fig. 5-5). A pinpoint nozzle can be added to concentrate the flow of hot air when spot heating. Alternatively, a paint remover gun, available from hardware stores, can be used. Spot heating is performed to smooth edges and make minor adjustments to the con-

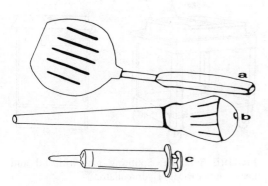

**FIGURE 5-3.**    *(a)* Spatula. *(b)* Baster. *(c)* Syringe.

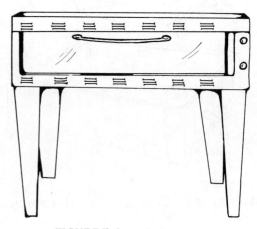

**FIGURE 5-4.**    Splinting oven.

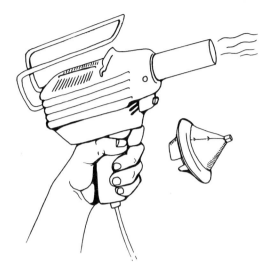

**FIGURE 5-5.** Silent heat gun with pinpoint nozzle to concentrate the heat.

tour of an orthosis or to dry heat materials that are to be bonded.

A hair dryer is required when molding heat-shrinking fiberglass precuts under the trade names of QuickCast or Dynacast Rapide.

Metal baking sheets sprinkled with cornstarch or talcum powder to prevent sticking are required for dry heat methods. Potholders or gloves protect the therapist's hands from hot surfaces and high-temperature thermoplastics.

## ● Cutting Low-Temperature Thermoplastics

Scissors are essential to the fabrication process, and therapy supply catalogs offer a wide range of designs (Fig. 5-6). For example, curved scissors of different sizes are useful for rounding material corners and cutting into small areas. Bandage scissors are ideal for cutting thermoplastic against the client's skin because the blunt tips prevent injury. For the therapist who has weak hands or inflamed joints or tendons, consider self-opening, cushion-handled scissors. Also available are scissors that are ergonomically angled and scissors for left-handed users.

To minimize hand stress, ensure that the blades are sharp and that materials ⅛ in. (3.2

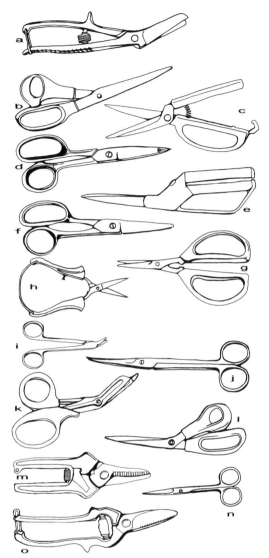

**FIGURE 5-6.** Various types of scissors. (*a*) EuroShears—self-opening, ergonomically angled handle. (*b*) Fiskars scissors—plastic, contoured handles, available in right- or left-handed models. (*c*) Good Grips by Oxo—self-opening, cushioned handles, ergonomically angled blades. (*d*) Large curved scissors—all metal. (*e*) Fiskars Softouch scissors—self-opening, padded handles. (*f*) Heavy duty scissors—rounded tips for safety. (*g*) Joyce Chen scissors—flexible handles, short blades. (*h*) Stirex curved scissors—self-opening, very short blades. (*i*) Serial cast cutter scissors—mini serrated blades for finger-based orthoses. (*j*) Curved Mayo scissors—medium-length curved blades. (*k*) Bandage scissors—blunt tip ensures safety when cutting thermoplastic against client's skin. (*l*) Razor Edge Fiskar scissors—adjustable blade tension. (*m*) All-purpose snip—cuts thermoplastic and wire, spring-loaded handles. (*n*) Surgical scissors—razor-sharp, short curved blades. (*o*) Heavy-duty shears.

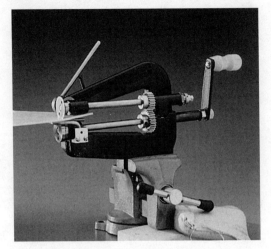

**FIGURE 5-7.** Rolyan® Cutting Tool.

mm) or thicker are heated before cutting or trimming. For cutting materials that have not been heated, use heavy-duty shears or the Rolyan® Cutting Tool mounted on a bench vise (Fig. 5-7). Designate one pair of scissors to be used exclusively for cutting adhesive-backed Velcro; the scissors used to cut warm thermoplastic must be kept free of Velcro adhesive residue that creates drag, making it difficult to cut a smooth edge. To remove adhesive residue, wipe the blades with an alcohol swab.

Knives are used to score thermoplastic sheets to break them into smaller sizes that fit into the heating pan. Rehabilitation suppliers carry utility knives (Fig. 5-8*a*). A better choice is a knife with retractable, break-off blades available from department, tool, or office supply stores (Fig. 5-8*b*). A metal-edged ruler facilitates scoring thermoplastic with a knife.

● **Bandage Wrapping**

Elastic bandage (e.g., Tensor, Ace) helps achieve contours when molding the low-confirming category A or B thermoplastics. Alternatively, Thera-Band or Orfiband can be used. To promote faster setup of the warm thermoplastic, soak the elastic bandage in ice water or store the Thera-Band or Orfiband in a freezer.

● **Edge Finishing**

This equipment is used to smooth the edges of polyethylene, category A or B materials, and foam thermoplastics (e.g., Plastazote, AliPlast, and Kushionsplint).

*Electric hand grinders (e.g., Dremel Moto-Tool) are versatile and portable, allowing one to smooth curved edges, such as the thumb hole of wrist orthoses (Fig. 5-8c). Cone-shaped grinding stones are best suited for this application. In addition, the grinding stone can be replaced with a drill bit, converting the tool into a power drill.*

Bench grinders, available from tool stores, are alternatives to hand grinders to smooth edges of larger orthoses. They are particularly useful for finishing the edges of Plastazote or AliPlast collars. Ideally, a vacuum attachment for the grinder should also be used to reduce the accumulation of dust in the work environment.

A plastic face shield is essential for protection from small pieces of thermoplastic flying from the grinder (Fig. 5-9*a*). Goggles or safety glasses provide eye protection but do not protect the lower face (Fig. 5-9*b*). Therapists with respiratory sensitivity should use a personal fil-

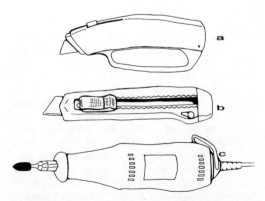

**FIGURE 5-8.** *(a)* Utility knife with knuckle guard and curved grip. Uses retractable, single blades that must be replaced when dull. *(b)* Retractable knife with break-off blades. *(c)* Electric hand grinder. The one shown here has a cone-shaped grinding stone.

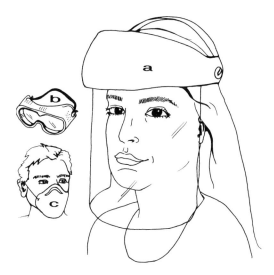

**FIGURE 5-9.** *(a)* Plastic face shield. *(b)* Safety goggles. *(c)* Filter mask.

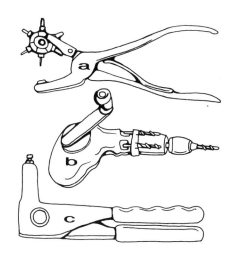

**FIGURE 5-10.** *(a)* Revolving hole punch. *(b)* Manual drill. *(c)* Rivet gun.

ter mask to avoid breathing dust particles, especially when grinding Plastazote or AliPlast (Fig. 5-9*c*). The filter mask can be used in combination with goggles or a face shield. These items are available from safety suppliers and hardware and tool stores. Again, install ventilation units to maintain air quality.

## Strapping

On occasion, a sewing machine is required for sewing straps and constructing a few fabric orthoses.

When it is necessary to punch a hole ⅛ in. (3.2 mm) or smaller within 1¼ in. (3 cm) from the edge of the orthosis, or through strapping material, use a revolving hole punch with different size holes (Fig. 5-10*a*). Some models are heavy duty but have only one size hole.

If a hole is required farther from the edge, use a manual drill (Fig. 5-10*b*). Another good choice is a power drill or a power hand grinder with a drill bit. Alternatively, create a hole by heating a scratch awl with a heat gun and then pushing through the material. Drills are also useful for removing metal rapid rivets.

Rivet guns (Fig. 5-10*c*) allow the therapist to use pop rivets, even in awkward places. Alternatively, the therapist could use metal rapid riv-

ets, which are secured with a rivet setter. If a rivet setter is not available, use a hammer and anvil clamped to a bench vise to hammer together the interlocking components.

## Wire Bending

These tools are used primarily for fabricating outriggers. Styles of pliers include round-nose, flat-nose, and needle-nose (Fig. 5-11*a, b,* and *c*). Round-nose pliers are particularly useful for

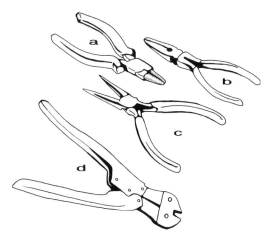

**FIGURE 5-11.** *(a)* Round-nose pliers. *(b)* Flat-nose pliers. *(c)* Needle-nose pliers. *(d)* Heavy-duty wire cutter.

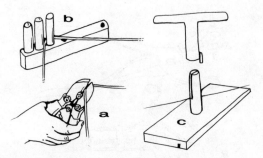

**FIGURE 5-12.** *(a)* 90° wire bender. *(b)* Wire-bending bar. *(c)* Wire-bending jig.

shaping arching spring wire or forming coils. Most pliers have an edge suitable for cutting spring wire. When cutting thick wire, use a heavy-duty wire cutter to minimize hand stress (Fig. 5-11*d*).

For tasks that require sharp-angle bends, a 90° wire bender makes the job easy and minimizes stress to the therapist's hands (Fig. 5-12*a*).

Alternatively, a wire-bending bar can bend wire to virtually any angle or curve required (Fig. 5-12*b*). A wire-bending jig allows the fabricator to create spring coils from spring wire (Fig. 5-12*c*).

## ● Tool Organizers and Carriers

A small, lightweight tool tote facilitates the transport of small tools when it is necessary to fabricate an orthosis on the ward (Fig. 5-13*a*). The tote is also useful in the orthotic education laboratory. We recommend one tote per pair of students. Another device for organizing and transporting small tools is a tool pouch (Fig. 5-13*b*). The Roylan® Port-A-Splint Kit comes with small heat pan, heat gun, cutting board, hole punch, scissors, utility knife, and samples of thermoplastics in a carrying case.

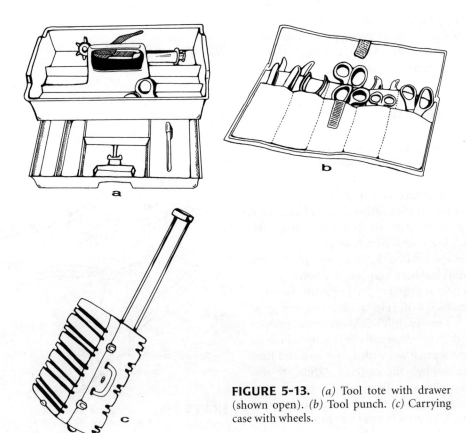

**FIGURE 5-13.** *(a)* Tool tote with drawer (shown open). *(b)* Tool punch. *(c)* Carrying case with wheels.

For the therapist who is traveling to clients' homes, consider a lightweight carrying case with wheels to hold the heat pan, thermoplastics, strapping materials, scissors, pliers, solvent, heat gun, and hand grinder. This is available from luggage stores (Fig. 5-13c).

## ● Spring Gauges

A spring gauge (also called an orthotic gauge or pinch meter) measures the force exerted by a dynamic or static-progressive outrigger. It is also used for torque-angle measurements. A spring gauge can measure force up to 150, 500, 600, or 1000 g, depending on the model (see Fig. 7-2).

CHAPTER **6**

# Ergonomic Considerations for Orthotic Fabrication

## ● Ergonomic Principles

Ergonomic principles, a common component of worker and workplace education by occupational therapists and physical therapists, should be applied during orthotic fabrication to minimize ergonomic risk factors contributing to injury. Possible injuries attributable to orthotic fabrication include sudden trauma, such as lacerations and burns, and cumulative trauma disorders (CTDs), such as joint strain, tendinitis, tenosynovitis, nerve compression, and back or neck strain.

Cumulative trauma disorders, commonly called repetitive strain injuries, are disorders of the tissues of the body caused by the cumulative effect of microtrauma.[1,2] In general, when the demands placed on the tissue exceed the ultimate adaptive limits of the tissue, microtrauma results.[1]

**Ergonomics,** derived from *ergon* meaning "work" and *nomos* meaning "laws of," literally means "the laws of work." Simply speaking, it is the science of fitting the task to the worker. The objective of ergonomics is to adapt the work and the elements of the work environment to match the worker's capacity, to reduce occupational injuries and enhance productivity. When principles of ergonomics are applied, worker productivity, comfort, and safety are increased.

To minimize ergonomic risk factors during orthotic fabrication, apply these key ergonomic principles:

- Decrease force
- Decrease repetition
- Optimize posture

## Workstation

To optimize the orthotic workstation the following should be considered:

- Lighting
- Noise
- Humidity/temperature
- Air quality
- Organization

To avoid eyestrain, ensure adequate task lighting and position work away from window glare.

Noise can be reduced by using silent heat guns instead of noisy models (see Fig. 5-5). Consider also the distracting influence of noisy bench and hand grinders, and try to operate these tools away from the client.

Air temperature and humidity should also be considered in the work environment, especially when heating thermoplastics. For example, in an operating room (OR) environment, thermoplastics should be heated outside the OR to avoid air contamination when using a moist heat method. Take into consideration how to counteract the effect of heating appliances on air temperature with ventilation, fans, open windows, and air conditioning.

Air quality in the fabricating environment can be contaminated by dust particles, solvents, and adhesives; ensure that there is an effective ventilation system and avoid using toxic solutions or sprays with chlorofluorocarbons whenever possible to avoid further ozone degradation. Consider using North Coast Medical's Quik-Freeze or Smith & Nephew, Inc.'s Cold Spray.[3,4] In addition, solvent-free contact cement is now available. To help prevent eye irritation or central nervous system (CNS) depression resulting from exposure to toxic agents, use a face shield or a filter mask (see Fig. 5-9a and c). Similarly, when operating a power grinder (especially with foam thermoplastics) it is important to attach a dust collection bag and use a face shield to protect the eyes and lungs.

Another concern is the possibility that thermoplastic materials or other orthotic products may emit toxic fumes during heating or use. The measured air concentration of commonly used orthotic products can reach levels from 165 to 1131 ppm (parts per million), depending on the solvent. This could adversely affect health, causing eye irritation, respiratory tract irritation, CNS depression, or headaches.[5] Thus, whenever possible, avoid using solvents when preparing surfaces of thermoplastic for bonding. If solvents must be used, wear gloves, avoid inhalation, close the bottle quickly after use, and ensure that the work area is well ventilated.

*Many thermoplastic surfaces can be primed for bonding with 100 percent isopropyl alcohol. Alternatively, the surface coating can be scraped off with scissors or a knife.*

Organization of the orthotic workstation should ensure that commonly used tools, equipment, and supplies are within a comfortable distance to avoid excessive reaching, bending, or twisting. These measures decrease the risk of back, neck, or shoulder pain and increase overall efficiency.[6,7] Lay out the workstation so that the client can be positioned near the heating appliance. In addition, the work area should be organized to avoid spills, tripping, and displacement of tools. For example, electric wires should be tucked away to avoid accidents. Storage for tools and supplies should ensure that they will not be a hazard for clients.

## Tools and Equipment

Stock your facility with tools that will make the fabrication process more efficient and safer. Increasingly, tools and equipment are being ergonomically redesigned to enhance the worker-environment fit and decrease stress on the therapist's joints and muscles. Ergonomically designed tables, chairs, keyboards (for computer charting), contoured hand tools (Fig. 6-1), and self-opening, cushion-handled, or left-handed scissors (see Fig. 5-6) are examples of such innovations. Some tools can greatly reduce the amount of force required to perform an activity, for example the 90° wire bender (see Fig. 5-12a). To enhance grip and dissipate vibrations, add slip-resistant, cylindrical foam

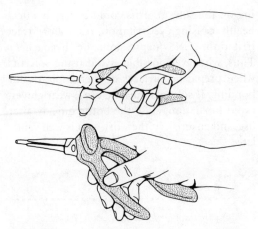

**FIGURE 6-1.** *(a)* Standard pliers promoting poor wrist positioning, in this case flexion and ulnar deviation. *(b)* Ergonomic pliers with contoured handles promoting good wrist alignment and better distribution of force.

tubing to build up tool handles. When using tools that vibrate, take periodic breaks and wear Sorbothane-lined gloves.

Maintain tools and equipment in proper working order and replace or repair when necessary. Doing so will prolong the life of the equipment and ensure that all parts are in good working order. For example, scissors should be kept sharp and free of any Velcro adhesive to ensure clean, smooth-cutting blades. To achieve this, keep a separate pair of scissors exclusively for cutting self-stick Velcro, or clean the blades as required with an alcohol swab. It is especially important to check the function of electrical equipment to prevent electrical malfunction and overheating.

Ensure that all electrical equipment is unplugged when not in use, especially at the end of the workday. Some heat guns operate so quietly that it is easy to accidentally leave them on. Consider purchasing a timer for the heating pan to avoid the possibility of forgetting to turn off the pan.

## ● Work Methods

Work methods that contribute to cumulative trauma include overexertion, repetitive movements, duration of the task, number of or-

thoses fabricated per day, and insufficient rest breaks.

Injuries caused by overexertion are the most common of all work-related injuries.[8] Keep cutting tools sharp to reduce exertion. When cutting 1/8 in. (3.2 mm) materials, always heat them first to prevent hand strain. Minimize trimming by taking the time to produce a precise custom pattern (as described in Chapter 7). The use of well-sized precuts decreases hand stress by eliminating the need to cut out patterns. Zipper precuts are particularly efficient because they eliminate cutting and strapping (see Fig. 4-1*b*). Similarly, prefabricated outriggers or preformed coil springs can eliminate wire bending (see Fig. 4-4).

*Rather than routinely using ⅛ in. (3.2 mm) thick low-temperature thermoplastics (LTTs), substitute thinner thermoplastics that are ³⁄₃₂ or ¹⁄₁₆ in. (2.4 or 1.6 mm) thick; they are easy and safe to cut cold and are strong enough for most orthotic applications (see Table 3 in Appendix A).*

Whenever possible, use the largest joints available to apply forces to prevent joint and muscle strain. For example, when "cold-adjusting" a molded orthosis to accommodate increased edema, avoid using the small joints of the fingers to apply the spreading force (Fig. 6-2). Instead, stabilize the orthosis on a tabletop and lean on the sides of the orthosis so that body weight applied through the palms will spread the edges of the trough apart to widen it (Fig. 6-3).

Traveling therapists may be required to lift equipment in and out of their vehicle. They can avoid injuries from overexertion and poor posture by employing safe lifting and carrying techniques. Using a carrying cart with wheels can enhance back safety and efficiency (see Fig. 5-13*c*). Therapists may also be required to assist a client to transfer before an orthosis can be molded. Learn and practice safe lifting and transfer techniques to avoid injury. Seek assistance when the task exceeds your capacity.

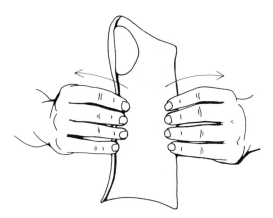

**FIGURE 6-2.** Incorrect method of widening the trough of an orthosis by using the small joints of the fingers.

The therapist who is required to do heavy lifting should develop and maintain strong muscles in the abdomen and back through regular exercise. During every activity, from lifting to operating a wire-bending jig, it is important to use the best biomechanical techniques. In addition, try to rotate your tasks so that you are not using the same joints or muscles for extended periods of time. Take the time to stretch muscles that have been exerted and schedule rest periods into your workday.

 ## Work Posture

Posture relates to positioning of all joints, but in orthotic fabrication, the positioning of the neck, back, and wrist is of particular concern. For example, keep the wrist and forearm in neutral alignment as much as possible; that is, avoid extremes of wrist extension, flexion, or radial or ulnar deviation, as well as pronation and supination, during work activities. Ergonomically designed hand tools (Fig. 6-1*b*) facilitate neutral alignment.

Awkward postures can cause muscle strain, joint strain, back pain, nerve compression, and other musculoskeletal stresses. Standing, sitting, and reaching can contribute to work-induced injury if proper techniques are not employed. Avoid excessive reaching, twisting, or bending.

For the therapist who prefers to stand to cut material or to mold the orthosis, bending over a standard 30 in. (76 cm) high table is not advisable because lumbar flexion puts strain on the intervertebral disks and back muscles (Fig. 6-4). To maintain an upright posture during molding, seat the client on an adjustable-height stool at a suitable work height (Fig. 6-5). For example, when molding a cervical collar, standing enhances the therapist's body mechanics. Seat the client in front of a mirror with the shoulder at

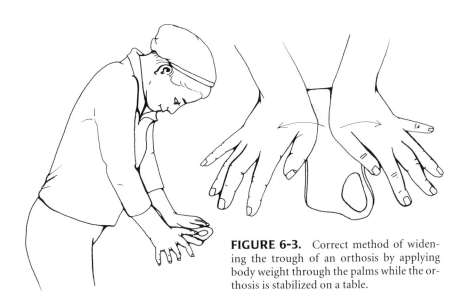

**FIGURE 6-3.** Correct method of widening the trough of an orthosis by applying body weight through the palms while the orthosis is stabilized on a table.

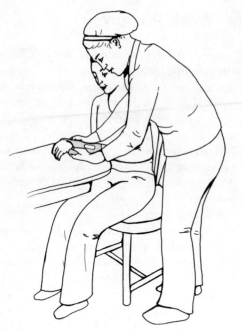

**FIGURE 6-4.**   Poor posture caused by standing to mold an orthosis on a client sitting at a standard-height table.

your elbow level so you can apply the most effective force for molding (Fig. 6-6). Similarly, when molding an orthosis to the lower extremity, a height-adjustable plinth enables the therapist to mold without excessive back bending.

For heavy work requiring upper body exertion, such as cutting thermoplastic or hammering in rapid rivets, the work surface should be about 6 in. (15 cm) below the elbow. If standing for prolonged periods, increase comfort by resting one foot on a footrest to flatten the curve of the lower back and reduce fatigue.

Whether standing or sitting, for precision work, a good work height is generally 2 to 4 in. (5 to 10 cm) above the elbow.[7] This position ensures elbow support to reduce the static load on the muscles of the back and brings the hands closer to the eyes. An elbow pad can be used to help protect the ulnar nerve when the therapist or client is resting the elbow on the table.

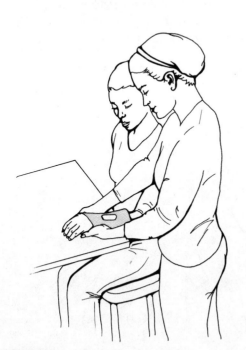

**FIGURE 6-5.**   Optimal positioning when molding a hand orthosis from a standing position. The client is seated on a height-adjustable stool at the corner of a high counter.

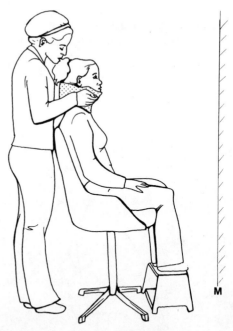

**FIGURE 6-6.**   Client-therapist positioning when molding a cervical collar. The therapist is standing and the client is seated on a height-adjustable stool (in front of a mirror) positioning the client's neck at the level of the therapist's elbow. The client's feet are supported on a footstool. Both the client and the therapist can observe the client's neck position in the mirror (M).

Sitting to work is generally preferred for most tasks because it decreases fatigue.[9] However, intravertebral disk pressure is greater in sitting than in standing,[10] although this is usually a concern only for therapists with disk pathology. The highest level of disk pressure occurs in unsupported sitting, when the spine is in a kyphotic (forward-slouched) position. However, chairs with lumbar supports and armrests decrease disk pressure and reduce fatigue.[11]

Many ergonomically designed chairs and stools are on the market. Therapists should consider the following principles when choosing seating for themselves and the client:

- The seat surface should be 1½ to 2 in. (3 to 5 cm) below the knee when standing: therefore, choose a height-adjustable chair.
- The width of the seat should allow 1 in. (2.5 cm) on either side at the widest part of the thigh.
- The depth of the seat should allow the user to rest against the seat backrest to reduce disk load and provide adequate thigh support. A seat that is too deep will press on the back of the knees.
- The backrest should have a well-formed lumber contour and be height adjustable so that it can be aligned with the user's lumbar curve.
- Armrests should be height adjustable to support the weight of the arms.
- Casters are helpful to move the chair around the room, but they make the chair less stable.
- Swivel is a useful function for both the therapist's and the client's chairs.

To optimize client-therapist positioning and permit easy access to the forearm and hand when molding from a seated position, support the client's arm on a small table or seat the client at the corner of a larger table.

## ● Early Identification and Remediation

Symptoms of CTDs can become irreversible if the individual persists with injurious activi-

ties.[12] Consequently, therapists should do the following:

- Promptly recognize symptoms of cumulative trauma in themselves.
- Apply a problem-solving approach to identify the factors contributing to the injury.
- Institute measures to minimize the risk factors before the problems become chronic.

## ● Safety and Environmental Considerations

It is important to comply with the safety standards set by your country, your workplace, and the equipment manufacturer. In North America, only purchase equipment with Underwriters Laboratories (UL) or Canadian Standards Association (CSA) approval to ensure the highest safety and quality. Before operating, read the owner's manual. Upon request, manufacturers or suppliers will provide a Material Safety Data Sheet (MSDS), which outlines pertinent safety information, for each of their thermoplastic materials.

Perform regular safety checks of the work area to ensure that fire extinguishers and a first-aid box are in good working order. Your workplace health and safety department or your local fire department will be able to advise you about safety standards.

Use caution when handling sharp objects or heating materials at high temperatures to avoid injuring one's own skin or that of the client. To prevent burns, a thermostatically controlled heating pan or a water thermometer can ensure that the water temperature is not too hot. Thoroughly dry perforated materials to remove hot water from the perforations. Always check the temperature of the heated thermoplastic on your own forearm and then the client's forearm before molding. For clients who lack adequate sensation or who are hypersensitive to heat, apply one or more layers of a cotton tubular bandage (e.g., Stockinette or Tubigrip) or a prefabricated splint liner over the limb before molding to prevent burns. This is particularly important when using thermoplastics that absorb a lot of heat (e.g., Synergy). Extra caution is required when using high temperature thermoplastics (see Chapter 7).

Exercise caution when using a knife to score thermoplastics. Always check your hand positions to ensure that the blade is not cutting toward your skin. To prevent injury from a piece of flying wire, cut the wire under a towel, pillowcase, or sheet.

# ● References

1. Pitner, MA: Pathophysiology of overuse injuries in the hand and wrist. Hand Clin 6:355, 1990.
2. Pulat, BM: Physical ergonomics. In Fabrycky, WJ, and Mize, JH (eds): Fundamentals of Industrial Ergonomics. Prentice Hall, Englewood Cliffs, NJ, 1992.
3. North Coast Medical: Hand Therapy Catalogue. San Jose, CA, 1997.
4. Rehabilitation Division, Smith & Nephew Inc: 1997 International Catalogue. Germantown, WI.
5. Yee, D: Exposure to toxic fumes while splinting handout. Unpublished material. Toronto Hand Therapy Group Meeting. Toronto, May 1995.
6. Keyserling, WM, et al: Trunk posture and back pain: Identification and control of occupational risk factors. Applied Industrial Hygiene 3:91, 1988.
7. Grandjean, E: Fitting the Task to the Man. Taylor and Francis, London, 1988.
8. Pheasant, S: Ergonomics Work and Health. Aspen, Gaithersburg, 1991.
9. Jacobs, K, and Bettencourt, CM: Ergonomics for Therapists. Butterworth-Heinemann, Boston, 1995.
10. Nachemson, A, and Morris, JM: In vivo measurements of intradiskal pressure. J Bone Joint Surg 46A:1077, 1964.
11. Anderson, GBJ, and Ortengren, R: Lumbar disk pressure and myoelectric back muscle activity during sitting: Studies on an office chair. Scan J Rehab Med 3:115, 1974.
12. Bertolini, R, and Drewczynski, A: Repetitive Motion Injuries. Canadian Centre for Occupational Health and Safety, Hamilton, Ontario, 1990.

# Orthotic Intervention Process

With the exception of the first section, which addresses assessment and analysis, we use the volar forearm-based static thumbhole-wrist orthosis to exemplify orthotic fabrication procedures, with occasional reference to the dorsal forearm-based static wrist orthosis and the volar forearm-based static wrist-hand orthosis. The attachment of outriggers is briefly discussed. The next five chapters have detailed fabrication instructions for numerous orthoses, including dynamic and static-progressive orthoses.

The student or therapist should not regard the fabrication techniques described in this and subsequent chapters as strict doctrine. Use them as guidelines and feel free to explore other methods for creating patterns, molding, and finishing orthoses. If the recommended materials and tools are unavailable, others can be substituted.

# ● Assessment and Analysis

The objective of this section is to discuss assessments that influence decisions concerning orthotic intervention. For a comprehensive description of condition-specific evaluation procedures, refer to texts specializing in hand or physical rehabilitation.[1-6]

Before providing an orthosis, conduct a thorough, well-documented assessment and analyze the findings to

- Identify the problem.
- Determine the suitability of orthotic intervention to address the problem.
- Define the objectives of orthotic intervention (see Chapter 1).
- Determine the orthotic design and suitable orthotic materials.

The following example illustrates this process. Clients with a stiff hand are commonly seen by therapists and often benefit from orthotic intervention. However, orthotic objectives and design cannot be determined without conducting thorough assessments to identify the factors limiting range of motion. Potential scenarios are outlined in Table 7–1.

To distinguish between contracted soft tissues and a bony block, evaluate the joint **end feel**.[1] A hard end feel indicates a bony block or resistant scar tissue, which will not respond to orthotic intervention and can be corrected only with surgery. A firm end feel indicates a soft tissue contracture that would likely respond to tensile forces applied by an orthosis. If a firm end feel is detected, the precise soft structures restricting **passive range of motion** must be determined through selective tissue tension testing.[2] Only by knowing the range-limiting

---

**TABLE 7-1.** **Orthotic Objectives and Design Options for Hand Stiffness**

| Possible Causes of Hand Stiffness | Orthotic Objectives | Design Options |
| --- | --- | --- |
| Joint effusion | Rest inflamed joints to reduce inflammation and pain | Static |
| Soft tissue swelling | Perhaps no orthosis; just institute measures to control edema If an orthosis is indicated, refer to Chapter 3, "Edema" | |
| Overstretched tendons | Unload slack tendons to promote resorption of redundant collagen fibers | Static |
| Ruptured or lacerated tendons | Protect healing tendons | Static (combine with passive range of motion of finger joints) |
| | Facilitate controlled, protected tendon excursion to promote tendon healing and minimize adhesions | Dynamic motion blocking |
| Reflex sympathetic dystrophy | Relieve pain and prevent contractures | Static |
| | Correct contractures | Serial-static Static-progressive Dynamic |
| Dupuytren's contracture | Maintain range of motion gained by surgical release | Static |
| | Correct residual contracture after surgical release | Serial-static Static-progressive Dynamic |
| Contracted soft tissues | Promote growth of contracted tissues | Serial-static Static-progressive Dynamic |
| Bony block | Not appropriate | Not appropriate |

structure(s) can the orthosis be designed to direct its tension appropriately. See Chapter 2 for a complete discussion.

In the hand, contracted or adherent soft tissues could include extrinsic flexor or extensor tendons, intrinsic muscles, metacarpophalangeal (MCP) collateral ligaments, interphalangeal (IP) joint ligaments, and scar tissue.

## ASSESSMENT CONSIDERATIONS SPECIFIC TO ORTHOTIC INTERVENTION

- Condition of the skin with attention to
  - Fragile skin caused by age, medication (e.g., steroids), disease
  - Quality of the circulation indicated by skin temperature and color and nail contour
  - Presence of wounds, incisions, skin grafts, amputations, or scars
- Sensation—hyposensitivity or hypersensitivity
- Bony prominences
- Pain
- Joint effusion (swelling)
- Joint posturing
- Muscle tone
- Protective positioning, guarding, or compensatory movement
- Ability to position the client for the fabrication procedure
- Age of client
- Cognition and comprehension of the client or caregiver
- Client's motivation and commitment to the orthotic process
- Psychosocial considerations
- Dexterity of the client or caregiver for application and removal of the orthosis
- Environments in which the orthosis will be worn (e.g., hot, cold, dirty, wet, isolation ward)
- Activities during which the orthosis will be worn (e.g., sports, work, child care)
- Presence of or potential for edema—fluctuating or consistent
- Torque-angle measurement

### Evaluation of Edema

Edema can be measured and monitored by circumferential measurements or volumetrics. The latter uses a volumeter, which is a water-filled container. As the hand, arm, or foot is lowered into the container, the submerged limb displaces water, which flows through the spout into a calibrated vessel (Fig. 7-1). The volume of displaced water represents the volume of the limb. To determine the extent of the edema, compare the affected limb with the unaffected side. Subsequent measurements show changes in edema.

Implications of edema to the fabrication process include the following:

- Mold the orthosis when edema is the greatest because it is better to have an orthosis that is too loose (after edema subsides) rather than too tight (if edema increases).
- Mold over tubular bandage or splint liner.
- Use a material that is somewhat flexible when cool so that the width of the trough can be manually adjusted to accommodate the changing size of the limb.
- Fixation with straps may be problematic, causing tissue fluid to become trapped be-

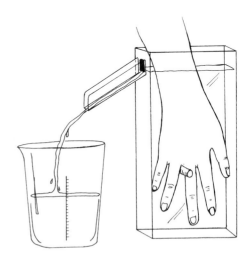

**FIGURE 7-1.** Hand volumeter measures the volume of water displaced by the hand to precisely measure the amount of hand edema. The hand is lowered into the container until the third web space meets the plastic dowel.

tween the straps (see Fig. 3-19). For solutions, see Chapter 3.

## Torque-Angle Measurement

Orthoses offer a safe, effective medium for applying gentle, prolonged stretch to reduce contractures.[7] To be safe, the tension exerted by the orthosis must be low enough to avoid undue stress to the tissues, which would cause counterproductive inflammation. A torque-angle measurement, described by Brand,[8,9] demonstrates how responsive the tissues will be to tensile forces; it also identifies the optimal joint angle to achieve the desired tissue tension within the elastic range (Fig. 7-2).

The forces and corresponding joint angles are plotted on a graph. When the points are joined, the result is a torque-angle curve, which is similar to a load-deformation curve. A gently sloping curve indicates a good prognosis for tissue growth (Fig. 7-3), and the orthosis should apply a force that positions the joint at an angle in the middle of the curve. This position will create tissue tension within the safe,

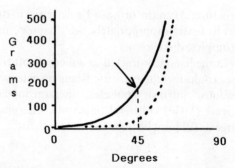

**FIGURE 7-3.** Torque-angle curves. The gently sloping curve (solid line) indicates a good prognosis for tissue growth through gentle, prolonged stress to resolve the joint contracture. The midpoint of the curve (arrow) identifies the desired joint position (45°) to create the optimal amount of tension to promote tissue growth. The steep curve (broken line) indicates a poor prognosis for tissue growth because of nonresponsive scar tissue.

elastic range, and prolonged application of the tension will promote tissue growth. If the curve is steep, the prognosis is poor for the tissues to grow in response to tension, and orthotic intervention is futile.

## ANALYSIS OF ASSESSMENT FINDINGS

Analysis helps the therapist determine the following:

- Optimal orthotic design (discussed later in this chapter)
- Suitable orthotic materials and paddings (see Chapter 4 and Appendix A)
- Desired joint positioning (discussed in relation to each orthosis in subsequent chapters)
- Preferred method of fixation
- Probable compliance

When a client has been referred for an orthosis, the therapist should apply professional judgment and seek input from the client, caregiver (where appropriate), and other team members to determine whether an orthosis is truly warranted. If so, estimate likely compliance and whether the orthosis will be used correctly. An in-depth discussion can be found in Chapter 3.

Bear in mind that an orthosis is part of a treatment program that often includes other

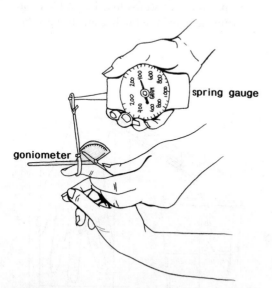

**FIGURE 7-2.** Torque-angle measurement. A series of increasing forces is applied to a joint (index proximal interphalangeal [PIP]) with a spring gauge and the corresponding joint angle is measured with a goniometer. Each force (*100g, 200g, 300g,* etc.) is applied through a lever arm (the perpendicular distance between the affected joint axis and the flexion crease of the next joint), creating a torque.

components such as strengthening, range-of-motion exercises, desensitization, joint protection, ergonomic intervention, gait training, and techniques to reduce muscle tone.

# ● Preparation

## POSITIONING THE CLIENT

*Client positioning for molding is not required until later in the process. However, the therapist should consider potential difficulties in positioning the client before making a final decision about the orthotic design and materials.*

Ensure that the client can be positioned near the heating appliance. This is especially important when using thermoplastics with a short working time, such as highly perforated or thin low-temperature thermoplastics (LTTs), foam thermoplastics, and high-temperature thermoplastics. If the client cannot be transported to the therapy department, the therapist must bring a portable heating appliance to the client's home, hospital room, or operating room.

If the limb has high tone, take the time to apply tone-inhibiting techniques before molding. If necessary, enlist the assistance of a second therapist to position the joints while the thermoplastic cools.

Three common techniques for positioning the client are described next.

### Gravity-Assisted Molding

With this technique, all or most of the thermoplastic is on the upper surface of the body part. It is particularly recommended for the highly conforming category C and D materials because gravity helps the warm material drape and conform to the body contours (Fig. 7-4).

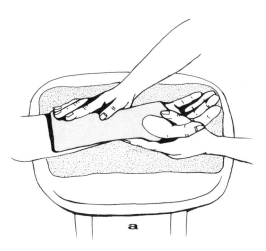

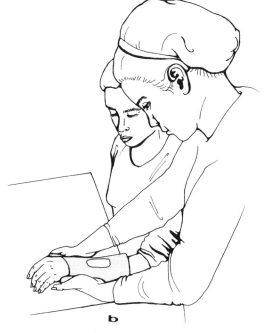

**FIGURE 7-4.** Gravity-assisted molding. *(a)* To mold a volar forearm-based orthosis, position the forearm and hand in supination. Seat the client at a small table (or at the corner of a larger table) and sit across from the client. Place a soft towel under the client's arm to enhance comfort. When molding to the client's right hand, the therapist's left hand controls the position of the wrist and the left thumb molds the contour for the distal transverse arch. The right hand strokes the material into the contours of the forearm. *(b)* To mold a dorsal forearm-based orthosis, position the forearm and hand in pronation. In this situation, the client is seated on a raised stool at an elevated work surface and while the therapist stands behind the client to mold from above. The hole in the dorsum of the thermoplastic is optional; removing this material reduces the weight of the orthosis. The dorsal hole is a signature of orthotic designs created by Paul Van Lede.

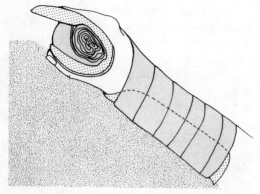

**FIGURE 7-5.** Gravity-resisted molding and bandage wrapping of a volar forearm-based hand orthosis. The forearm and hand are supported in pronation on a soft foam wedge (or pillow) so that weight bearing against the warm material does not create a flat surface. The unrolled portion of the bandage is placed in the palm of the hand to position the wrist in extension.

## Gravity-Resisted Molding

With this technique, all or most of the thermoplastic is on the underside of the body part being molded. This method is more challenging and is used when it is difficult to position the client for gravity-assisted molding. Usually it is necessary to wrap the material with an elastic bandage to achieve contour and conformity (Fig. 7-5). If this is the case, select a category A thermoplastic because it will resist being marked by the bandage texture; the second choice is from category B, but these materials are more impressionable (see Tables 1 and 2 in Appendix A). Categories C and D are generally unsuitable because they are highly impressionable. Alternatively, lightly wrap the material with Thera-Band or Orfiband, which will leave less impression than elastic bandage. (See "Bandage Wrapping" later in this chapter.)

## Vertical Molding

With this technique, the body part is held vertically. Vertical molding is commonly used to mold circumferential orthoses for the humerus, forearm (Fig. 7-6a), and leg (see Fig.

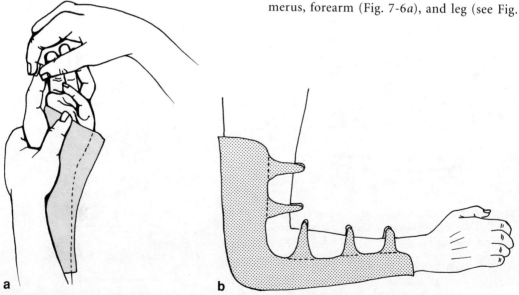

a                    b

**FIGURE 7-6.** *(a)* Vertical molding of a circumferential forearm-based wrist orthosis. The thermoplastic is pinched together along the ulnar border of the limb to secure it and leave both hands free for molding and positioning of the joints. The therapist's left hand is controlling the wrist position and forming the contours in the palm while the right hand is positioning the client's thumb. *(b)* Stretch-and-pinch method of molding an orthosis. When cooled, the trim lines (broken lines) are marked, the pinched material is pulled apart, the orthosis is removed from the limb, and the stretched material is cut off.

12-7). Ideal materials are somewhat tacky when warm. Opaque category D materials should not be used for large orthoses because they will stretch in length. Opaque category C materials are suitable because of its resistance to stretch when warm and its flexibility when cool. Opaque category A or B and translucent category B or C materials are also appropriate for this technique.

*When using translucent materials for either gravity-resisted or vertical molding, small pieces of the warm thermoplastic can be stretched from each side and pinched together to contour the orthosis. When cooled, mark the trim lines, pull the pinched material apart, remove the orthosis from the limb, and trim off the stretched material (Fig. 7-6b). This technique leaves the therapist's hands free to mold material and control the position of the joints.*

## THE DESIGN

The therapist should apply creative problem solving and critical thinking and involve the client or caregiver in choices regarding the orthotic design because each client has unique requirements and attitudes. If possible, the therapist should have samples of different designs for the client to view.

For each orthotic application, several design options usually exist. For example, various orthoses can be used for a client with a radial nerve injury (Table 7-2). A fully dynamic orthosis facilitates the most functional prehension by providing dynamic assistive-extension forces to the wrist and MCPs; however, it is more conspicuous because of the outrigger mechanism. Therefore, a static wrist orthosis may be preferable for some social situations. Similarly, a more complex dynamic orthosis may not be appropriate for a young child because it requires more handling caution to prevent damage than does a static design. For some clients, it may be appropriate to fabricate two or more styles of orthoses because one may not be adequate for all applications.

## PATTERNS, PRECUTS, PREFORMED, AND PREFABRICATED ORTHOSES

The therapist has five basic choices, ranging in price, time, and effort, as demonstrated in Table 7-3.

- Custom-designed pattern
- Standard pattern
- Precut thermoplastic
- Preformed thermoplastic orthosis
- Prefabricated orthosis (soft)

A **custom** pattern is designed by the therapist directly from the client's limb dimensions. The pattern is transferred to the thermoplastic sheet, cut out, and then heated and molded to the client. Using this method, the unit cost for the thermoplastic is lowest, but it is the most labor intensive. Methods for producing a custom pattern are described later in this chapter.

A standard pattern is a pattern obtained from a book or a supplier of LTTs. This method eliminates the time and effort required to create a custom pattern; however, the pattern may need adjustment to fit the client. Standard patterns are provided with the fabrication procedures for many orthoses in Chapters 8 through 12.

Precuts, or splint blanks, are flat pieces of precut thermoplastic available in a variety of styles, materials, and adult sizes (Fig. 7-7a and b). A few precuts are also available in pediatric sizes. The unit cost for the orthosis appears to be greater than cutting a custom pattern from a sheet of thermoplastic. However, there is little or no thermoplastic waste. As a result, the overall cost of thermoplastic used in the clinic may be no greater than cutting the pattern from the thermoplastic sheet. Furthermore, any additional cost is often justified because the effort to design and cut a pattern is eliminated, reducing fabrication time and stress to therapists' hands. However, if a precut is oversized, extensive trimming is required and waste material is generated. Some suppliers will provide custom precuts designed and sized to the specifications of the therapist. Precuts are also available in a variety of kits complete with outrigger components and straps for dynamic or static-progressive orthoses.

*Objectives for peripheral nerve injuries*
- To enhance prehension by substituting for weak or paralyzed muscles
- To prevent stretching of denervated (paralyzed) muscles
- To prevent shortening of innervated muscles
- To prevent the development of maladaptive prehension patterns

| Orthotic Objectives for Radial Nerve Injury | Orthotic Design |
|---|---|
| | 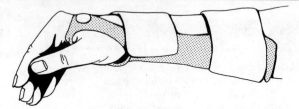<br>Volar forearm-based static thumb-hole wrist orthosis |
| Static wrist support | 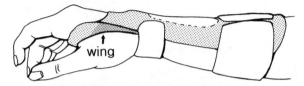<br>Dorsal forearm-based static wrist orthosis |
| | 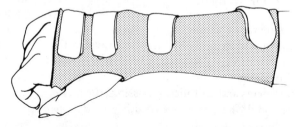<br>Circumferential forearm-based static wrist orthosis |
| Dynamic wrist extension assist | 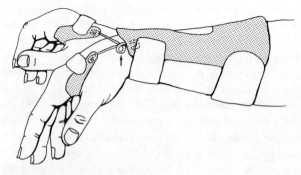<br>Dorsal forearm-based dynamic joint-aligned coil-spring wrist assistive-extension orthosis |

*(continued)*

| Orthotic Objectives for Radial Nerve Injury | Orthotic Design |
|---|---|

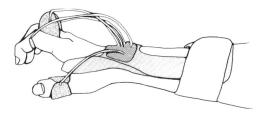

Dorsal forearm-based dynamic arching spring-wire D1-5 MCP assistive-extension orthosis

Combination of
  Static wrist support
  Dynamic finger MCP
    extension assist
  Dynamic thumb extension and
    abduction assist

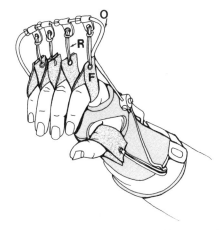

Volar forearm-based dynamic high-profile D1-5 MCP assistive-extension orthosis (prefabricated Rolyan® High-Profile Outrigger splint[10])

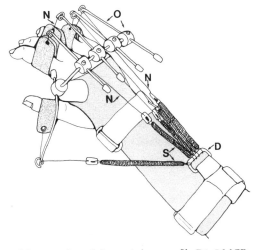

Dorsal forearm-based dynamic low-profile D1-5 MCP assistive-extension orthosis (using a Rolyan® Adjustable Outrigger Kit for extension[10])

*(continued)*

**TABLE 7-2.** Orthotic Design Options after a Radial Nerve Injury at Mid-humeral Level—Lacking Wrist Extension, Finger Metacarpophalangeal Extension, and Thumb Extension (Continued)

| Orthotic Objectives for Radial Nerve Injury | Orthotic Design |
|---|---|
| Combination of  Dynamic wrist extension assist  Dynamic finger MCP extension assist  Dynamic thumb extension and abduction assist | 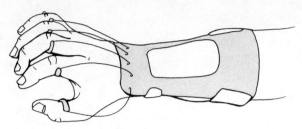 Dorsal forearm-based dynamic arching spring-wire wrist and D1-5 MCP assistive-extension orthosis  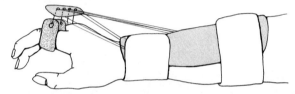 Dorsal forearm-based dynamic low profile wrist and D2-5 MCP assistive-extension orthosis |

Preformed orthoses are mass-produced, premolded low-temperature thermoplastic shells (Fig. 7-7*d*). They are available from several suppliers in various styles, materials, and sizes. Although the material cost is highest with this product, it may be justified by the time saved in fabrication, provided that spot heating and trimming are minimal. They are also par-

**TABLE 7-3.** Comparison of Different Orthotic Approaches

| | Material Cost | Therapist's Time and Effort |
|---|---|---|
| Custom pattern | $ |  |
| Standard pattern | $ | |
| Precut | $ to $$ | |
| Preformed orthosis | $$$ | |
| Soft prefabricated orthosis | $$$ | |

$ = least expensive; $$$ = most expensive.

*Precuts include two distinctive designs: zipper precuts and heat-shrink fiberglass precuts. Zipper precuts, available in Aquaplast and Orfit, produce a circumferential orthosis with a zipper closure that facilitates molding (Fig. 7-7c) (see Table 6 in Appendix A). They require no pattern, are easy to mold, and require no additional fixation. Heat-shrink fiberglass precuts, marketed under the names QuickCast or Dynacast Rapide, produce circumferential non-removable casts or removable orthoses (see Fig. 4-1). The finishing requires the addition of straps. The heat-shrink orthoses are bulky because of their plush terry cloth liner. In contrast, the zipper orthoses fit close to the limb.*

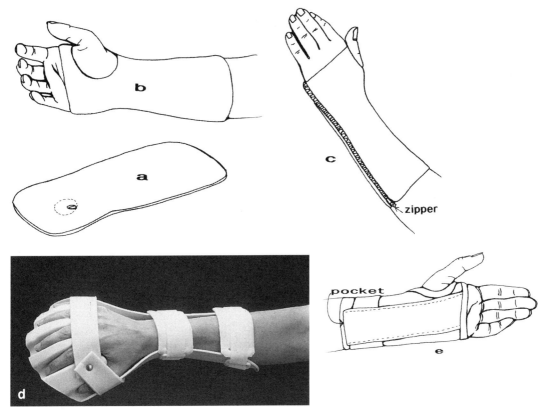

**FIGURE 7-7.** *(a)* Precut for a volar forearm-based static thumb-hole wrist orthosis. The thumb hole is about ½ in. (1 cm) wide. To prevent a bulky roll of thermoplastic around the thumb and to ensure full mobility of the thumb, enlarge the opening to the about 1 ½ in. (3 cm) as indicated by the broken line. *(b)* The orthosis molded from the precut after trimming. *(c)* Circumferential forearm-based static wrist orthosis molded from a zipper precut. *(d)* Preformed volar forearm-based static tone-reducing hand orthosis. Pictured is Smith & Nephew Inc's preformed Anti-Spasticity Ball Splint.[10] (courtesy of Smith & Nephew, Inc.) The wrist and proximal forearm straps have D-ring closure and a splint pad. *(e)* Prefabricated circumferential forearm-based static wrist orthosis with dorsal opening. A strip of flexible metal that slips into a pocket on the volar surface can be contoured to adjust the position of the wrist.

ticularly useful when it is difficult to mold an orthosis on a spastic limb. Preformed orthoses tend to fit loosely but can be spot heated and trimmed to customize the fit. Alternatively, elastomer can be poured into the shell to create an insert with precise conformity to the contours of the limb. Most preformed orthoses come complete with straps to add to the shell.

Prefabricated orthoses are fully finished devices that are intended to fit with little or no adjustment. They are made from soft materials, LTTs, or high-temperature thermoplastics. As the range of soft prefabricated orthoses expands, their popularity increases as an alternative to custom-fabricated orthoses molded from LTTs (Fig. 7-7e). Those made from soft materials are particularly popular because they are semiflexible and provide support without complete joint immobilization. In comparison to thermoplastic orthoses, perspiration is less of a problem and pressure points are less likely to develop. As a result, soft orthoses are preferred in settings where they are unlikely to be closely monitored by a therapist, for example, in a nursing home.

## SELECTING A SUITABLE SOFT PREFABRICATED ORTHOSIS

There is a wide range of prefabricated soft, circumferential orthoses for the hand, the most popular being the thumb-hole wrist orthosis. Numerous styles are available, and suggestions to guide the therapist's decision about what to stock include the following:

- If wrist immobilization is desired, select an orthosis with a volar pocket containing a strip of malleable metal or low-temperature thermoplastic (Fig. 7-7*e*).
- Unlike the orthosis in Figure 7-7*e*, ensure that the distal edge permits full MCP flexion and that the thumb hole permits full thumb opposition.
- If the client has limited finger dexterity, select a design with easy fastening straps.
- Select a design that is tapered at the wrist to conform to the contours of the limb.
- Consider the ease of washing the orthosis.

## THERMOPLASTIC SELECTION

If the decision is to fabricate a custom orthosis, the next consideration is what thermoplastic to use. Selection is based on the therapist's familiarity with the materials, their availability, and their cost, as well as many factors outlined in Chapter 4. Some considerations are outlined in Tables 1 through 4 in Appendix A. If options are available, optimize compliance by including the client in decisions regarding color of thermoplastic and Velcro and method of fixation.

## PRODUCING A CUSTOM PATTERN

The landmarks for hand orthoses are illustrated in Figure 7-8.

Three methods for producing a custom pattern use paper towels, plastic bags, or tape measurements. Techniques are described in relation to specific orthoses in later chapters. The first two are particularly well suited for hand orthoses.

### Paper Towel Custom Hand Pattern

1. Position the client's hand and forearm in pronation on the paper towel. If the client's limb is too long for a single sheet of toweling, tape two pieces together. The

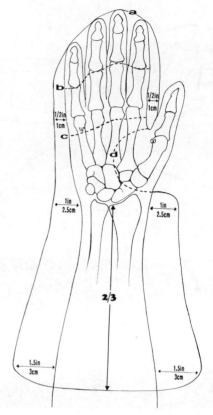

**FIGURE 7-8.** Landmarks for hand orthoses. For forearm-based orthoses—the proximal edge is at the ⅔ point between the wrist and the elbow. (*a*) For orthoses that support the fingers—terminate at the tips of fingers. (*b*) For orthoses that support the MCPs and leave the IPs free—terminate at the PIP joint creases. (*c*) For orthoses that support the wrist and leave the fingers free—use the proximal palmar crease as landmark for the distal edge; for more precise identification of the distal edge, mark the proximal edge of the second MC head and ¼ in. (½ cm) proximal to the base of the fifth MC head. (*d*) For orthoses that leave the thumb free—use the thenar crease as a landmark to ensure full thumb mobility. Approximate trough widths of half-shell orthoses for the adult hand are ½ in. (1 cm, 1 finger width) wider than the ulnar and medial borders of the hand; 1 in. (2 cm, 2 finger widths) wider than the ulnar and medial sides of the wrist; and 1½ in. (3 cm, 3 finger widths) wider than the ⅔ point on the forearm.

forearm portion of the orthosis should be two thirds the length of the forearm for adequate leverage. The trough of a half-shell orthosis should extend slightly more than halfway up the sides of the limb. Therefore, the width of the forearm portion should be slightly more than half the circumference of the limb.

2. Trace around the areas of the client's hand and forearm where the orthosis will be molded and note any pertinent landmarks on the paper outline (Fig. 7-8).

3. Remove the client's limb from the paper towel and add guide marks (Fig. 7-8). For half-shell orthoses, the trough should be
   ○ ½ in. (1 cm; 1 finger width) wider than the ulnar and medial borders of the hand
   ○ 1 in. (2 cm; 2 finger widths) wider than the ulnar and medial sides of the wrist
   ○ 1½ in. (3 cm; 3 finger widths) wider than the two-thirds point on the forearm

The distal end of the orthosis varies according to the joints that are incorporated:

   ○ For hand orthoses at the tips of fingers
   ○ For MCP orthoses at proximal interphalangeal (PIP) joint creases
   ○ For wrist orthoses, use the proximal palmar crease as a landmark. For more precise positioning of the distal edge, use the proximal edge of the second metacarpal (MC) head and ¼ in. (½ cm) proximal to the base of the fifth MC head. This ensures full mobility of the MCPs.
     ○ To ensure good mobility of the thumb, use the thenar crease as a landmark.

4. Connect the guide marks to create the custom pattern outline and then cut out the paper pattern (Fig. 7-9*a*).

5. To check the fit, apply the pattern to the client's limb and position the joints as they will be when the orthosis is molded. Trim off or add extra paper as necessary (Fig. 7-9*b*) to generate a precise custom pattern that will eliminate the need for trimming after molding.

## Plastic Bag Custom Pattern

1. Select clear, flexible plastic that is large enough to wrap circumferentially around the hand and forearm. The plastic bags

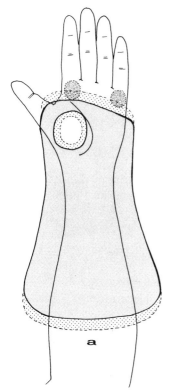

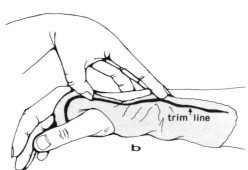

**FIGURE 7-9.** (*a*) Paper towel pattern for a volar forearm-based static thumb-hole wrist orthosis. The solid outline represents the pattern when using ³⁄₃₂ or ⅛ in. (2.4 or 3.2 mm) thick materials. The distal edge terminates at the base of the second MC head and about ¼ in. (½ cm) proximal to the fifth MC head. The thumb hole is about 1½ in. (3 cm) wide. If ¹⁄₁₆ in. (1.6 mm) thickness is used, enlarge the pattern to the broken lines to allow about ¼ to ½ in. (½ to 1 cm) extra to fold over proximal and distal edges and around the thumb hole to strengthen the orthosis. (*b*) Paper towel pattern applied to client's limb with trim lines marked to adjust the fit.

used to package thermoplastic sheets are ideal.

2. Cut a hole to slip over the thumb and wrap the material circumferentially around the hand and forearm.

3. Secure the plastic with straight pins, a stapler, or tape. For a volar-based orthosis, secure the plastic along the middorsum of the forearm and hand; for a dorsal-based orthosis, secure the plastic along the midvolar aspect.

4. Use a permanent medium-point marker to mark the outline of the orthosis. All landmarks can be easily viewed through the clear plastic. Mark the depth of the trough two thirds along the sides of the forearm and the length two thirds up the forearm from the wrist.

5. Remove the pins or tape, or tear open the stapled seam, and then remove the plastic from the client's limb.

6. Cut out the plastic pattern with scissors.

7. To check the fit, apply the pattern to the client's limb and position the joints as they will be when the orthosis is molded. Trim off or add extra plastic as necessary to generate a precise custom pattern.

## TRANSFERRING THE PATTERN TO THE THERMOPLASTIC

Transfer the custom pattern to the thermoplastic sheet. Position the pattern near the edges of the thermoplastic to conserve material and reduce costs. Yellow or white grease pencils are ideal because they leave little pigment on the plastic. For opaque thermoplastics, lay the pattern on top of the thermoplastic and trace around it. For lightly tinted translucent thermoplastics, lay the material on top of the pattern and trace the outline that can be viewed through the material.

If a darker-pigmented grease pencil or ballpoint pen is used, cut off all pattern lines because they detract from the cosmesis of the orthosis. Dark grease markings can be erased if the material has not been heated. To remove the remaining markings, use alcohol or chlorine bleach. The completed orthosis should be

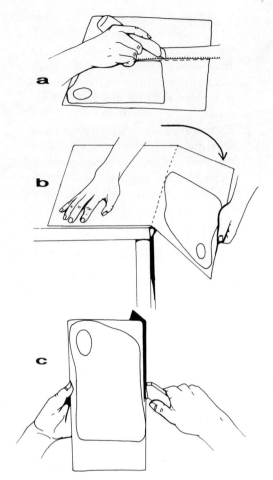

**FIGURE 7-10.** Sizing the material. *(a)* Score the material with a knife blade, using a metal-edged ruler as a cutting guide. *(b)* Bend the material over the edge of a table at the score line. *(c)* If the material does not break at the score line, cut through the remaining material with a knife.

free from all pattern or trim markings to optimize compliance and to create a professional-looking product.

## SIZING THE MATERIAL

Using a metal-edged ruler, score the thermoplastic with a knife blade to form a rectangle slightly larger than the pattern (Fig. 7-10a). Then fold the material over the edge of a table to break it into a smaller size (Fig. 7-10b). If necessary, cut through the fold with the knife (Fig. 7-10c). This procedure prevents warming of excess material and ensures easy fit of the thermoplastic into the heating pan. Relabel the unused part of the thermoplastic so the material can be identified at a later date.

## PROTECTING BONY PROMINENCES

Tissues over bony prominences are vulnerable to being compressed and irritated by the orthosis. As discussed previously, inspect the limb for any bony prominences that should be accommodated in the molding process. The more "bony" the limb, the greater the risk of pressure points.

The most susceptible prominences in the hand are shown in Figure 7-11*a* and *b*. Other sensitive areas are

- The medial epicondyle, with elbow orthoses
- The clavicles and mandible, with cervical collars
- The ribs and iliac crests, with some shoulder-positioning orthoses
- The medial and lateral femoral condyles and malleoli, with knee and ankle orthoses

To prevent pressure points, special allowance must be made. Two common techniques are as follows:

- Flare or dome the material away from the bony prominence during the molding process. This technique is described later in this chapter under "Molding the Material."
- Pad the bony prominence(s) *before* molding the thermoplastic. Do not add padding *after* the molding because it will compress the tissue over the bony prominence.

To pad a bony prominence, cut a circular piece of ⅛ in. (3.2 mm) thick self-adhesive padding to apply to the skin over the bony prominence (Figs. 7-12 and 7-13*a*). Alterna-

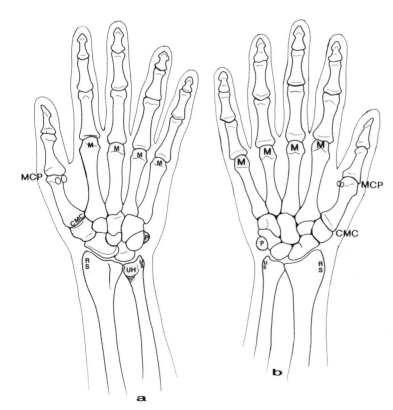

**FIGURE 7-11.** Bony prominences in the hand that require padding or flaring to prevent pressure areas. (*a*) Dorsal view. (*b*) Volar view. UH = the ulnar head (especially vulnerable with dorsal, ulnar, or circumferential forearm-based orthoses); US = the ulnar styloid; RS = the radial styloid. P = the pisiform; CMC = carpometacarpal joint of the thumb (especially vulnerable in osteoarthritis); MCP = metacarpophalangeal joint of the thumb; M = the metacarpal heads (especially vulnerable with dorsal-based hand orthoses).

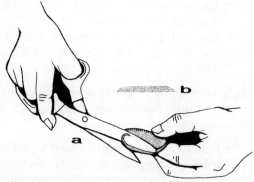

**FIGURE 7-12.** Cutting a circle of ⅛ in. (3.2 mm) self-adhesive padding to protect a bony prominence. (*a*) For the best cosmetic result, hold the scissors at a 45° angle while cutting to create a beveled edge. (*b*) Cross-sectional view of pad with beveled edge.

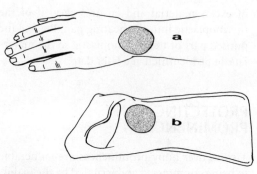

**FIGURE 7-13.** (*a*) Padding applied to the ulnar head before molding. (*b*) Inside view of a dorsal forearm-based static wrist orthosis with padding for the ulnar head.

tively, select a circular, self-adhesive gel dot or disc, available in diameters of 1, 2¼, and 4 in. (2.5, 3, and 10 cm). Thero-Gel Dots and Discs are available from Sammons Preston (see Table 9 in Appendix A). Padding is particularly important when using materials with memory because flaring and doming efforts are counteracted by the material's inherent tendency to return to its original form (i.e., without contours). If padding is to be used, enlarge the size of the pattern accordingly.

*After molding, remove the pad from the skin and either adhere it to the adjacent inner surface of the thermoplastic to become part of the finished orthosis (Fig. 7-13b) or discard the pad. If you intend to discard the pad, reduce its adhesiveness by applying it to your clothing before applying it to the client's skin. This will reduce the discomfort of pulling the pad off the skin after molding. The space that the padding occupied during the molding creates a small gap or "bubble" between the skin and the orthosis to prevent pressure. If you wish to incorporate an asymmetric pad into the finished orthosis, cut two pieces that are mirror images—one to use during molding and one to adhere to the orthosis after molding.*

## PROTECTING THE SKIN

Some clients are particularly heat sensitive and cannot tolerate the heated thermoplastic against the skin. To increase the client's comfort and to reduce the risk of burns, apply a splint liner or one or two layers of Stockinette or Tubigrip to the limb before molding (see Figs. 3-17 and 3-18). Use 2 or 3 in. (5 or 7.5 cm) width for the arm and 3 or 4 in. (7.5 or 10 cm) width for the leg. For forearm-based orthoses, cut a length of Stockinette or Tubigrip and then cut a small hole at the location of the base of the thumb. The hole will stretch to permit the thumb to protrude through the opening. The thumb is unprotected, but it rarely poses a problem. If the thumb needs protection, cover it with cohesive tape or a finger sleeve. When an orthosis is molded over a liner, it will fit more loosely than an orthosis molded directly to the skin. However, this poses no problem because the orthosis is usually worn over a perspiration-absorbing liner. When molding circumferential orthoses from LTTs with memory, it is desirable to allow a safety margin to compensate for shrinkage.

Materials such as Orfit Classic are sticky when warm and will adhere to hairy skin. To avoid discomfort when removing the newly formed orthosis, mold over a liner as described above, or apply lotion to lubricate the client's skin before molding. The Stockinette will adhere to warm Orfit Classic; however, it can be peeled off the cooled thermoplastic. It is also

To protect fragile skin or prevent an orthosis from migrating, adhere a strip of very thin, self-adhesive gel padding to the inside of the orthosis. Some gel padding moisturizes the skin by releasing mineral oil. It can be used as an isolated pad or to line the entire inner surface if it is very thin. Alternatively, self-adhesive Dycem strips will also prevent migration, but they do not moisturize the skin.

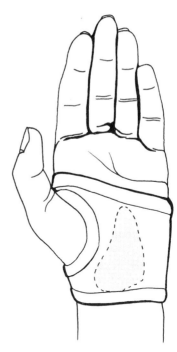

**FIGURE 7-14.** Prefabricated Rolyan® Gel shell Splint[10] with gel padding on the inside against the skin to cushion the carpal tunnel and soften incision scar.

easier for the therapist to manipulate the warm Orfit with lubricated hands. Another technique to reduce surface stickiness is to add liquid disinfectant to the water of the heating pan.

Skin lubrication is particularly important when molding materials with memory circumferentially around a thumb or finger. As the material cools, it will contract around the proximal phalanx and make it become difficult to slide off over the more bulbous distal joints. To avoid this problem, apply lotion to the skin before molding. If the problem occurs, apply lotion to the skin and allow the client to pull the orthosis off.

## SCAR TISSUE MANAGEMENT

When an orthosis is to be applied over a surgical incision (e.g., for carpal tunnel or de Quervain's release) or hypertrophic burn scar, incorporate gel padding or an elastomer conformer into the design. Elastomer is not suitable for an open wound. It requires time to set before molding can begin. Once it has cured, mold the warm thermoplastic over top of the conformer. Thoroughly wash the molded insert to remove any catalyst that could irritate the skin. If using gel padding, apply it to the scar tissue, and then mold the warm thermoplastic over top of the conformer. Some gel sheets are better suited to open wounds than others. Check the manufacturer's specifications.

Some prefabricated orthoses have built-in gel pads, for example, Smith & Nephew Inc.'s Rolyan® Gel Shell® Thumb Spica Splint, which cushions the first dorsal compartment (site of de Quervain's release), and the Rolyan® Gel Shell® Splint, which cushions the carpal tunnel (Fig. 7-14).[10]

## HEATING THE THERMOPLASTIC

Materials thicker than $\frac{3}{32}$ in. (2.4 mm) should *not* be cut cold because this creates undue stress on the therapist's hands. To reduce the risk of repetitive strain injuries, partially heat the material until it is soft enough to cut easily. After the pattern has been cut out, return the thermoplastic to the heating appliance and heat the material until it is malleable enough to mold.

### Moist Heating

The most common heating method for LTTs is immersion in water heated in a splinting pan or other water-heating appliance. Some heating pan manufacturers recommend distilled water to extend the life of the pan.

*The addition of a liquid disinfectant to the water will reduce the risk of cross-infection and help prevent accidental adherence of thermoplastics as they are heating.*

When using a thermostatically controlled heating pan, set the temperature between 135° and 180°F (57° and 82°C) as recommended for that specific thermoplastic. When using a skillet on a stove, the water should be just steaming and not forming any bubbles. To monitor the water temperature, use a cooking thermometer. LTTs can also be heated in water that has been boiled in a kettle and poured into a deep-dish pan. The heating time is generally between 30 and 60 seconds.

*To heat a piece of thermoplastic that is too long for a heating pan, dip in whatever amount readily fits and heat until it can be folded over. Several folds may be necessary to accommodate a long piece of thermoplastic in a small pan. Place a paper towel between the layers of thermoplastic to prevent accidental adherence.*

## Microwave Heating

As mentioned in Chapter 5, LTTs can be softened in a microwave oven.[11] Place the material in a nonmetal container of water and heat on high for 1 to 2 minutes, depending on the size and thickness of the material and the output of the oven.

## Dry Heating

Foam thermoplastics (e.g., Plastazote, AliPlast, Kushionsplint, PE-LITE) and high-temperature thermoplastics (e.g., polyethylene) require the dry heat of an oven at 250° to 300°F (120° to 140°C). A heat gun can be used for small pieces no larger than about 4 in. (10 cm) and for spot heating. Heat them for a few minutes in an oven on a baking sheet covered with sili-

cone release paper, cornstarch, or talcum powder to prevent sticking. Check the malleability of the material periodically and remove when it has absorbed sufficient heat for molding. These materials have a short working time (about 30 seconds), so position the client near the oven.

Isoprene rubber-based materials such as SanSplint, Orthoplast, Kay-Prene, and Orthoform can be either moist heated or oven heated at 225°F (110°C). This option is useful for pieces of thermoplastic that are too large for a heating pan.

## CUTTING THE THERMOPLASTIC

Cut out the pattern, removing all pattern marks. Use long, smooth strokes rather than

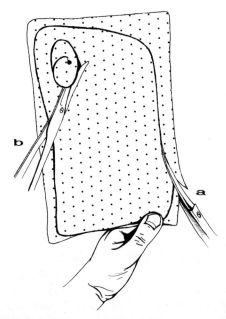

**FIGURE 7-15.** Cutting out the pattern. (*a*) Use long, even strokes to create a smooth edge and cut off the pattern lines, leaving no marks on the material before molding. When using curved scissors, orient the concave side of the blade toward the orthosis. For materials with well-spaced perforations, try to cut between the holes. Cutting through the perforations would create sharp points along the edge. (*b*) To cut out an interior circle for the thumb, punch a hole in the material with a hole punch, heat the material, then use medium or small curved scissors and poke the blade through the hole and cut out the circle about 1½ in. (3 cm) in diameter.

short snips. To prevent a jagged edge, do not completely close the blades of the scissors with each stroke. Careful cutting will eliminate the need for edge finishing later. All corners must be rounded for cosmesis and comfort; square corners could injure the client's skin. When cutting material with well-spaced perforations, try to cut between the holes (Fig. 7-15). When cutting most maxi/superperforated materials, the perforations will create an unavoidable irregular edge that will require a covering. Edge-covering techniques are described later under "Finishing the Edges." Smith & Nephew, Inc.'s Optiperf Aquaplast (introduced in 1997) is superperforated but does not require edge covering.

Choose the correct style of scissors for the cutting task (see Fig. 5-6). When cutting the edges with large, curved scissors, orient the blades with the concave edge toward the orthosis (Fig. 7-15). Keep the blades sharp and free from the adhesive that accumulates from cutting self-adhesive Velcro. Use isopropyl alcohol to remove adhesive residue.

*When using a thumb-hole wrist precut, enlarge the hole to 1½ in. (3 cm) diameter (Fig. 7-7a). If this material is not cut away before molding, it will be difficult to adequately enlarge the thumb hole without creating a bulky border.*

## Molding and Adjusting the Fit

### HANDLING THE MOIST-HEATED MATERIAL

After cutting out the pattern, ensure that the client is optimally positioned for the molding process, then return the material to the heating pan and heat it until it is malleable. For a volar forearm-based static wrist orthosis, position the client with forearm supported in supination (Fig. 7-4a). To promote even heating of the thermoplastic, stir the water as it heats. The heating time and the working time are directly proportional to the thickness of the thermoplastic. Perforations will shorten the heating and cooling time.

Translucent materials will become more translucent or fully transparent when completely heated. This property of translucent materials eliminates the need to test the malleability as it heats. To test the malleability of an opaque material, lift a corner of the material out of the water with a spatula to check the flexibility (Fig. 7-16).

Many materials have a nonstick coating to prevent accidental self-adherence during heating and molding. (Check the material's specification sheet.) However, the edges are uncoated and will stick to any thermoplastic that they contact. Furthermore, when coated materials are stretched, the coating "breaks up" and the nonstick quality is compromised.

When the material is fully heated, use the spatula to raise a corner of the material out of

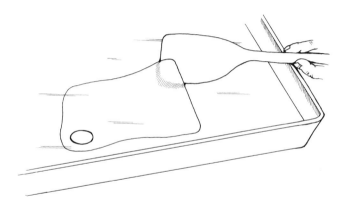

**FIGURE 7-16.** Checking the malleability of the heated thermoplastic by testing the flexibility of a corner lifted out of the water with a spatula.

the water. Then lift the material out of the water, cradling it across outstretched hands and forearms (Fig. 7-17a). This technique is particularly important for the more conforming category C and D materials because they stretch easily. Do *not* lift a conforming material with the spatula while it is warm, as shown in Figure 7-17b; the impressionable material will drape over the edges of the spatula, embossing them into the material. Furthermore, do *not* hold category D material vertically because it will stretch in length (Fig. 7-17c). For the same reason, it is unwise to heat highly conforming materials by suspending them vertically in a hydrocollator. Instead, heat them horizontally on a shelf fitted to the hydrocollator or on a piece of plastic mesh covered with a paper towel. The paper towel prevents the mesh from leaving impressions in the warm thermoplastic.

Place the moist-heated material onto smooth, absorbent fabric to dry. It is especially important to dry materials with perforations; otherwise, the holes will hold hot water that could burn the client. Do *not* use a terry towel to dry category C and D materials because the texture of the towel will become embossed in the impressionable material; instead use a folded sheet or pillowcase.

## MOLDING THE MATERIAL

For the volar forearm-based wrist orthosis, fold back about ¼ to ½ in. (½ to 1 cm) around the thumb hole to enlarge the opening and create a smooth edge (Fig. 7-9a). Blend the folded material into the outer surface of the orthosis to eliminate crevices.

Test the temperature of the material on your forearm, especially if it is to be molded directly against the client's skin. For babies, test the temperature on your neck, which is more heat sensitive than the forearm. If it is too hot, wait until the material has cooled to a more tolerable temperature. Then test it on your client's skin, keeping in mind that some people are more heat sensitive than others. Some initial shaping can be done on your own body.

When the temperature is tolerable, position yourself across from the client and then apply and mold the material to the hand, as shown in Figure 7-4a. For a volar forearm-based static thumb-hole wrist orthosis, slip the thumb through the thumb hole and then gently pull the material ulnarly to uncover the thenar eminence. Do not roll back the edge of the thumb hole any farther because this creates bulk and interferes with prehension. Gently stroke the material until it stretches and conforms to the body contours. Use broad surfaces of the hand to smooth the material (Fig. 7-4a). Never use a static grip (Fig. 7-18a) or fingertips because impressions will be left in the material. Use the pad of your thumb to mold the material to the contour of the distal transverse arch. Control the position of the wrist

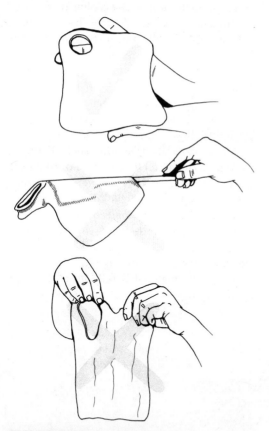

**FIGURE 7-17.** Handling the heated thermoplastic, especially if category C or D. *(a)* Correct way of carrying heated thermoplastics: on outstretched hands. *(b)* Incorrect way of carrying: on a spatula. The impressionable material will drape over the edges of the spatula, embossing them into the material. *(c)* Do not hold a category D material vertically because it will stretch in length.

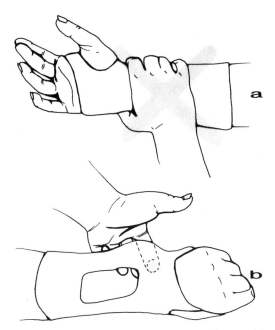

**FIGURE 7-18.** Molding the thermoplastic. *(a)* Never use a static grip or the fingertips because impressions will be left in the material. *(b)* Dome the material of a dorsal forearm-based static wrist orthosis away from the ulnar head to prevent a pressure point.

with consideration of flexion/extension and ulnar/radial deviation (Fig. 7-4*a*).

If the pattern was not precisely designed to terminate proximal to the MC heads, the excess material must be dealt with. One method is to fold back the material to clear the MC heads. This technique produces a smooth distal edge and eliminates the need for trimming. As discussed in Chapter 3, this technique is suitable for materials ⅟₁₆ and ³⁄₃₂ in. (1.6 and 2.4 mm) but not recommended for materials ⅛ in. (3.2 mm) thick because it creates extra bulk and weight. We prefer to mark and trim the distal edge of ⅛ in. (3.2 mm) materials as shown later.

In general, if molding to the client is difficult and precise contouring is not required, the orthosis can be molded on a "model" who is approximately the same size as the client.

If bony prominences have not been padded, flare or dome the material as it cools (Fig. 7-18*b*). When using materials with memory, it may be necessary to flare or dome repeatedly while the material cools because it may not readily retain the desired contours.

When molding translucent thermoplastic circumferentially around the thumb, apply a strip of ⅟₁₆ in. (1.6 mm) self-adhesive foam around the metacarpal and proximal phalanx of the thumb to prevent excessive shrinkage. Another technique is to run the tip of a pen or pencil between the proximal phalanx and the thermoplastic to keep it stretched out as it cools (see Fig. 10-10e). Similarly, when molding translucent thermoplastic circumferentially around a finger, wrap it first with cohesive tape or apply a finger sleeve.

## Working Time

The working time for ⅛ in. (3.2 mm) thick LTTs is generally 3 to 5 minutes. Translucent materials and isoprene-based opaque materials are workable for 4 to 6 minutes. Thinner or perforated materials cool more quickly.

Foam thermoplastics (e.g., Plastazote, Aliplast, Kushionsplint) and polyethylene have a working time of about 30 seconds, so position the client near the oven and have all necessary tools close at hand.

## Bandage Wrapping

When molding a large orthosis or when using gravity-resisted positioning of the client, it may be useful to wrap a bandage (elastic, Thera-Band, or Orfiband) over the warm material to help form the contours (Fig. 7-19*a* and *b*). Support the bandage-wrapped body part on soft foam so that weight bearing against the warm material does not create a flattened surface (Fig. 7-5). To facilitate the process, ensure that the bandage unrolls around the limb, as shown in Figure 7-19*a*. Bandage wrapping helps retain the heat of the warmed thermoplastic and thus extends the working time, a quality that may or may not be desirable. If quick cooling is preferred, soak the elastic bandage in ice water or store Thera-Band or Orfiband in the freezer.

Elastic bandage wrapping works well with opaque category A and B materials because their impressionability is low. For opaque category C or D and translucent materials, Thera-Band or Orfiband is recommended because they leave less impression than an elastic bandage. Use 2 or 3 in. (5 or 7.5 cm) wide bandage

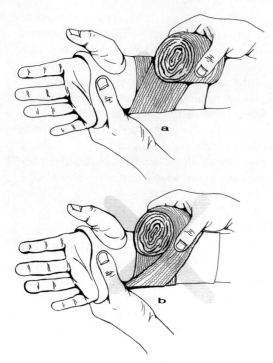

**FIGURE 7-19.** *(a)* The right way to unroll the bandage over the warm thermoplastic. The bandage unrolls in the same direction as it is being wrapped. *(b)* Inefficient way to unroll the bandage. The bandage unrolls in the opposite direction to the wrapping.

for hand orthoses and 4 or 6 in. (10 or 15 cm) wide bandage for larger body parts.

## Quick Cooling

It may be desirable to hasten the cooling of the material if it is difficult to maintain the position of the joints until the material sets. Techniques include the following:

- Remove the orthosis when partially set and dip into a bowl of cold water or place under cold running water.
- Apply a cold pack to the thermoplastic. Take care not to distort the contours of the orthosis with the pressure of the cold pack.
- Wrap low-conforming material with an elastic bandage that has been soaked in ice water.
- Wrap thermoplastic with Thera-band or Orfiband that has been stored in a freezer.

- Use an environmentally friendly cold spray such as North Coast Medical's Quik-Freeze or Smith & Nephew, Inc.'s Cold Spray.

## Reheating and Remolding

If the first molding attempt does not achieve satisfactory contours and joint positioning, you can either reheat and remold the entire orthosis or spot heat the problem area. To spot heat a section of the orthosis:

- Use a heat gun.
- Apply hot water with a baster or syringe.
- Dip the section in the heating pan.

*Spot heating can leave a ridge, or hot-cold line, between the heated and unheated thermoplastic. To avoid this occurrence, gently move the submerged part of the orthosis through the water to create a gradual transition between the heated and the unheated thermoplastic. Similarly, when using a heat gun, move the nozzle to avoid a hot-cold line.*

If two or more areas need adjustment, it is often less time-consuming to completely reheat and remold the orthosis. The LTTs can be reheated many times without affecting the quality of the material. However, foam thermoplastics lose some resiliency with each heating, becoming stiff and resistant to molding after three or four times.

Remolding is also required to adjust a serial-static orthosis. Either spot heat or reheat the entire orthosis.

## ADJUSTMENTS AND TRIMMING

While the material is setting, add any additional flaring over bony prominences. For a volar forearm-based orthosis, the most vulnerable prominence is the ulnar styloid, whereas the ulnar head is more vulnerable to pressure with a dorsal forearm-based orthosis (Fig. 7-20*a* and *b*). If the material is too cool, spot heat the area to relieve the pressure point. Check and adjust the

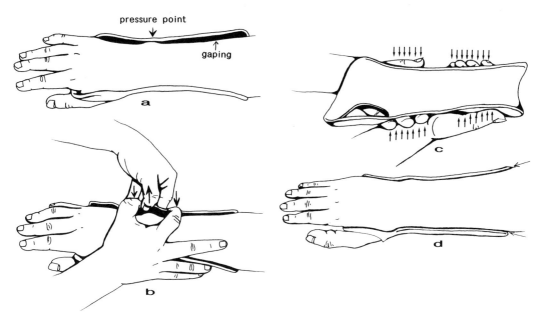

**FIGURE 7-20.** Checking and adjusting the fit after molding. *(a)* Potential pressure point beside the ulnar styloid (arrow). Trough is gaping along the ulnar side of the forearm. *(b)* While the material is still somewhat warm, use 3-point pressure to flare away from the ulnar styloid. *(c)* Correct a gaping trough by squeezing in the sides of the orthosis. *(d)* Well-fitting trough with a slight, uniform gap between the limb and the orthosis.

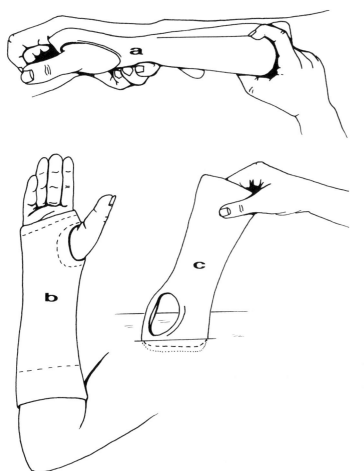

**FIGURE 7-21.** Trim Lines. *(a)* Marking trim line with a fingernail to adjust the depth of the trough to ⅔ up the sides of the forearm. *(b)* Trim lines to ensure freedom of the MCPs, thenar eminence, and elbow. *(c)* Spot heating the distal edge by submersion in hot water to trim to clear the MCPs.

conformity of the trough. If the trough is too wide, squeeze in the sides (Fig. 7-20c) or expand the trough to achieve the desired fit (see Fig. 6-3). Try to adjust the width of the trough before the material is fully cooled. A well-fitting trough should have a slight gap between the limb and the material (Fig. 7-20d).

If a precise custom pattern is made and low-conforming material (category A or B) is used, trimming should be unnecessary. Category C or D materials are more likely to stretch during the molding process. Thus trimming might be necessary.

Check the depth of the trough and ensure that all joints excluded from the orthosis are free to move. For example, a wrist orthosis should allow unrestricted movement of the MCPs, thumb, and elbow. A half-shell trough should extend slightly more than halfway up the sides of the limb. Mark trim lines using a marking utensil or a fingernail (Fig. 7-21a and b).

Remove the orthosis and cut away the excess material. The material can be readily cut if not fully cooled. If it becomes too hard, spot heat the edges to facilitate trimming using a heat gun, baster, or syringe or by submerging the trim line (Fig. 7-21c). Cutting the material when it is warm produces a neater, smoother edge and prevents undue stress to the therapist's hands.

Return the trimmed orthosis to the body part and check the fit once again. Re-mark and trim again if necessary. After trimming, a well-fitting volar forearm-based static thumb-hole wrist orthosis demonstrates full freedom of the MCPs and thumb (see Fig. 3-12).

## ● Finishing Procedures

### FLARING THE PROXIMAL EDGE

If left unflared, the proximal edge of volar fore-arm-based orthoses and posterior knee or ankle orthoses will create a pressure line in the skin (see Fig. 3-2a). To flare the proximal edge, heat it with a heat gun or by submersion into a heating pan (Fig. 7-22a). Once heated, the edge can be gently flared using the palm of the hand (Fig. 7-22b). Avoid overflaring (see Fig. 3-3c). For posterior knee or elbow orthoses, do not flare the medial side of the proximal edge be-

cause a medial flare will irritate the other thigh or chest wall.

## FINISHING THE EDGES

After trimming and flaring to accommodate bony prominences, smooth any rough edges. This procedure is unnecessary if the edges were carefully cut when warm. To finish the edges:

- Reheat and recut the edge with long, smooth strokes to remove irregularities.
- Reheat and smooth the edges of category C and D materials with the hand.
- Grind the edges.
- Cover the edges.

### Edge Smoothing with Heat

The edges can be heated with a heat gun, by submersion, or by hot water applied with a baster or

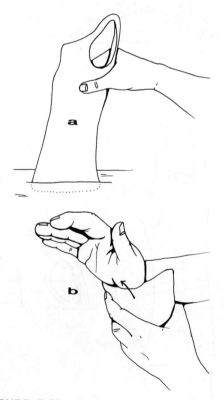

**FIGURE 7-22.** Flaring the proximal edge. *(a)* Spot heating by submersion. *(b)* Gently flaring the warmed proximal edge with the thenar eminence.

syringe. Once the orthosis is malleable, stroke the edge with the palm or thumb to blend it smooth. Lubricating the hand with lotion reduces friction and facilitates the smoothing process.

## Edge Grinding

If the material is category A or B, the edges may be difficult to smooth with heat. Instead, reheat the edges and carefully cut them smooth. Alternatively, once the material has fully cooled, grind the edges with a hand grinder (Fig. 7-23a and b). The spinning stone creates friction against the material, causing it to heat up. If the material heats too much, it will become gummy and the edges will actually become rougher. Avoid smoothing the same edge for too long; before it overheats, move to another edge. Return to the first edge once it has cooled to smooth it further if necessary. Do not use small back-and-forth strokes because this will roughen the edge. Use long, smooth strokes, moving the grinding stone along the edge toward you.

*Edge grinding is a time-consuming process that a busy therapist may not have time to do. However, the task may be unnecessary if the edges are carefully cut with long strokes when initially cutting the pattern from the warm thermoplastic. Edge grinding is not appropriate for maxi- or superperforated materials.*

## Edge Covering

A common but usually inappropriate method of edge finishing is to use a strip of adhesive moleskin. On first impression, the moleskin-edged orthosis looks neater and the edge feels soft. However, in time the moleskin becomes dirty, smelly, and rough, especially on a hand orthosis. Unlike thermoplastics, the moleskin does not wash or dry easily, and it retains moisture. Furthermore, it is difficult to remove moleskin from an orthosis to replace it, and often a sticky residue from the adhesive backing remains. Similarly, open-cell padding is unsuitable.

If maxi- or superperforated material is used, the edge will be rough and irregular because of the cut perforations. To produce a smooth, nonirritating, washable edge, use a strip of

- $\frac{1}{16}$ in. (1.6 mm) thick self-adhesive Plastazote (Fig. 7-24)
- Aquaplast Ultra Thin Edging Material (specially designed for this purpose)
- Microfoam tape—ultrathin, closed-cell, and stretchy tape to conform to contours; a 3M product available from Smith & Nephew Inc.

## ATTACHMENT OF OUTRIGGERS AND THERMOPLASTIC BONDING

To form spring wire coils, either use round-nose pliers or even better, a wire-bending jig (Fig. 7-25) (see Fig. 5-12c). When cutting outrigger wire or spring wire, use appropriate wire cutters or pliers. To prevent injury from a piece

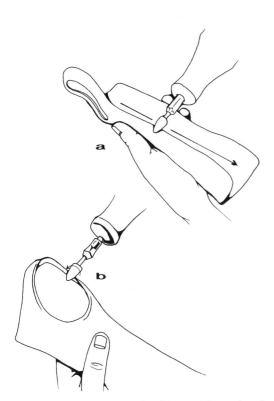

**FIGURE 7-23.** Edge finishing with a hand grinder. *(a)* Draw the spinning stone along the edge in a long, continuous stroke, toward you if you are right-handed and away from you if you are left-handed. *(b)* Smoothing the edge of the thumb hole.

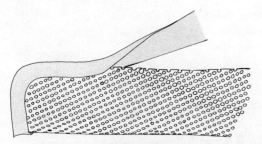

**FIGURE 7-24.**  Edge covering. Covering the rough edge of a maxi-perforated thermoplastic with a smooth, washable, non-irritating covering.

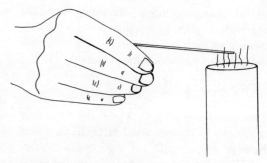

**FIGURE 7-26.**  Heating spring wire over the nozzle of the heat gun to imbed it into the thermoplastic.

of flying wire, cut the wire under a towel, pillowcase, or sheet.

When wire or metal outriggers are used, they must be anchored to the orthosis. Heat the wire over a heat gun (Fig. 7-26) and then press the heated wire into the thermoplastic base with pliers to prevent burns. Reinforce the attachment by bonding a layer of thermoplastic over the imbedded wire. When using coated thermoplastics, prime the surfaces by applying alcohol or solvent to the adjacent surfaces or scrape off the surface coating with scissors or a knife (Fig. 7-27a and b). Then thoroughly heat the anchor piece and warm the receptor site on the orthosis with a heat gun. Dry heating produces a more secure bond than moist heating (see Fig. 10-13d).

Use the same technique to bond a reinforcement strip if the orthosis is too flexible and unable to maintain the position of the joints. Similarly, if a tube outrigger is used, bond it to the

thermoplastic base using the aforementioned method (see Fig. 3-11c).

## SEALING THE CREVICES

Wherever thermoplastic is bonded or folded over, a crevice is created that is difficult to clean

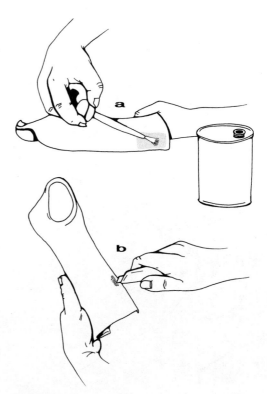

**FIGURE 7-27.**  Surface preparation for bonding or secure adhesion of hook Velcro patches. *(a)* Application of solvent to dissolve the surface coating. *(b)* Scraping off the coating with a knife.

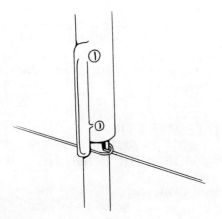

**FIGURE 7-25.**  Forming a coil spring with a wire-bending jig.

and that becomes a breeding ground for bacteria (see Fig. 3-13). To enhance resistance to soiling and to maintain a healthy environment, seal these crevices by spot heating. The application of solvent or isopropyl alcohol to the crevice may facilitate the procedure.

## METHODS OF FIXATION

The most common method of fixation uses Velcro strapping. Alternative methods, such as sterile gauze or elastic bandage, are discussed later in this chapter.

### Strap Location and Width

First, determine the optimal location and width of the straps. Most orthoses have a key strap that applies the key force to secure the orthosis and usually one or more stabilizing straps (see Chapter 3, "Fixation").

For volar forearm-based orthoses, the key strap crosses the dorsum of the wrist, over the axis of rotation. If this strap is positioned too proximally, greater force is required to secure it and prevent the wrist from flexing out (see Fig. 3-7). A stabilizing strap is located at the proximal end of the orthosis, across the dorsum of the forearm. Optional straps are located distal to the key strap depending on the orthotic design (Figs. 7-28 and 7-29*a*).

For dorsal forearm-based orthoses, the key strap is located at the proximal end of the orthosis, across the volar aspect of the forearm, and an optional strap is located across the volar aspect of the wrist (Fig. 7-29*b*).

For the adult, the key strap of a hand orthosis should be 2 in. (5 cm) wide to distribute the securing force over a large area. Stabilizing and optional straps can be narrower if desired. For finger orthoses, use ½ in. (2.5 cm) wide loop Velcro (see Fig. 11-14). If possible, use a low-plush version, ideal for finger orthoses called R-Thin (from Smith & Nephew Inc.) or Extra-Thin (from North Coast Medical).

### Dedicated Velcro-Cutting Scissors

Typically, Velcro strapping uses self-adhesive (sticky-back) hook patches and a nonadhesive

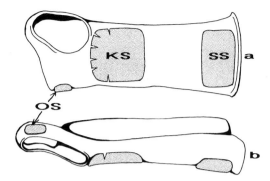

**FIGURE 7-28.** Self-adhesive hook Velcro patches for volar forearm-based static thumb-hole wrist orthosis. Center patches for the key strap (KS) and stabilizing strap (SS) and side patches for the optional strap (OS) over the dorsum of the hand. A center patch cannot be used for the dorsal hand strap because it would interfere with thumb mobility. *(a)* Volar view. *(b)* Radial view.

loop (hook-sensitive) strap. When cutting self-adhesive Velcro we recommend a dedicated pair of scissors. Otherwise the residue left on the scissors from the adhesive backing will impede smooth cutting of warm thermoplastic. The residue can be removed from scissors with alcohol or solvent. Self-adhesive hook patches can be either a center patch or two side patches.

### Center Hook Patch Method

Either cut a 2 in. (5 cm) length of self-adhesive hook Velcro off the roll or use a suitable precut tab. The width of the hook Velcro should match

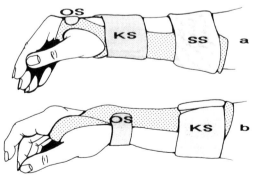

**FIGURE 7-29.** Straps for *(a)* Volar forearm-based wrist orthosis, *(b)* Dorsal forearm-based static thumb-hole wrist orthosis. KS = key strap; SS = stabilizing strap; OS = optional strap.

the width of the loop strap. Round the corners with scissors because square corners make the patch more susceptible to peeling away from the thermoplastic base. Position the center patch in the middle of the trough. To make the patch conform to a concave or convex contour, "notch" the edges (Fig. 7-28). Secure one end of the loop Velcro strap to the midpoint of the center patch; the other end wraps around the limb and is secured to the remaining portion of exposed hook. Center patches are generally more durable than side patches.

*Ensure that the loop strap completely covers the hook Velcro because exposed hook Velcro is abrasive to the skin and catches on clothing.*

## Double Side Hook Patch Method

Either cut two pieces of 1 in. (2.5 cm) long self-adhesive hook Velcro off the roll or use two suitable precut tabs. Match the width of the hook to the loop Velcro, round the corners, and position the side patches on either side of the trough (Figs. 7-28 and 7-29). Secure each end of the loop Velcro strap to one of the side patches.

The challenge of the double side patch method is to ensure long-lasting adherence of the hook Velcro patches to the thermoplastic base. Every time the loop Velcro is detached from the hook patch, the edge of the patch is subjected to a force that eventually causes it to peel off the thermoplastic base. This is especially troublesome with coated thermoplastics. Many strategies will counteract peeling Velcro. First, use the center patch method whenever possible. However, if side patches are required (e.g., for straps over the dorsum of the hand or fingers), ensure better adhesion of side patches through the following methods:

- Remove the coating on the thermoplastic at the side patch location by scraping it off with scissors or knife or by dissolving it with solvent or alcohol (Fig. 7-27a and b).
- Dry heat the adhesive backing of the hook Velcro patch with a heat gun to enhance its

adhesive qualities (Fig. 7-30a and b). Avoid overheating the Velcro to prevent it from melting.
- Dry heat the attachment site on the orthosis (Fig. 7-30c).
- Embed one edge of the patch into preheated translucent material (Fig. 7-31). Remove the paper backing from the hook Velcro patch and fold over one edge of the patch ¼ in. (½ cm). Using a heat gun, warm the recipient area of the thermoplastic orthosis until it is translucent, and then attach the self-adhesive backing to the translucent material, embedding the folded back hook into the warm plastic.
- Refrain from detaching the loop Velcro strap until the adhesive hook patch has

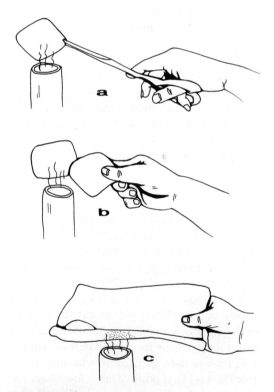

**FIGURE 7-30.** Enhancing self-stick qualities of hook Velcro patch. (*a*) Heat the adhesive over the nozzle of a heat gun, holding the patch with the blades of Velcro-designated scissors. (*b*) Remove the paper backing of the self-stick Velcro. (*c*) Use a heat gun to spot heat the orthosis before attaching Velcro or bonding thermoplastic. Full heating is not required and is undesirable because the orthosis will lose its shape.

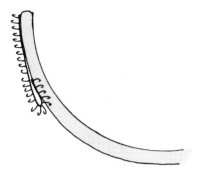

**FIGURE 7-31.** Embedding the edge of a hook Velcro patch. ½ in. (1 cm) of the self-adhesive hook patch has been folded back and imbedded into the warm translucent thermoplastic.

been in place for a few hours to ensure firm adherence to the thermoplastic.

## The Detachable Loop Strap

With the center patch or side patch method, the loop strap is fully detachable so that it can be washed or replaced as needed. A considerable disadvantage is that the strap can be lost, especially in the white linen of a client's hospital bed. To minimize this possibility, use brightly colored Velcro straps. Alternatively, secure the loop Velcro to one side of the orthosis as described next.

## Securing the Loop Strap

Before securing one side of the loop Velcro to the orthosis, determine which side the strap should open from to facilitate donning and doffing of the orthosis. Several methods can secure the strap:

- Attach the strap with a metal rivet (also called speedy or rapid rivet) or pop rivet. Rivet attachment is highly secure. The only way to remove the riveted strap is to drill through the rivet with a power drill. Alternatively, plastic finger rivets can be snapped together to secure straps (see Fig. 4-3).
- Use metal or nylon screws for a secure, nonpermanent attachment (Fig. 7-32).

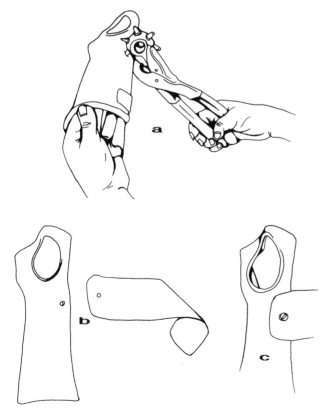

**FIGURE 7-32.** Securing the loop strap. *(a)* Using the setting that matches the size of the rivet or screw, place a hole about ½ in. (1 cm) from the edge of the loop strap and the orthosis. *(b)* Holes in the thermoplastic and the loop strap for a metal rivet, pop rivet, finger rivet, Chicago screw, or nylon screw. *(c)* Loop strap secured with a Chicago screw.

They can be unscrewed to remove the strap for washing or replacing. If spontaneous loosening of the screw is a problem, apply Loctite or Vibratite (available from hardware stores) to the screw before fastening.

- Replace the rivet with a thermoplastic plug formed from category C or D thermoplastic (Fig. 7-33*a* and *b*). Use the largest hole setting on a revolving hole punch to place a hole about ½ in. (1 cm) from the edge of the loop Velcro strap. Prepare the thermoplastic base for bonding by scraping off or dissolving the coating of the recipient surface. Make the thermoplastic plug by heating a small piece of thermoplastic until it is malleable. Form it into a narrow plug and pass it through the hole in the loop Velcro strap to secure it to the thermoplastic base. It is difficult to remove if it has been firmly attached.

- Another approach is to embed one edge of the loop Velcro strap into the thermoplastic. This technique is most appropriate for translucent materials because heating causes the molecules to separate, allowing the plush loop to be embedded. Warm the thermoplastic at the attachment site until it is translucent (Fig. 7-30*c*). Then firmly press the plush loop into the warm plastic. When the plastic is cool, the Velcro will be firmly attached (Fig. 7-34*a*). To remove the embedded strap, see Figure 7-34*b*.

- Use a prefabricated overlap strap that has a plain loop Velcro or padded material, available in varying lengths and widths, with a 3 in. (7.5 cm) length of self-stick hook Velcro attached at one end. Alternatively, use a prefabricated D-ring strap that has a length of loop Velcro with a hook portion attached at one end and a D-ring sewn to the other end. Such straps are

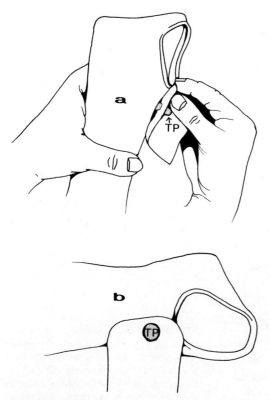

**FIGURE 7-33.** (*a*) A warm thermoplastic plug (TP) secured to the orthosis and passed through the hole in the loop strap. (*b*) The thermoplastic plug has been flattened to secure the loop strap.

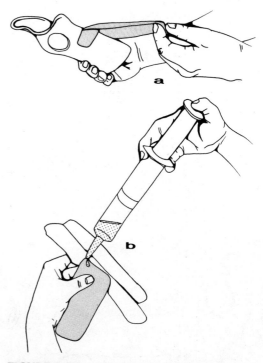

**FIGURE 7-34.** (*a*) One end of the loop strap has been embedded into translucent thermoplastic, creating a secure attachment. (*b*) Removal of the embedded loop strap is achieved by heating the attachment site with hot water administered by a baster or syringe. As the material heats, gently pull the strap away.

available in self-stick and nonstick versions.

### Preventing Irritation by the Edge of the Velcro Strap

The edge of the standard loop Velcro is somewhat sharp and may irritate the client's skin. This is particularly a problem with volar forearm-based wrist orthoses because the edge of the wrist strap often rubs against the dorsum of the hand. One solution is to substitute a conforming cushioned strap for the standard loop Velcro. (See Chapter 4, "Loop Strap Alternatives.") Alternatively, a strap pad can be added to the loop strap (Fig. 7-7*d*). Other solutions are illustrated in Figure 7-35.

Another approach is to reverse the placement of the hook and loop Velcro, applying a patch of self-adhesive loop Velcro to the orthosis and using nonadhesive hook Velcro for the strap. Line the hook Velcro that crosses the skin with a padded loop alternative (Fig. 7-35*d*).

## FACILITATING STRAP MANIPULATION

If the assessment identified that the client might have a problem with strap manipulation because of dexterity limitations, the therapist can provide easy-fastening straps, as shown in Figure 3-16. D-ring straps are easier than overlap straps to achieve a secure fixation.

## GAUZE BANDAGE FIXATION

This method is appropriate when the orthosis is applied over burned skin or other open wound. The used sterile bandage is discarded and replaced with a new one each time the orthosis is removed. The bandage should be wrapped from distal to proximal to promote venous return.

## FIXATION FOR THE EDEMATOUS LIMB

If edema is present or likely to develop, fixation of an orthosis with straps may be problematic because the tissue fluid tends to become trapped between the straps (see Fig. 3-19). To counteract this tendency, one or more of the following strategies can be used:

- Apply a sleeve of elasticized tubular bandage (e.g., Tubigrip), or a compression garment, to be worn under the orthosis to provide circumferential compression.
- Wrap each finger with self-adherent (cohesive) tape—Coban (from Sammons Preston), Co-Flex or Flex Power (from Sammons Preston), Rol-Flex (from Smith & Nephew, Inc.), or Medi-Rip (from North Coast Medical)—or cover each finger with

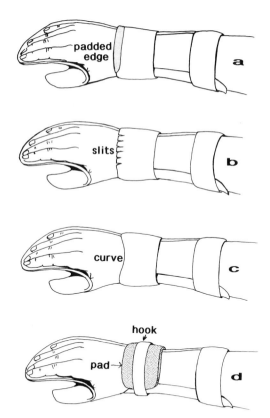

**FIGURE 7-35.** Preventing irritation by the edge of the Velcro strap. (*a*) Cover the edge of the standard loop strap with a soft, self-adhesive padding such as 1/16 in. (1.6 mm) Plastazote. (*b*) Cut small slits into the wrist edge of the strap to create a fringe so that it will conform to the dorsum of the hand. (*c*) Cut the distal edge of the strap to form a curve that conforms to the dorsum of the hand. (*d*) Attach self-adhesive loop Velcro to the thermoplastic. Replace the loop strap with a hook strap with a padded loop alternative (e.g., Velfoam) against the skin.

¾ in. (2 cm) wide tubular compression bandage.

- Use a wide, soft, conforming strap material such as CushionStrap, Velfoam, AlphaStrap, or SoftStrap.
- Replace strap fixation with elastic bandage (e.g., Tensor or Ace), wrapping the orthosis in place from distal to proximal, in the direction of venous blood flow.
- Educate the client about strategies to control edema, as discussed in Chapter 3, emphasizing the importance of elevating the edematous limb.

# ● Final Instructions, Evaluation, and Follow-Up

*A final evaluation should be done after the client has worn the device for at least 20 minutes. For example, an outpatient can go for coffee and return after 15 to 30 minutes.*

Once all the adjustments have been made and straps have been attached, provide a splint liner or tubular bandage (Stockinette or Tubigrip) to be worn under the orthosis to absorb perspiration, if appropriate. While the client removes the orthosis and liner, observe the technique used and make suggestions to facilitate the process. Check carefully for red areas on the skin and adjust the contours to relieve pressure points as required. Also, recheck the freedom of uninvolved joints and trim the orthosis if necessary. As the client reapplies the orthosis, observe the method again and clarify the technique that should be used.

Provide the client, caregiver, or nursing staff with written instructions about how to apply and remove the orthosis, wearing schedule, care of the orthosis and splint liner, and how to recognize fitting problems and what to do. Refer to the sample information sheet provided at the end of the chapter. If you provide written information, make a copy to keep in the client's file for documentation and future reference.

Ensure that the client understands the objectives of the orthosis and the implications of noncompliance. For the inpatient, provide clear application and care instructions to hospital staff; where permitted, place a labeled illustration or Polaroid photograph of the orthosis above the bed. If the client is not an inpatient, make a follow-up appointment within 1 week to check the fit and adherence to the prescribed wearing schedule. If it is not possible to see the client in person, follow up with a telephone call. Provide a contact telephone number and encourage the client to call if there are any questions or possible fitting problems.

Clients with serial-static or static-progressive orthoses may require appointments as often as every 2 or 3 days to make adjustments. Similarly, frequent contact with the client is important if noncompliance would have serious consequences, for example, when providing an orthosis for a fracture or tendon injury.

Following the Orthosis Information Sheet are guidelines for the final evaluation.

# Orthosis Information Sheet

Name: _____ Date: _____

Orthosis: _____

Purpose of the Orthosis: _____

Therapist: _____ Contact telephone number: _____

Next Appointment: _____

**Wear your orthosis:**

☐ all the time      ☐ night and rest periods      ☐ when activity causes pain

☐ during these activities _____

☐ remove every_____ hours for cleaning

☐ remove every_____ hours for exercising the joints as instructed by your therapist

☐ discontinue the orthosis_____

☐ other_____

**Do NOT wear your orthosis:**

☐ when driving a car      ☐ when operating machinery      ☐ other_____

**How to care for your orthosis:**

- Avoid exposing the orthosis to heat sources such as stoves, radiators, heat vents, direct sunlight (e.g., window ledge or car dashboard), very hot water, or clothes dryer because the material is heat-sensitive and will lose its shape.
- Do not attempt to make adjustments or add padding to your orthosis.
- Hand wash the orthosis in lukewarm water with a mild soap. For difficult spots use a scouring powder or an all-purpose spray cleaner. Straps may be scrubbed with a brush. Rinse well and dry thoroughly before reapplying.
- Cornstarch may be applied to the skin to absorb perspiration (exception: open wounds or if sutures have not been removed).
- Wash liner in cold water with mild soap, rinse well, and lay it flat to dry.
- Other _____

**Special Instructions:** _____

_____

**PRECAUTIONS:** **If any of the following problems are noted, report them to your therapist immediately:**

- Swelling, pain, excess tension, pressure, or tightness
- Burning, tingling or numbness
- Red areas or rash
- The orthosis becomes damaged, needs adjustment, or fits poorly
- Other _____

**Note:** **It is not uncommon for an orthosis to feel awkward for the first few days. If you have difficulty adjusting, contact your therapist.**

## Evaluation Form for Upper Extremity Orthoses

**Desired Quality** | **Deficits**

☐ **Good cosmesis**
- ☐ pattern or trim marks
- ☐ rough edges
- ☐ square corners
- ☐ imprints

☐ **Conformity to contour**
- ☐ gaping
- ☐ flat transverse arch in the hand
- ☐ proximal edge too flared
- ☐ lacks conformity at: _____

☐ **Free from pressure points and irritation**

*Poor contour, tightness, or redness over:*
- ☐ MC heads
- ☐ ulnar head
- ☐ ulnar styloid
- ☐ radial styloid
- ☐ pisiform
- ☐ thumb CMC joint
- ☐ transverse arch (too high)
- ☐ thumb web space
- ☐ radial/ulnar side of palm and fingers
- ☐ edges of straps or finger loops/slings
- ☐ webspaces from arching spring wire
- ☐ medial/lateral epicondyle
- ☐ ribs/iliac crest
- ☐ proximal edge—unflared or overflared
- ☐ edges of trough (tight)
- ☐ other: _____

☐ **Correct width and depth of trough**
- ☐ too deep
- ☐ too shallow
- ☐ too short
- ☐ too long—restricts movements at:

☐ **Correctly positioned joints**
- ☐ Poor positioning of: _____ _____

*Restriction of:*

☐ **No unnecessary restriction of uninvolved joints**
- ☐ wrist
- ☐ thumb opposition
- ☐ finger MCPs
- ☐ IPs
- ☐ elbow
- ☐ shoulder
- ☐ other: _____

☐ **Correct location of straps**
- ☐ wrist strap too proximal
- ☐ key strap too narrow
- ☐ other: _____

☐ **Self-adhesive Velcro patches securely attached**
- ☐ self-adhesive Velcro peels away easily
- ☐ square corners

☐ **No client discomfort after 20–30 minutes of continuous wear**
- ☐ pain, excess tension
- ☐ burning, tingling, numbness
- ☐ circulation impeded
- ☐ skin reaction to material
- ☐ swelling between the straps
- ☐ pressure point redness

☐ Incisions, scars, skin grafts and edema accommodated by appropriate padding/lining and fixation

☐ Client/caregiver can apply and remove orthosis easily and correctly

☐ Client/caregiver received oral and written instructions as well as demonstration regarding:

- Name and contact number of therapist
- Purpose of orthosis
- Wearing schedule
- Care of the orthosis
- Special instructions
- Precautions

## Evaluation Form for Lower Extremity Orthoses

| Desired Quality | Deficits |
|---|---|

**Good cosmesis**
- [ ] pattern or trim marks
- [ ] rough edges
- [ ] square corners
- [ ] imprints

**Conformity to contour**
- [ ] gaping
- [ ] proximal edge too flared
- [ ] lacks conformity at: _____

**Free from pressure points and irritation**

*Poor contour, tightness, or redness over:*

- [ ] metatarsal heads
- [ ] medial longitudinal arch of the foot
- [ ] medial/lateral malleolus
- [ ] head of fibula
- [ ] tibial plateau
- [ ] femoral condyles
- [ ] proximal edge—unflared or over-flared
- [ ] edges of trough (tight)
- [ ] other:_____

**Correct width and depth of trough**
- [ ] too deep
- [ ] too shallow
- [ ] too short
- [ ] too long—restricts movement at: _____

**Correctly positioned joints**
- [ ] Poor positioning of: _____

**No unnecessary restriction of uninvolved joints**

*Restriction of:*

- [ ] hip
- [ ] knee
- [ ] ankle
- [ ] other:_____
- [ ] other:_____

**Correct location of straps**
- [ ] poor location of straps
- [ ] straps too narrow

**Self-adhesive Velcro patches securely attached**
- [ ] self-adhesive Velcro peels away easily
- [ ] square corners

**No client discomfort after 20–30 minutes of continuous wear**
- [ ] pain, excess tension
- [ ] burning, tingling, numbness
- [ ] circulation impeded
- [ ] skin reaction to material
- [ ] swelling between the straps
- [ ] pressure point redness

- [ ] Incisions, scars, skin grafts and edema accommodated by appropriate padding/lining and fixation
- [ ] Client/caregiver can apply and remove orthosis easily and correctly
- [ ] Client/caregiver received oral and written instructions as well as demonstration regarding:

- Name and contact number of therapist
- Purpose of orthosis
- Wearing schedule
- Care of the orthosis
- Special instructions
- Precautions

## Evaluation Form for Head and Neck Orthoses

| **Desired Quality** | **Deficits** | |
|---|---|---|

☐ *Good cosmesis*
  ☐ pattern or trim marks      ☐ square corners
  ☐ rough edges                ☐ imprints

☐ *Conformity to contour*
  ☐ gaping                     ☐ proximal edge too flared
  ☐ flat transverse arch in the hand   ☐ lacks conformity at:

  _____

☐ *Free from pressure points and irritation*

*Poor contour, tightness, or redness over:*

  ☐ facial contours            ☐ mandible
  ☐ larynx                     ☐ clavicles
  ☐ sternum

☐ *Correctly positioned cervical spine*
  ☐ too flexed                 ☐ laterally flexed
  ☐ too extended               ☐ rotated

*Restriction of:*

☐ *No unnecessary restriction of uninvolved joints*
  ☐ cervical spine             ☐ shoulders
  ☐ other:_____

☐ *Correct location of straps*
  ☐ specify problem:_____

☐ *Self-adhesive Velcro patches securely attached*
  ☐ self-adhesive Velcro peels away easily   ☐ square corners

☐ *No client discomfort after 20–30 minutes of continuous wear*
  ☐ pain, excess tension       ☐ skin reaction to material
  ☐ burning, tingling, numbness   ☐ redness
  ☐ circulation impeded

☐ Incisions, scars, skin grafts, and edema accommodated by appropriate padding/lining and fixation.

☐ Client/caregiver can apply and remove orthosis easily and correctly

☐ Client/caregiver received oral and written instructions as well as demonstratation regarding:

- Name and contact number of therapist
- Purpose of orthosis
- Care of the orthosis
- Special instructions

# References

1. Magee, DJ: Orthopedic Physical Assessment, ed 2. WB Saunders, Philadelphia, 1992.
2. Nicholson, B: Evaluation of the hand. In Stanley, BG, and Tribuzi, SM (eds): Concepts in Hand Rehabilitation. FA Davis, Philadelphia, 1992.
3. Tan, AM: Sensibility testing. In Stanley, BG, and Tribuzi, SM (eds): Concepts in Hand Rehabilitation. FA Davis, Philadelphia, 1992.
4. Totten, PA, and Flinn-Wagner, A: Functional evaluation. In Stanley, BG, and Tribuzi, SM (eds): Concepts in Hand Rehabilitation. FA Davis, Philadelphia, 1992.
5. O'Sullivan, SB, and Schmitz, TJ: Physical Rehabilitation: Assessment and Treatment, ed 3. FA Davis, Philadelphia, 1994.
6. Clarkson, HM, and Gillewich, GB: Musculoskeletal Assessment: Joint Range of Motion and Manual Muscle Strength. Williams & Wilkins, Baltimore, 1989.
7. Fess, EE, and Philips, CA: Hand Splinting Principles and Methods. Mosby, St. Louis, 1987.
8. Brand, PW, and Hollister, A: Clinical Mechanics of the Hand, ed 2. Mosby, St. Louis, 1993.
9. Brand, PW: Mechanical factors in joint stiffness and tissue growth. Hand Ther 8:91, 1995.
10. Smith & Nephew Inc.: Rehabilitation Division Catalogue, 1997. Rolyan® and Gel Shell® are trademarks of Smith & Nephew, Inc.
11. Afor, JD: Microwave proves effective for softening low temperature splinting materials. Advance for Occupational Therapists, June 26, 1989.

# Midline Orthoses for Head, Face, Neck, and Back

## Chapter Outline

Beginning with this chapter, the format of the book changes to a tabular presentation of fabrication procedures for 67 custom orthoses, organized regionally from head to toe. Chapter 8 contains eight orthoses for the midline of the body—head, face, neck, and back. Chapter 9 has 11 orthoses for the axilla, shoulder, elbow, and forearm. Chapter 10 describes 21 forearm-based orthoses. Chapter 11 presents 19 hand-, finger-, and thumb-based orthoses, and Chapter 12 has eight lower extremity orthoses. In each of Chapters 9 through 12, the content is organized from proximal to distal.

The fabrication instructions for the orthoses in Chapters 8 through 12 are brief. As a result, the student or inexperienced therapist is encouraged to read Chapter 7, which describes the fabrication process in detail. Before attempting more complex designs, develop some basic skills by making a volar or dorsal forearm-based static wrist orthosis.

Each orthosis is named according to the terminology described in Chapter 1 and summarized in Table 1-3. Common names for each orthosis are listed, along with objectives and suggested indications or conditions. Where appropriate, the therapeutic rationale of the orthosis is provided. Recommended materials, equipment, tools, and positioning of the client and therapist are outlined, as well as specific joint positioning, where appropriate. Usually the category of thermoplastic is identified, rather than a specific material. To select a thermoplastic from the suggested category, refer to Tables 1 and 2 in Appendix A. To select a supplier from whom to order orthotic materials, equipment, or tools, refer to Appendix D. Procedures for generating a custom pattern and fabricating each orthosis are described, along with suggested wearing regimens, precautions, options, and alternatives, including precuts and prefabricated orthoses.

Throughout Chapters 9 through 11, the **Splint Classification System (SCS)** name is also included. This naming system was developed by the Splint Classification Task Force of the American Society of Hand Therapists for upper extremity orthoses, describing the function but not the appearance of each orthosis. Both the SCS and our system identify the target joint, bone, or region, and both use the same descriptors for the direction of forces (e.g., flexion, extension, rotation). Although both systems describe the primary purpose, or objective, the terminology for each is different. In the SCS, the primary purpose is described as immobilization, mobilization, or restriction. The term *immobilization* corresponds to our *static* design category, and *mobilization* corresponds to our terms *assistive* or *corrective*, for which the design category could be serial-static, static-progressive, or dynamic. The SCS uses the term *restriction*, whereas we use the term *motion-blocking*.

Unlike our naming system, the SCS has no description of the base (e.g., volar forearm-based). However, it identifies the number of secondary or nontarget joints and the total number of joints included in the orthosis. For example, Figure 10-10*a* depicts the radial forearm-based static wrist-thumb orthosis for which the SCS name is "thumb MP extension immobilization; type 2[3]." Type 2 means that in addition to the target thumb MP (metacarpophalangeal joint), there are two secondary joints, and the illustration shows that they are the thumb carpometacarpal joint and the wrist. Because the SCS describes function but not appearance, the same name can apply to other orthoses with a different appearance. For example, the same SCS name is also used for the volar forearm-based static wrist-thumb orthosis in Figure 10-11*a*. The SCS names have not been included in Chapters 8 and 12 because that terminology pertains only to the upper limb.

Although Chapters 8 through 12 document a wide range of orthoses, the possibilities for orthotic design extend far beyond this book. New challenges and new orthotic materials, combined with the therapist's creative and problem-solving skills and client input, lead to the ongoing development of new designs. The therapist is encouraged to use these chapters as a guideline and not as strict doctrine. If the recommended materials, equipment, or tools are not available, substitute another thermoplastic or modify the fabrication procedures. Feel free to adapt the pattern to meet the individual requirements of the situation. The orthoses described for the various conditions should not be regarded as the only suitable design to use. As Table 7-2 illustrates, for any condition, there are often numerous design options, and we surely have not documented all of them.

Orthoses that are custom molded to the body contours of one person should not be used by another person. However, some metal components such as prefabricated outriggers can be salvaged and used on a different orthosis.

An evaluation form for head and neck orthoses can be found at the end of Chapter 7. It can be used as a guideline for designing, fabricating, and evaluating many of the orthoses in Chapter 8.

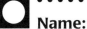
## Name:    Nonarticular Plastazote Protective Helmet (Fig. 8–1*a*)

| | |
|---|---|
| *Common Name* | Helmet |
| *Objectives* | To protect the brain, skull, or skin graft |
| *Indications* | • Potential for head injury from |
| | ○ Self-destructive behavior |

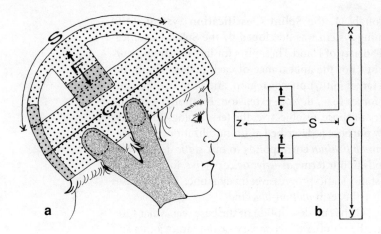

**a**      **b**

**FIGURE 8-1.** Nonarticular Plastazote protective helmet. *(a)* Lateral view showing location of measurements. Thermoplastic reinforcements (shaded areas) are attached with contact cement. *(b)* Pattern: all pieces are 2 to 3 in. (5 cm to 7.5 cm) wide, depending on size of head. C = circumference around forehead plus 1 in. (2.5 cm). S = sagittal measurement; F = frontal measurement.

- ○ Repeated falls
- ○ Seizures
- **Craniotomy** or skull fracture (proceed cautiously to avoid applying force over area of skull injury)
- **Skin graft** of scalp

**Materials**

- ½ in. (1.2 cm) thick foam thermoplastic—#1 pink perforated Plastazote or 4E AliPlast
- 1½ in. (3 cm) wide padded Velcro strapping and self-adhesive hook
- Contact cement—100 percent solvent free (no toxic fumes)
- Any ⅛ in. (3.2 mm) thick low-temperature thermoplastic for reinforcement pieces
- ¹⁄₃₂ in. (0.8 mm) thick self-adhesive, very thin gel sheeting to help cling to the hair (optional)

**Equipment and Tools**

- Splinting or kitchen oven with good ventilation
- Mirror
- Height-adjustable stool
- Metal sheet lined with silicone release paper, talcum powder, or cornstarch
- Marking utensil
- Heat gun
- Scissors
- Bench or hand grinder to finish edges (optional)

**Client's Position**

- Seated on a stool, next to the oven, in front of a mirror; the top of the client's head is at the therapist's midchest level.

**Therapist's Position**

- Standing beside or behind the client.
- Assistance from a second therapist may be required.

**Pattern**

- Figure 8-1*b*

**Fabrication**

1. Preheat oven to 250°F (140°C).
2. Heat the foam thermoplastic for 3 to 4 minutes on a metal sheet.
3. Check the temperature on your skin.
4. Mold to the client's head, avoiding pressure on the injury site. Bring

edges x, y, and z (shown in Fig. 8-1*b*) together at back of head forming a T-shaped seam. Working time is 20 to 30 seconds.

5. Remove from the client.

6. If desired, adhere gel sheeting to the inside of the Plastazote or Ali-Plast after molding to prevent migration.

7. Trim edges to meet without overlap.

8. Apply contact cement to all the edges to be glued together. Allow cement to dry (10 to 15 minutes—drying can be hastened with the heat gun) and then join the edges.

9. To reinforce the back seam and two side seams, apply contact cement over the seam areas (Fig. 8-1*a*—shaded areas) and allow to dry as described previously.

10. If the thermoplastic for reinforcements has been surface treated, remove the coating by applying solvent or by scraping. Heat with a heat gun to enhance adhesive properties. Press firmly onto the areas with contact cement. There is no need to apply contact cement to the thermoplastic. Warm thermoplastic will adhere directly to contact cement.

11. Apply two side patches of hook Velcro to each side of the helmet. Attach a padded Velcro strap for fixation.

| | |
|---|---|
| *Wearing Regimen* | • As needed for protection |
| *Precautions* | • Avoid pressure over injury site during molding. |
| *Options* | • Cover entire helmet with ⅛ in. (3.2 mm) thick thermoplastic, following steps 9 and 10.<br>• Span uncovered areas with Hexcelite to protect a skin graft while allowing good air flow. Apply contact cement to attachment sites on the helmet, allow to dry, and adhere the warm Hexcelite. |
| *Alternatives* | • Mold the helmet entirely out of a category C thermoplastic with a foam or Plastazote or AliPlast lining.<br>• Other custom designs.[1–3]<br>• Prefabricated baseball or bicycle helmets.<br>• Prefabricated helmets for special needs populations.[4] |

## Name: Nonarticular Scar-Controlling Face Mask (Fig. 8-2)

| | |
|---|---|
| *Common Name* | Face mask |
| *Objectives* | To apply pressure in order to<br>• Prevent or soften **hypertrophic** scar<br>• Prevent or correct contractures and prevent facial distortion<br>• Maintain or restore facial contours, cosmesis, and mobility |
| *Indications* | • Burn scar hypertrophy<br>• Skin graft<br>• Laceration<br>• Excision of tumor |

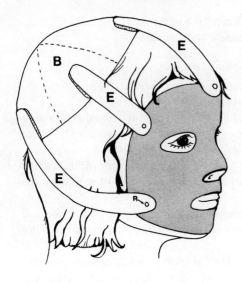

**FIGURE 8-2.** Nonarticular scar-controlling face mask. Side view showing elastic Velcro straps (E) attached by rivets (R) to face mask and anchored to hook Velcro tabs on skullcap or beanie (B).

| | |
|---|---|
| ***Rationale*** | • See Chapter 2, "Scar Management" |
| ***Materials*** | • Unperforated ⅟₁₆ or ³⁄₃₂ in. (1.6 or 2.4 mm) thick thermoplastic—try to match the color of thermoplastic to the skin color<br>　○ Opaque category C or D<br>　○ Orfit Classic (clings to skin better than other translucent thermoplastics with memory)<br>• Elastic Velcro straps<br>• Beanie (match color to hair color, if possible) with hook Velcro tabs<br>• Chicago screws/nylon screws/rivets<br>• Elastomer putty/gel padding (optional) |
| ***Equipment and Tools*** | • Heating pan<br>• Hammer and anvil if metal rapid rivets are used<br>• Sewing machine<br>• Scissors<br>• Flexible clear plastic for pattern |
| ***Client's Position*** | • Supine on an elevated plinth with the client's head at a comfortable work height for the therapist.<br>• For client comfort, support the natural extension curve of the cervical spine with a small rolled towel. |
| ***Therapist's Position*** | • Standing behind the client's head |
| ***Custom Pattern*** | 1. Use clear plastic to define the borders of the face and location of the nostrils.<br>2. Transfer the pattern to the thermoplastic and cut it out, including a breathing hole for the nostrils.<br>3. It is easier to mold the thermoplastic over the mouth and eyelids then cut out the areas after molding. |
| ***Fabrication*** | 1. If desired, mold elastomer putty or apply a piece of gel padding over the concave areas of face before molding.<br>2. Heat and check the temperature of the thermoplastic. |

3. Mold the thermoplastic, gently stroking into the facial contours.
4. When the contours are set, mark trim lines (border of face, around eyes and mouth) (Fig. 8-2).
5. Remove the thermoplastic from the face, and trim.
6. Attach elastomer or gel padding, if used, with double-stick tape.
7. Smooth all the edges with heat or a grinder.
8. Attach four or five elastic Velcro tabs to the face mask with screws or rivets (Fig. 8-2).
9. Sew a beanie to fit the contours of the head. Sew hook Velcro tabs to the beanie.

*Wearing Regimen*

- Wear directly against the skin. If there are open areas, apply over antibiotic mesh dressing.
- Wear continuously except for bathing, eating, facial massage, and stretching exercises.
- Remove as required to wipe off perspiration.
- Use for up to 2 years after the burn, until the scar has matured and is no longer amenable to pressure (i.e., no further softening or flattening of scar can be achieved), as determined by the therapist or physician.

*Precautions*

- Ensure grafts are stable before molding, usually 7 days after grafting.
- Monitor the skin for maceration, wound deterioration, and adverse reaction to the thermoplastic. If pressure area develops, spot heat and relieve the pressure point, or temporarily discontinue.
- Monitor children closely for sleep apnea. If this occurs, discontinue night use and substitute gel sheeting alone, although this provides less effective scar control.

*Adjustment*

- For children, remold periodically to accommodate growth.
- As scar tissue flattens, remold to restore pressure on the contours.

*Client Education*

- Educate client about
  ○ How pressure influences scar tissue
  ○ How to adjust tension in the straps to exert the desired amount of pressure
  ○ How to clean with mild cleanser, rinse, and dry well

*Options*

- If desired, add ½ in. (0.8 mm) thick self-adhesive, very thin gel padding, but nothing thicker because conformity to contour will be disturbed.

*Variations*

- Partial face mask applying pressure to isolated area of scar tissue

*Alternatives*

- Custom-fabricated Lycra face masks (e.g., Jobskin, with or without elastomer or thermoplastic conformer against the concave areas).
- Transparent plastic face mask molded from high-temperature thermoplastic (e.g., Uvex) over a positive plaster impression of the face. May be more acceptable to the client than an opaque low-temperature thermoplastic mask, and the amount of pressure exerted by the mask can be monitored by observing the degree of skin blanching.[5–7]
- Substitute gel sheeting over scar tissue for situations in which the client is reluctant to wear a mask (see Chapter 2, "Scar Management").

● ● ● ● ● ● ● ● ● ● ● ● ● ● ● ● ● ● ● ● ● ● ● ● ● ● ● ● ● ● ● ● ● ● ● ● ● ● ● ● ● ● ● ● ● ● ● ●

⬤ **Name:**       **Static Microstomia Prevention Orthosis**  (Fig. 8–3)

| | |
|---|---|
| *Common Names* | • Vancouver Microstomia Orthosis[8–10] |
| | • Microstomia splint/appliance prosthesis (This device is sometimes incorrectly called a "prosthesis," which actually denotes a device that replaces a body part.) |
| *Objective* | • To maintain or increase the opening of the mouth |
| *Rationale* | • See Chapter 2, "Promoting Tissue Growth to Reduce Contractures" |
| *Advantages over Other Designs* | • Will not dislodge into the mouth to cause choking |
| | • Lips can close |
| | • Adjustable |
| *Disadvantages of This Design* | • May cause drooling |
| | • Interferes with speech |
| | • Conspicuous |
| *Indications* | • Microstomia resulting from |
| | ○ Perioral scar contracture secondary to electrical, thermal, or chemical burns around the mouth |
| | ○ Scleroderma[11,12] |
| *Materials* | • Unperforated opaque category C or D thermoplastic—⅛ in. (3.2 mm) thick |
| | • 1 Kirschner wire, 0.045 in. (1.1 mm) diameter, 4 in. (10 cm) long, or use a large paper clip unfolded |
| | • For the crossbar—³⁄₃₂ in. (2 mm) diameter outrigger wire, 1½ to 2 in. (3 to 5 cm) long |
| | • ¹⁄₃₂ in. (0.8 mm) thick self-adhesive, very thin gel padding (optional) |

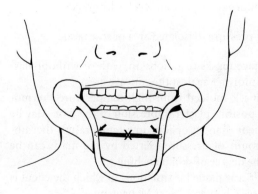

**FIGURE 8-3.**  Static microstomia-prevention orthosis. X = crossbar. Arrows point to location of holes to insert crossbar.

**Equipment and Tools**
- Heating pan
- Heat gun with pinpoint nozzle
- Wire cutter
- Pliers
- Hand grinder with ³⁄₃₂ in. (2 mm) drill bit or use a manual drill
- Scissors

**Pattern[8]**
- Figure 8-4*a* and *b*.
- The proportions can be reduced for a small child.

**Fabrication[8]**
1. Follow the steps in Figure 8-4*a* through *f*.
2. Place the orthosis in the client's mouth and mark just under the lower lip on each of the vertical components of the U-shaped covered wire (indicated by arrows in Fig. 8-3).
3. Remove from the mouth. Using the manual drill or hand grinder with drill bit, drill a hole about ⅛ in. (3 mm) deep at these two marks.
4. Reapply the orthosis and cut a length of outrigger wire to span between holes, forming the crossbar (Fig. 8-3).
5. If desired, apply very thin gel padding to inside of commissure pieces.

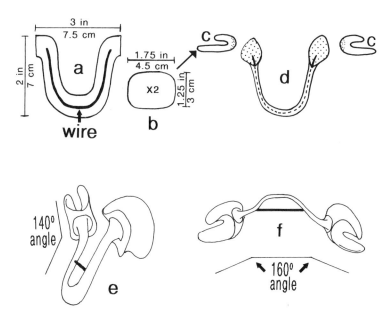

**FIGURE 8–4.** Fabrication steps for static microstomia-prevention orthosis. *(a)* Pattern for U-shaped thermoplastic, 3 × 2.5 in. (7.5 × 7 cm). Kirschner wire has been bent and superimposed. *(b)* Pattern for commissure piece 1.75 × 1.25 in. (4.5 × 3 cm). Cut two pieces with rounded corners. *(c)* Heat the commissure pieces and form one to fit each corner of the mouth with at least 1 in. molded to the inside of the mouth for secure fitting. Gently flare the top and bottom edges to prevent irritation of lips. *(d)* Heat the U-shaped thermoplastic and mold it over the Kirschner wire, except for the ends, which are left flat. Scrape or dissolve the coating on the surfaces to be bonded and spot heat with heat gun (stippled areas). Bond the pieces together, angling the commissure pieces *(e)* 140° upwards and *(f)* 160° backward (as shown in top view).[8]

| | |
|---|---|
| ***Application and Removal*** | 1. If there are any open wounds, spread antibiotic ointment over inside of commissure piece on the affected side(s). |
| | 2. To apply, squeeze the sides together, place in the mouth, and then insert the crossbar. |
| | 3. To remove, lift out the crossbar, squeeze the sides together, and then extract. |

***Wearing Regimen[8]***

- Remove for eating, oral hygiene, and active exercises.
- For facial burns involving the mouth, fit as early as 3 days after injury, or delay up to 4 weeks after injury.
- Begin with 10 minutes every 2 hours and increase to 30 minutes of every waking hour or as tolerated.
- Correction of established microstomia may be achieved after about 8 weeks. However, continue wearing regimen until scar tissue is mature (up to 2 years after the burn).
- For scleroderma, use at night only.

***Precautions***

- During first the few days after fitting, check lips twice daily for pressure sores. If necessary, narrow the U bar and shorten the crossbar to relieve pressure.

***Adjustments***

- For serial-static correction, widen the U bar to increase the horizontal force to accommodate growth. Lengthen the crossbar accordingly.

***Options***

- The crossbar can be omitted to convert the orthosis into a dynamic design.
- Substitute an Aquatube or Orfitube for the U-shaped component.
- If desired, add ½2 in. (0.8 mm) thick self-adhesive, very thin gel padding, but nothing thicker because conformity to contour will be disturbed.

***Alternatives***

- Static custom orthoses.[11–15]
- Prefabricated static Microstomia Prevention Appliance.[16]
- External traction hooks mounted to a neck conformer[17] or head gear.[18–21]
- Custom toothborne intraoral orthosis, either removable[22–24] like a dental bridge or attached to the teeth[25–27] like orthodontic braces. These devices are fitted by dentists or related professionals.
- Dynamic microstomia-prevention orthosis.

---

● • • • • • • • • • • • • • • • • • • • • • • • • • • • • • • • • • • • • • • • • •

■ **Name:**    **Dynamic Microstomia-Prevention Orthosis** [28]    (Fig. 8-5a)

| | |
|---|---|
| ***Common Names*** | Microstomia splint/appliance/prosthesis |
| ***Objective*** | To maintain or increase the opening of the oral cavity |
| ***Rationale*** | • See Chapter 2 "Promoting Tissue Growth to Reduce Contractures" |

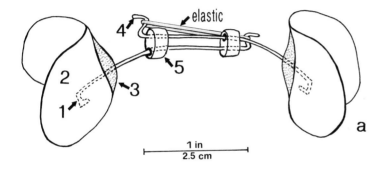

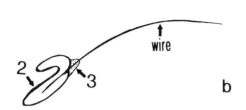

**FIGURE 8-5.** Dynamic microstomia-prevention orthosis. *(a)* Completed orthosis viewed from the inside with an orthodontic elastic spanning between the two central S-shaped hooks (4). *(b)* Top view showing gently arced wire imbedded in one of the commissure pieces. The numbers in (a) and (b) refer to fabrication step numbers.

| | |
|---|---|
| ***Advantages of a Dynamic Design*** | • Interferes less with speech than a static design<br>• Allows the client to exercise the muscles around the mouth |
| ***Disadvantages of This Design*** | • May cause drooling<br>• Interferes with speech<br>• Conspicuous<br>• Cannot be readily adjusted to accommodate growth<br>• Unable to close the mouth |
| ***Indications*** | • Microstomia resulting from<br>  ○ Perioral scar contracture secondary to electrical burns of the mouth<br>  ○ Scleroderma[11,12] |
| ***Materials*** | • Unperforated opaque category C or D thermoplastic—⅛ in. (3.2 mm) thick<br>• 0.045 in. (1.1 mm) diameter unthreaded Kirschner wires or 0.9 mm gauge spring wire<br>• Orthodontic elastics<br>• ¹⁄₃₂ in. (0.8 mm) thick self-adhesive, very thin gel padding (optional) |
| ***Equipment and Tools*** | • Heating pan<br>• Heat gun<br>• Two pairs of pliers |

- Wire cutter
- Scissors

**Pattern**
- Two pieces of thermoplastic 2.25 × 1.25 in. (6 × 3 cm) with corners rounded

**Fabrication (Fig. 8-5 a and b)**

The fabrication step numbers are shown in Figure 8–5*a* and *b*.
1. Form a U-shaped bend at one end of each wire with pliers.
2. Heat the thermoplastic piece and fold around bent end of the wire. Then form to one side of the mouth with at least 1 in. (2.5 cm) molded to inside of the mouth for secure fitting. Gently flare the top and bottom edges to prevent irritation of the lips. Repeat steps 1 and 2 on the other side.
3. To reinforce the wire attachment, apply solvent at the wire site and bond a small piece of dry-heated thermoplastic (stippled). Blend in the bonded pieces to eliminate any crevices. Apply a small amount of hand cream to fingers and heat smooth all edges and surfaces.
4. Measure the mouth opening from one commissure to other when mouth is stretched horizontally (e.g., 3 in. [7.5 cm]). Divide measurement in half (1½ in. [3.75 cm]). Using this length less ½ in. (1 cm), measure from lateral edge of commissure piece and form an S-shaped hook. Cut off the extra wire with the wire cutter. Repeat steps 3 and 4 on other side, creating a mirror-image component.
5. Lay the paired components side by side. Dry heat two small pieces of thermoplastic and mold around wires to maintain their parallel arrangement while allowing them to slide over each other. Then apply an orthodontic elastic over the two central hooks so that the orthosis opens to its maximum width.

**Application and Removal**
1. If there are any open wounds, spread antibiotic ointment over the inside of the commissure piece on the affected side(s).
2. To apply, squeeze the commissure pieces together to narrow the orthosis. First position the affected side, then the unaffected side. Gently release the orthosis, allowing it to expand.
3. To remove, squeeze together the anterior edges of commissure pieces to narrow the orthosis. Remove from the unaffected side first.

**Wearing Regimen**
- See Static Microstomia-Prevention Orthosis.

**Precautions**
- Contraindicated for small children because of the risk of choking.
- If significant bleeding occurs from the affected commissure, apply pressure immediately and seek medical attention.

**Options**
- If desired, add ½₂ in. (0.8 mm) thick self-adhesive, very thin gel padding, but nothing thicker because conformity to contour will be disturbed.

**Alternatives**
- Static microstomia-prevention orthosis
- Dynamic custom orthoses[29–31]

● **Name:**  ### Circumferential Static Plastazote Stabilizing Collar
(Fig. 8-6)

*Common Names*   Collar; neck brace

*Objectives*
- To relieve pain
- To prevent deformity
- To limit joint movement
- To support the weight of the head
- To compensate for weak neck extensors
- To stabilize, protect, and align the cervical spine

*Indications*
- **Vertigo**
- **Torticollis**
- Cervical pain
- Disk herniation
- Nerve root impingement

- Degenerative joint disease (**osteoarthritis**)
- Soft tissue injury, often resulting from whiplash
- Rheumatoid arthritis—pain or C1-2 subluxation
- Postsurgery—**laminectomy**, fusion, mandibular advancement

*Materials*
- ½ in. (1.2 cm) thick foam thermoplastic—#1 pink perforated Plastazote or 4E AliPlast. (AliPlast has a smoother surface than Plastazote and is less irritating to the skin.)
- For a small child, use ¼ in. (0.6 cm) thick foam thermoplastic.
- 1 or 1½ in. (2.5 to 4 cm) D-ring strap.

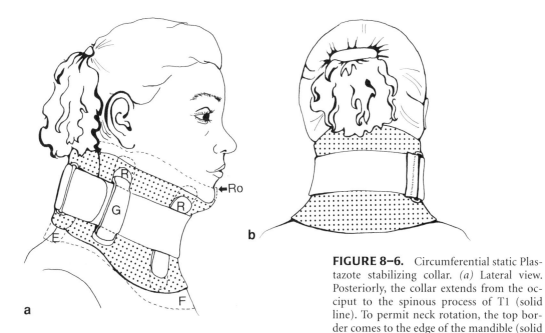

**FIGURE 8–6.** Circumferential static Plastazote stabilizing collar. *(a)* Lateral view. Posteriorly, the collar extends from the occiput to the spinous process of T1 (solid line). To permit neck rotation, the top border comes to the edge of the mandible (solid line). To restrict neck rotation, top border extends 1 in. (2.5 cm) above edge of mandible (Ro). To enhance flexion control, increase the area over the anterior chest (F). To enhance extension control, increase the area over the upper back (E). R = reinforcement; G = strap guide. *(b)* Posterior view.

- For reinforcement strips: ⅛ in. (3.2 mm) thick thermoplastic, 1½ in. (4 cm) wide.
- Solvent-free contact cement.
- 3 or 4 in. (7.5 or 10 cm) wide Stockinette (optional).

*Equipment and Tools*
- Dry heat source— kitchen or splinting oven
- Metal sheet lined with silicone release paper, talcum powder, or cornstarch
- Solvent or 100 percent isopropyl alcohol
- Heat gun
- Marking utensil
- Scissors
- Bench or hand grinder or belt sander
- Sewing machine

*Client's Position (see Fig. 6-6)*
- The client is seated, in front of a mirror, on a height-adjustable stool beside the oven, with the neck at the level of the therapist's elbow. If a mirror is not available, the assistance of a second therapist is required to control the client's neck position.
- Ensure easy access to neck, upper chest, and back. Secure long hair with elastics or hair clips above the level of the occiput. The client should wear an open-neck T-shirt, tank top, or hospital gown.
- Remove earrings and necklaces.
- Ideally, the neck should be in neutral alignment—no flexion, extension, rotation, or lateral flexion. However, contracture or muscle spasm may prevent ideal positioning, and the collar should be molded to the best-tolerated position. The collar can be remolded to improve neck alignment when contracture or spasm is reduced.

*Therapist's Position (see Fig. 6-6)*
- Standing behind client.
- Assistance from a second therapist positioned in front of the client is warranted if a mirror is unavailable or if help is required to stabilize the client's head during the molding.
- The molding procedure requires the therapist to stabilize the client's head and neck against the therapist's body. To avoid any misunderstanding of intentions, explain the molding procedure and the therapist's positioning before the fabrication process begins.

*Pattern*
- Create a rectangular pattern. The length is the circumference of the neck plus 4 in. (10 cm). The height is the measurement from the tip of the chin to the sternal angle (junction between manubrium and sternum).

*Fabrication*
1. For postsurgical applications, mold before surgery if possible.
2. Preheat the oven to 250°F (140°C).
3. Heat the foam thermoplastic on a metal sheet for 3 to 4 minutes. The working time is 20 to 30 seconds.
4. Check the temperature on your skin and then on the client's skin before molding.
5. If the client is heat sensitive or in pain, quickly stretch the foam thermoplastic around your own neck to establish general contours.

6. When the client can tolerate temperature, center the foam thermoplastic on client's chin. If the collar is to extend above the edge of the mandible to control rotation, position the top border just under the lower lip (Fig. 8-6). If the collar is to extend to the edge of the mandible, position the top border at this location. Confirm the location by looking in the mirror or with the help of a second therapist.

7. Ask the client to clench the teeth so that the lower jaw is not pushed backward, creating stress on the temporomandibular joint.

8. Work quickly to stretch the material around neck and mandible. While the assisting therapist controls the position of the head from the front, the primary therapist overlaps the back edges. If the overlap exceeds 3 in. (7.5 cm), trim the excess.

9. Stabilize the client's head and neck against your body to block neck extension, but guard against pushing the neck into flexion. Firmly mold around the mandible to achieve an accurate chin contour.

10. Watch the client's face for signs of distress, and do not press on larynx. Ask the client to swallow during the molding process to accommodate the contours of the larynx. Form the contours to accommodate the clavicles.

11. If insufficient contouring was achieved or the neck was poorly positioned, reheat and remold. However, Plastazote and AliPlast can only be reheated 3 or 4 times before becoming stiff and unmoldable.

12. If contracture or muscle spasm prevents optimal positioning, finish the collar and remold when the spasm has subsided or the contracture has reduced.

13. When the material has cooled, wrap a temporary D-ring strap around the collar to hold it in place and mark the trim lines.

14. Remove the collar and use the scissors to trim. Cut back the overlap to 2 in. (5 cm). Reapply and trim further if necessary.

15. Remove the collar and use scissors or knife, followed by a grinder, to bevel the outer edges of the upper and lower borders and the posterior overlap so that the collar will blend in with the contours of the head and trunk (Fig. 8-7).

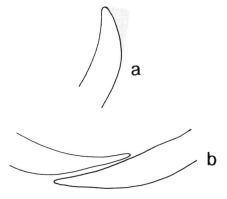

**FIGURE 8-7.** *(a)* Cross section of the top border of Plastazote collar showing the material that has been removed (shaded) to create a beveled edge. *(b)* Superior view of the beveled posterior edges.

16. Reapply the collar and mark the location of four 1½ in. (4 cm) wide reinforcement strips—one below each ear and one to either side of larynx (Fig. 8-6).
17. Remove the collar and apply contact cement at these locations. Allow the cement to dry (10 to 15 minutes—drying can be hastened with the heat gun).
18. Cut out reinforcement strips and remove the coating by scraping or applying solvent or alcohol. Heat in water, dry, and then heat further with the heat gun to enhance adhesive properties. Press firmly to areas with contact cement. No cement needs to be applied to the warm thermoplastic.
19. Measure the circumference of the collar on the neck. Add 4 in. (10 cm) to this measurement and cut webbing to this length. Sew Velcro and a D-ring to the webbing (Fig. 8-8).
20. Bond a thermoplastic strap guide to each of the reinforcements under the ears (Figs. 8-6 and 8-9). Pass the strap through the guides on the reinforcements.

***Wearing Regimen***

- Recommended for upright use only. For sleeping, stabilize the neck with a prefabricated soft foam collar, ruffs (described next), or a hand towel (folded lengthwise in thirds, wrapped around neck, and secured with safety pins).
- If the collar is for short-term use during the healing period after injury or surgery, provide guidelines about how and when to discontinue.

***Precautions***

- Do not mold if the cervical spine is unstable or there is a possibility of vertebral fracture.
- Driving a car and operating other machinery may be dangerous while wearing the collar because of restricted neck rotation.
- Monitor the skin for maceration, adverse reaction to the foam thermoplastic, and pressure points over the mandible, clavicles, and sternum.

***Client Education***

- Teach the client how to apply and remove. Also provide cleaning instructions using mild soap, water, and nail brush. A hair dryer can be used to thoroughly dry the interior.

***Options***

- If limited mobility or muscle weakness interferes with fastening the strap posteriorly, modify the design to have a side instead of a back opening.
- Cut a hole in front over the larynx to accommodate a tracheotomy.
- Enclose the orthosis in 3 or 4 in. (7.5 or 10 cm) wide Stockinette to absorb perspiration. This cover can be removed for washing in cold water. The strap is secured over the top of the Stockinette.

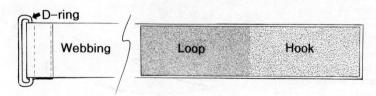

**FIGURE 8-8.**  D-ring strap.

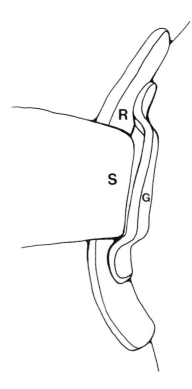

**FIGURE 8-9.** Close-up view of the strap (S) passing under thermoplastic guide (G), which has been bonded to thermoplastic reinforcement (R).

- Fabricate the collar in two pieces, which overlap at the sides, to create a bivalved design.

*Alternatives*
- Prefabricated bivalved version: Philadelphia Collar with optional thoracic stabilizer, available in a tracheotomy design.
- Canadian Collar[32]—custom orthosis kit—circumferential open design made of flexible tubing. The open design is less conspicuous and retains less heat than an enclosing collar.
- Prefabricated Headmaster Collar—adjustable, padded tubular, open design.
- Custom thermoplastic halo splint.[5,33]
- Numerous other prefabricated collars.

---

⬤ **Name:** **Static Cervical-Stabilizing Ruffs** (Fig. 8-10)

*Common Names* Ruffs; ruff collar; padded rolls

*Objectives* See Circumferential Static Plastazote Stabilizing Collar—however, ruffs offer less cervical stabilization than a collar.

*Indications*
- See Circumferential Static Plastazote Stabilizing Collar—good for night wear when a more rigid Plastazote collar is worn during the day.

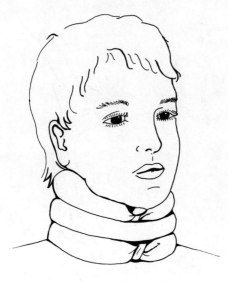

**FIGURE 8-10.** Static cervical-stabilizing ruffs. The top and bottom ruffs are tied at the front. The middle ruff is tied at the back.

| | |
|---|---|
| *Materials* | • 2 in. (5 cm) wide Stockinette<br>• Abdominal padding or quilt batting |
| *Equipment and Tools* | • Scissors |
| *Client's Position* | • Sitting with the neck in neutral alignment, if possible. See Circumferential Static Plastazote Stabilizing Collar. |
| *Therapist's Position* | • Standing or sitting beside the client |
| *Fabrication* | 1. Measure the neck circumference.<br>2. Add 8 in. (20 cm) to this measurement and cut the Stockinette to this length.<br>3. Cut the abdominal pad to the neck circumference less 2 in. (5 cm).<br>4. Roll the abdominal pad and insert into the Stockinette, leaving 5 in. (12.5 cm) unfilled at each end.<br>5. Create one to four ruffs to match the height of the client's neck. |
| *Wearing Regimen* | • Tie the ruffs at the front, back, or alternating to achieve the desired neck position. Front knots promote flexion; back knots promote neck extension. Tuck in the ends.<br>• Wear during the day or night or both. |
| *Alternatives* | • See Circumferential Static Plastazote Stabilizing Collar. |

⬤ • • • • • • • • • • • • • • • • • • • • • • • • • • • • • • • • • • •

**Name:** **Anterior Static Cervical Scar-Controlling Orthosis**[5,6,34–38] (Fig. 8-11)

| | |
|---|---|
| *Common Name* | Neck conformer |
| *Objectives* | To apply pressure in order to<br>• Prevent or soften hypertrophic scar |

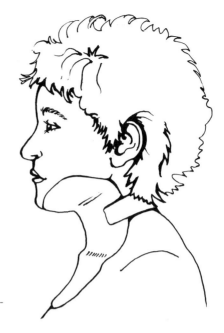

**FIGURE 8-11.** Anterior static cervical scar-controlling orthosis.

|  |  |
|---|---|
|  | • Prevent or correct contractures (e.g., flexion or lateral flexion)<br>• Maintain or restore cosmesis, skin mobility, and contours of chin and neck |
| *Indications* | • Acute burns (for positioning)<br>• Burn scar hypertrophy (for scar control) |
| *Rationale* | • See Chapter 2, "Scar Management." |
| *Materials* | • Unperforated ³⁄₃₂ or ⅛ in. (2.4 or 3.2 mm) thermoplastic depending on the size of the neck—try to match the thermoplastic color to the skin color<br>　◦ Opaque category C<br>　◦ Orfit Classic—clings to skin better than other translucent thermoplastics with memory<br>• Padded Velcro strap<br>• Elastomer putty/gel padding/foam padding (optional)<br>• Chicago screws/nylon screws/rivets (optional) |
| *Equipment and Tools* | • Heating pan<br>• Hammer and anvil if metal rapid rivets are used<br>• Sewing machine (to sew D-ring to Velcro)<br>• Measuring tape<br>• Marking utensil |
| *Client's Position* | • Supine (see "Face Mask") or seated (see "Circumferential Static Plastazote Stabilizing Collar") |
| *Therapist's Position* | • If the client is supine (see "Face Mask"); if the client is seated (see "Circumferential Static Plastazote Stabilizing Collar")<br>• The molding procedure in standing requires the therapist to stabilize the client's head and neck against the therapist's body. To avoid any misun- |

derstanding of intentions, explain the molding procedure and the therapist's positioning before the fabrication process begins.

**Custom Pattern**

- Rectangular piece with rounded corners
  - Width—measure from earlobe to earlobe, along the edge of the mandible.
  - Height—measure from the edge of the chin to the sternal angle (junction between manubrium and sternum).

**Fabrication**

1. If appropriate, apply padding to the clavicles. If desired, mold elastomer putty or apply a piece of gel sheeting over concave areas of the neck before molding.
2. Heat the thermoplastic. Check the temperature on your skin and then on the client's skin.
3. Center the thermoplastic on the chin with the top edge along the mandible.
4. Stroke the material into contours. Stabilize the head to prevent extension. Ask the client to clench the teeth so that the lower jaw is not pushed backward, creating stress on the temporomandibular joint.
5. Do not press on the larynx or apply force to cause chin retraction. Ask the client to swallow during the molding process to accommodate the contours of the larynx.
6. When set, secure a temporary strap around the orthosis and mark trim lines.
7. Remove the orthosis and trim the edges with scissors to restore symmetry because the material will have stretched during molding.
8. Smooth and gently flare all edges.
9. Apply an overlap or D-ring strap.

**Wearing Regimen**

- Wear directly against the skin or over antibiotic mesh dressing or antibiotic cream if appropriate.
- Wear continuously, except for bathing, eating, massage, and stretching exercises.
- Remove as needed to wipe off perspiration or to clean.

**Precautions**

- If necessary, add ½₂ in. (0.8 mm) thick self-adhesive, very thin gel padding, but nothing thicker because conformity to contour will be disturbed.
- Ensure grafts are stable before molding, usually 7 days after grafting.
- Monitor the skin for maceration, wound deterioration, adverse reaction to the thermoplastic, and pressure points over clavicles or mandible. If a pressure area develops, spot heat to relieve the pressure point or temporarily discontinue.
- Monitor children closely for sleep apnea. If this occurs, discontinue at night and substitute gel sheeting for night use.

**Client Education**

- Educate the client or caregiver about
  - How to adjust the tension in the straps to exert the desired amount of compression
  - Cleaning the inner surface with mild cleanser frequently to remove perspiration—rinse and dry well
- If worn over an open wound, clean with an antibacterial cleanser

*Options*
- For adults, the orthosis can extend over the edge of the mandible to prevent lower lip eversion. For extended use by young children, do not mold above the mandible because of adverse effects on the developing mandible[5]; instead, trim the orthosis to edge of mandible as described in the fabrication section.

*Alternatives*
- Postoperative splint for the lower face and neck.[39]
- Triple-component neck splint.[40]
- Multiring (Watusi) collar—fabricated from flexible rubber tubing.[5,6]
- Custom-fabricated, circumferential Plastazote collar as described previously. (Substitute AliPlast, which has a smoother surface than Plastazote and is less irritating over burn scars.)
- Custom-fabricated, Lycra chin strap (e.g., Jobskin).
- Custom-fabricated, transparent plastic neck orthosis molded from high-temperature thermoplastic (e.g., Uvex) over a positive plaster impression of the neck. It may be more acceptable to the client than an opaque low-temperature thermoplastic orthosis, and the amount of pressure exerted by the mask can be monitored by observing the degree of skin blanching.
- Substitute gel sheeting over the scar tissue for situations in which the client is reluctant to wear the orthosis, although scar control is less effective. Gel sheeting clings to the skin without need for additional fixation.

● ● ● ● ● ● ● ● ● ● ● ● ● ● ● ● ● ● ● ● ● ● ● ● ● ● ● ● ● ● ● ● ● ● ● ● ● ● ●

## ⬤ Name: Circumferential Static Lumbosacral-Stabilizing Maternity Orthosis (Fig. 8-12)

*Common Name*     Maternity support

*Objectives*
- To reduce pain
- To stabilize pelvic joints with ligamentous laxity
- To partially support the weight of the fetus to reduce compensatory low back extension, which compresses the facet joints

*Indications*
- Pregnancy

*Materials*
- 6 in. (15 cm) wide elastic
- 1 in. (2.5 cm) wide, nonadhesive, hook and loop Velcro
- Four D-rings

*Tools and Equipment*
- Sewing machine
- Scissors
- Measuring tape
- Straight pins

*Client's Position*
- Standing

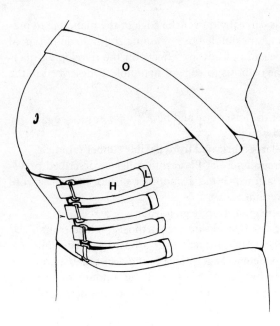

**FIGURE 8-12.** Anterolateral view of circumferential static lumbosacral-stabilizing maternity orthosis. O = optional strap; H = hook Velcro; L = loop Velcro.

*Therapist's Position*   • Sitting beside client

*Fabrication*

1. Measure circumference at the largest part of the abdomen.
2. Add approximately 10 in. (25 cm) to this measurement to accommodate the anticipated growth during the remainder of the pregnancy. Cut the elastic to this length.
3. Sew D-rings and Velcro at the front opening (Fig. 8-12).
4. Apply the orthosis and pin along the center back conforming to contours, taking up the excess material. Sew up the 10 in. (25 cm) growth allowance as "let-out seams" (Fig. 8-13).
5. Attach an optional 2 in. (5 cm) wide nonelastic strap over the top of the belly to prevent slipping (Fig. 8-12).

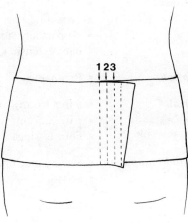

**FIGURE 8-13.** Posterior view of circumferential static lumbosacral-stabilizing maternity orthosis. 1, 2, and 3 are the first, second, and third let-out seams, respectively.

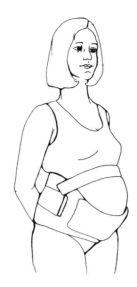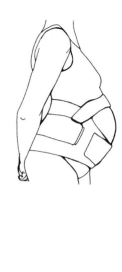

**FIGURE 8-14.** Prefabricated Rolyan® Maternity Support.

| | |
|---|---|
| *Adjustment* | • Instruct the client how to unstitch the let-out seams to accommodate growth (Fig. 8-13). |
| *Wearing Regimen* | • For day or night. |
| *Alternative* | • Prefabricated Rolyan® Maternity Support[41] with or without a pocket for optional custom-moldable thermoplastic insert (Fig. 8-14). |

In addition, there is a wide range of prefabricated back supports designed to relieve back pain or prevent back injury. We have included the maternity orthosis to make therapists aware of a very effective device to relieve pain and enhance function during pregnancy.

## ● References

1. Belgian G, et al: Further development of a protective helmet for persons with disabilities. J Assoc Child Prosthet Orthot Clin 26:23, 1991.
2. Clench, M: The fabrication of a protective helmet. Fracture Mag 10:7, 1994.
3. Emery, E, et al: Fracture of the occipital condyle: Case report and review of the literature. Eur Spine J 4:191, 1995.
4. Danmar Products, Inc., Special Products for Special Needs Catalog, no. 909.
5. Malick, MH, and Carr, JA: Manual on Management of the Burn Patient. Harmarville Rehabilitation Centre, Pittsburgh, 1982.
6. Staley, MJ, and Richard, RL: Scar management. In Richard, RL, and Staley, MJ (eds): Burn Care and Rehabilitation: Principles and Practice. FA Davis, Philadelphia, 1994.
7. Shriners Hospital for Children, Cincinnati Burn Institute: Face Mask Instructional Video. 3229 Burnet Ave., Cincinnati, OH, 45229, USA Tel: 513-872-6200. Fax: 513-872-6999.
8. Carlow, D, et al: Fabrication of a removable microstomia orthosis. Can J Occup Ther 55:206, 1988.
9. Carlow, DL, Conine, TA, Stevenson-Moore, P: Static orthoses for the management of microstomia. J Rehabil Res 24(3):35, 1987.
10. Conine, TA, Carlow, DL, Stevenson-Moore, P: The Vancouver microstomia orthosis. J Prosthet Dent 61(4):476, 1989.
11. Naylor, WP, and Manor, RC: Fabrication of a flexible prosthesis for the edentulous scleroderma patient with microstomia. J Prosthet Dent 50:536, 1983.
12. Weismann, RA, and Calcaterra, TC: Hand and neck manifestations of scleroderma. Ann Otol Rhinol Laryngol 87:332, 1978.
13. Cain JR, Greasley, JW: Prosthetic management of electrical burns to the oral commissure. Quintessence of Dental Technology 9:249, 1985.
14. Khan, Z, Banis, JC: Oral commissure expansion prosthesis. J Prosthet Dent 67:383, 1992.
15. Pitanguy, I, et al: Electric burns of the lip. Compendium 10:30, 1989.
16. MPA Co.: Microstomia Prevention Appliance. 6526 Meadowcreek Drive, Dallas, TX, 75240, 972-458-0757.
17. Daugherty, MB, Carr-Collins, JA: Splinting techniques for the burn patient. In Richard, RL, and Staley, MJ

(eds): Burncare and Rehabilitation: Principles and Practice. FA Davis, Philadelphia, 1994.

18. Cheuk, SL, Kirkland, JL: Splint for burns to lip commissures. J Prosthet Dent 52:563, 1984.
19. Denton, BG, Shaw, SE: Mouth conformer for prevention and correction of burn scar contracture. Phys Ther 56:683, 1976.
20. Josell, SD, et al: Extraoral management for electrical burns of the mouth. ASDC J Dent Child 51:47, 1984.
21. Reisberg, DJ, et al: Electrical burns of the oral commissure. J Prosthet Dent 49:71, 1983.
22. Port, RM, Cooley, RO: Treatment of electrical burns of the oral and perioral tissues in children. J Am Dent Assoc 112:352, 1986.
23. Sadove, AM, et al: Appliance therapy for perioral electrical burns: A conservative approach. J Burn Care Rehabil 9:391, 1988.
24. Vorhies, JM: Electrical burns of the oral commissure. Angle Orthod 57:2, 1987.
25. Salman, RA, Glickman, RS, Super, S: Splint therapy for electrical burns of the oral commissure in children. ASDC J Dent Child 54:161, 1987.
26. Silverglade, D: Splinting electrical burns utilizing a fixed splint technique: A report of 48 cases. ASDC J Dent Child 50:455, 1983.
27. Walters, C: Splinting the Burn Patient. Maryland, Ramsco, 1987.
28. Smith & Nephew Inc.: Fabrication of a Microstomia Splint with Sans-Splint XR. Ref. #10. Smith & Nephew Inc., 2100, 52nd Avenue, Lachine, Quebec, H8T 2Y5, Canada.
29. Cheuk, SL, Kirkland, JL: Splint for burns to lip commissures. J Prosthet Dent 52:563, 1984.
30. Josell, SD, et al: Extraoral management for electrical burns of the mouth. ASDC J Dent Child 51:47, 1984.
31. Madjar, D, Shifman, A, Kusner, W: Dynamic labial commissure widening device for the facial burn patient. Quintessence International 18:361, 1987.
32. Hannah, RE, and Cottrill, SD: The Canadian collar: a new cervical spine orthosis. Am J Occup Ther 39:171, 1985.
33. Apfel, LM: Halo neck splint. JBCR 8:140, 1987.
34. Orfit Industries: Orfit Splinting Guide. Antwerp, Belgium, 1990.
35. Orfit Industries: Orfit Catalogue—Orthotic Products. Antwerp, Belgium, 1992.
36. Smith & Nephew Inc.: Smith & Nephew: Splinting Guidelines. Smith & Nephew Inc., Lachine, Quebec, 1986.
37. Willis, BA: Splinting the Burn Patient. Shriners Burns Institute, Galveston, ND.
38. Willis, BA: The use of orthoplast isoprene splints in the treatment of the acutely burned child. Am J Occup Ther 25:187, 1970.
39. Parrish, NE: Postoperative splinting for the lower face and neck. JBCR 7:148, 1986.
40. Leman, CJ: The triple component-neck splint. JBCR 7:387, 1986.
41. Smith & Nephew, Inc.: Rehabilitation Division Catalogue, 1997. Rolyan® is a trademark of Smith & Nephew, Inc.

# *Orthoses for Shoulder and Elbow*

## *Chapter Outline*

This chapter describes the fabrication process for 11 proximal upper extremity orthoses. The content is organized from proximal to distal, beginning with the axilla and proceeding to the shoulder, elbow, and forearm. Some of these orthoses are large and elaborate, requiring the assistance of a second person to manage large pieces of thermoplastic and position the client's joints.

An evaluation form for upper extremity orthoses can be found at the end of Chapter 7. It can be used as a guideline for designing, fabricating, and evaluating many of the orthoses in Chapter 9. Refer to the introduction to Chapter 8 for more information and to Appendix A to select orthotic materials.

 **Name:**   **Figure-Eight Nonarticular Axilla Orthosis** (Fig. 9-1)

| | |
|---|---|
| *Common Names* | Axilla wrap; clavicle strap brace |
| *SCS Name** | Nonarticular splint—axilla |

---

*SCS = Splint Classification System, which is described in Chapter 8.

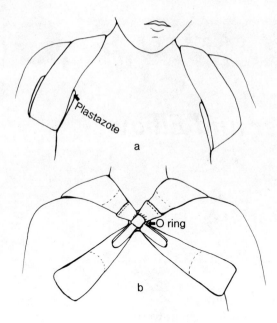

**FIGURE 9-1.** Figure-eight nonarticular axilla orthosis. *(a)* Anterior view. *(b)* Posterior view.

| | |
|---|---|
| *Objectives* | • To retract the scapulae<br>• To apply pressure to the axilla to prevent or correct hypertrophic scarring and thus maintain or restore shoulder mobility<br>• To stretch contracted tissues across the anterior chest<br>• To prevent or correct **kyphotic** posture |
| *Indications* | • Axilla burns or skin grafting<br>• Shoulder adduction contracture<br>• Kyphotic posture<br>• Fracture of the clavicle |
| *Rationale* | • See Chapter 2, "Scar Management" |
| *Materials* | • 2, 3, or 4 in. (5, 7.5, or 10 cm) wide Stockinette (depending on the size of the client)<br>• 1½ in. (3 cm) wide O-ring<br>• ¼ in. (6.4 cm) thick #1 Plastazote or 4E AliPlast (optional)<br>• 1 in. (2.5 cm) wide nonadhesive hook and loop Velcro<br>• Firm density foam—3 in. (7.5 cm) wide, 1½ in. (3 cm) thick, 8 to 10 in. (20 to 25 cm) long<br>• Self-adhesive gel sheeting (optional) |
| *Equipment and Tools* | • Sewing machine    • Scissors    • Measuring tape |
| *Client's Position* | • Seated or standing |
| *Therapist's Position* | • Seated or standing |
| *Fabrication* | 1. Measure the length from the location of the O-ring between the scapulae, over the shoulder, through the axilla, and back to the O-ring. Add 2 in. (5 cm) and cut the Stockinette to this length (× 2).<br>2. Cut two pieces of foam to this measurement, less 6 in. (15 cm). |

3. Sew one end of each foam-stuffed Stockinette strap to the O-ring.

4. Sew the hook and loop Velcro to each of the other two Stockinette ends.

| | |
|---|---|
| *Wearing Regimen* | • For scar control, wear all the time, except for bathing and exercises.<br>• Can be worn over compression garments. |
| *Precautions* | • Adjust the tension of the Velcro straps to avoid compression of the neurovascular structures in the axilla. Educate the client regarding the signs of nerve or vascular compression.<br>• Monitor closely for skin irritation in the axilla. |
| *Options* | • To increase compression, dry heat and mold a strip of Plastazote or Ali-Plast—approximately 3 in. (7.5 cm) wide—to the axilla to be positioned under the axilla straps.<br>• Line the inside surface with self-adhesive gel padding. |
| *Alternative* | • Prefabricated versions[1] |

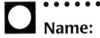

| | |
|---|---|
| **Name:** | **Lateral Trunk-Based Static Shoulder-Elbow-Wrist Orthosis** (Fig. 9-2) (see Fig. 1–4)[2] |

Usually the shoulder is the target joint; sometimes the elbow is also a target joint. Regardless, shoulder, elbow, and wrist are included in the orthosis. Originated at Victoria General Hospital, Halifax, Nova Scotia, and refined at St. Michael's Hospital, Toronto, Ontario.

Developed by occupational therapists in consultation with orthopedic surgeons.

| | |
|---|---|
| *Common Names* | Shoulder/gunslinger splint[3] |
| *SCS Name* | Shoulder adduction (or abduction) immobilization; type 3[4]—i.e., 3 secondary joints (elbow, forearm, and wrist) + shoulder = 4 joints |
| *Objectives* | • To fully immobilize the shoulder (and sometimes the elbow) to promote healing of surgically repaired bony or soft tissues.<br>• The elbow and wrist are immobilized to maintain full control of the shoulder. |

| *Indications (and Duration of Orthotic Requirement)* | *Shoulder Position* | *Elbow and Forearm Position* |
|---|---|---|
| • Posterior stabilization—to tighten the shoulder capsule in the case of posterior glenohumeral instability (4–6 weeks) | • Adducted<br>• Slight extension<br>• Rotation: neutral to slight external rotation | • 100°–110° flexion<br>• Neutral forearm rotation |
| • L'Episcopo procedure (transfer of latissimus dorsi and teres major to the external rotators)—for partial brachial plexus injury or brachial neuritis (full-time first 4 weeks; part-time next 4 weeks) | • As per posterior stabilization, with slightly more external rotation | • 90° flexion<br>• Neutral forearm rotation |

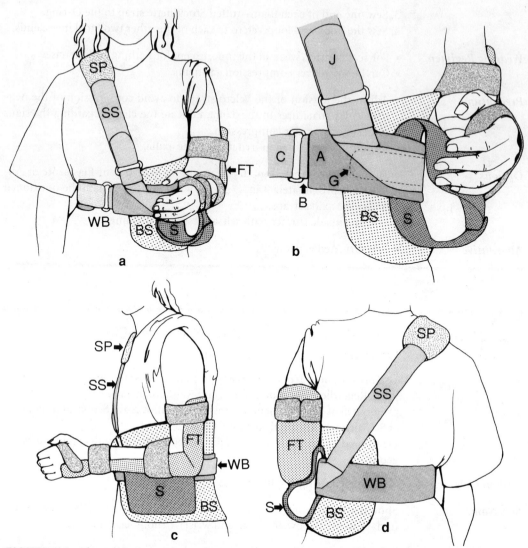

**FIGURE 9-2.**    Lateral trunk-based static shoulder-elbow-wrist orthosis. *(a)* Anterior view. *(b)* Close-up view of stay attaching forearm trough to body shell. *(c)* Lateral view. *(d)* Posterior view. BS = body shell; FT = forearm trough; WB = waist belt; SS = shoulder strap; SP = shoulder pad; S = stay.

| *Indications (and Duration of Orthotic Requirement)* | *Shoulder Position* | *Elbow and Forearm Position* |
| --- | --- | --- |
| • Shoulder fusion—for flail shoulder, e.g., brachial plexus injury (6–8 weeks) | • 30° abduction<br>• 30° flexion<br>• 30° internal rotation | • 90° flexion<br>• Neutral forearm rotation |
| • Elbow **flexorplasty**—performed with a shoulder fusion (6–8 weeks) | • As above | • At least 110° flexion<br>• Forearm neutral to slight supination |
| • Rotator cuff repair (6 weeks) | • 45° abduction<br>• Neutral rotation | • 90° flexion<br>• Forearm rotated for the client's comfort |

| Component | Materials | Measurements |
|---|---|---|
| • Body shell (BS) | a. ⅛ in. (3.2 mm) category A or B thermoplastic—preferably uncoated to facilitate bonding<br>b. ⅛ in (3.2 mm) thick self-adhesive foam or gel padding | a. Length: half of the waist circumference; height: from midchest to 2 in. (5 cm) below the iliac crest<br>b. Same as above, to line the inside of the thermoplastic |
| • Forearm trough (FT) | c. ⅛ in. (3.2 mm) thick self-adhesive foam or gel padding<br>d. ⅛ in. (3.2 mm) category A or B thermoplastic—preferably uncoated to facilitate bonding<br>e. 2 in. (5 cm) wide self-adhesive hook Velcro<br>f. 2 in. (5 cm) wide padded Velcro strap | c. 1½ in. (4 cm) wide strip to pad the olecranon process, ulnar ridge, and ulnar head/styloid<br>d. From the midhumerus proximally to the fifth MC head distally—3/5 circumference (pattern: Fig. 9-3)<br>e. Side patches<br>f. To span the limb |
| • Stay (S) | g. ⅛ in. (3.2 mm) category A or B thermoplastic—preferably uncoated to facilitate bonding | g. 15 to 18 in. (37.5 to 45 cm) long; 8 in. (20 cm) wide |
| • Waist belt (WB)<br>The letters A, B, C, etc., refer to the letters in Fig. 9-4. | A. 6 in. (15 cm) wide cotton webbing<br>B./C. 2 in. (5 cm) wide webbing<br>D. 1½ in. (3 cm) wide hook Velcro<br>E./F. 1½ in. (3 cm) wide loop Velcro<br>G. 2 in. (5 cm) wide self-adhesive hook Velcro<br>• 2 in. (5 cm) wide D-ring | A. Circumference of waist plus 1 in. (2.5 cm)<br>B. 4 in. (10 cm) long for D-ring<br>C. 11 in. (27.5 cm) long<br>D. 6 in. (15 cm) long<br>E. 8 in. (20 cm) long<br>F. Half the length of waist belt<br>G. Half the length of waist belt |

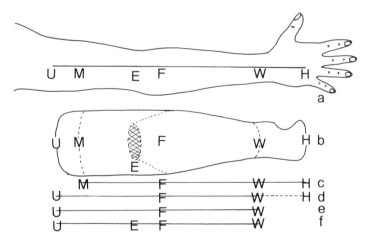

**FIGURE 9-3.** Patterns for the forearm trough of the lateral trunk-based static shoulder-elbow-wrist orthosis and for various elbow orthoses. (*a, b*) Measure the distances between the landmarks and take three fifths of the circumferences, as appropriate for the orthosis being made. (*c*) Forearm trough for lateral trunk-based static shoulder-elbow-wrist orthosis from midhumerus to the metacarpophalangeal joints (MCPS) in the hand. (*d*) Posterior static elbow orthosis from upper arm to wrist or MCPs. (*e*) Anterior static elbow orthosis from upper arm to wrist. (*f*) Bisurfaced static elbow orthosis from upper arm to wrist; for this orthosis only, the hole at the elbow (cross-hatched) is cut out. The fold lines (dotted) are used for this orthosis only. U = upper arm; M = midhumerus; E = elbow; F = widest part of forearm; W = wrist; H = hand.

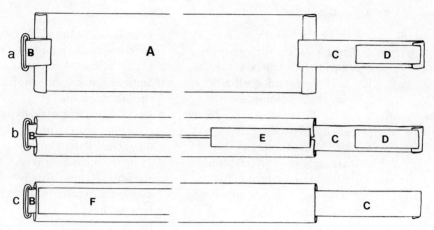

**FIGURE 9-4.**   Fabrication of waist belt. A through F refer to materials for the waist belt identified in the body of the text. *(a)* Outside view. Fold over and sew down 1 in. (2.5 cm) at each end of webbing A. Use webbing B to attach the D-ring to one end of webbing A. Sew webbing C to the other end. Sew hook Velcro D on top. *(b)* Outside view. Fold webbing A into the middle, creating a 3 in. (7.5 cm) wide belt. Sew down the folds. Sew loop Velcro E over center seam, opposite hook Velcro strap. *(c)* Inside view. Flip the strap over and sew the loop Velcro F at the end with the D-ring.

| Component | Materials | Measurements |
|---|---|---|
| • Shoulder pad (SP) | H. Fabric—cotton or cotton-polyester blend | H. 8 × 22 in. (20 × 55 cm) |
|  | I. ½ in. (1 cm) thick soft or medium-density foam | I. 7 × 10 in. (17.5 × 25 cm) |
| • Shoulder strap (SS) | J. 2 in. (5 cm) wide heavy cotton webbing<br>• 2 in. (5 cm) wide D-ring | J. Measure from the anterior midline at the waist, over the opposite shoulder to the posterior midline at the waist plus half of the waist circumference plus 12 to 18 in. (30 to 45 cm) for folding and the Velcro closures |

**Equipment and Tools**
- Sewing machine
- Large heating pan (or oven for Isoprene-based materials)
- Heat gun
- Scissors
- Elastic bandage, Thera-Band, or Orfiband
- Solvent or alcohol for bonding

**Client's Position**
- Seated on the front edge of a chair to have space behind the client to measure and mold to the back; the arm is supported at all times on a table beside the client.
- Remind the client to keep the shoulder relaxed (not shrugged), especially when molding and bonding the stay.

**Therapist's Position**
- Seated or standing. Assistance from a second person is essential to support the arm and maintain the desired shoulder and elbow positions.

**Fabrication**

The letters a, b, c, etc., refer to the materials

1. If possible, take measurements and mold the body shell and forearm trough before surgery and then attach the stay after surgery.

listed on page 169.

*Body shell:*

2. Heat the thermoplastic (a), apply the foam padding (b) to the inside, and mold the body shell to the trunk, wrapping it in place with a bandage.
3. Gently flare the top and bottom edges of the body shell.

*Forearm trough:*

4. Apply padding (c) to the client's olecranon, ulnar ridge, and ulnar styloid/head.
5. Heat the thermoplastic (d), check the temperature, and then mold it to the client's limb.
6. To form the elbow seam, pinch the excess material together and cut off, forming a sealed, mitered seam (Fig. 9-5). Alternatively, a seamless elbow can be achieved during gravity-resisted molding by stretching and pinching together the corresponding edges about every 4 in. (10 cm) (see Fig. 7-6*b*).
7. If the stretch-and-pinch method is not used, wrap the orthosis in place with a bandage, Thera-Band, or Orfiband to help form the contours.
8. Gently flare the distal edge.
9. When the material is almost cool, unwrap the bandage, mark the trim lines, remove the orthosis, and trim. Any thermoplastic that was stretched along the edges is cut off.

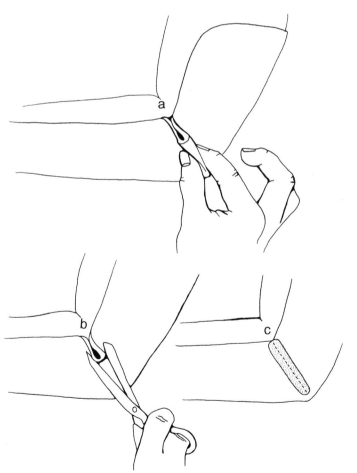

**FIGURE 9-5.** Formation of a mitered seam. *(a)* Pinch excess material together. *(b)* Cut off excess material flush with the limb. *(c)* Bond a strip of thermoplastic (stippled) over the seam.

10. Ensure full freedom of the MCPs and thumb.
11. Using solvent or alcohol and a heat gun, bond a strip of thermoplastic about 1 in. (2.5 cm) wide to reinforce the elbow seam (Fig. 9-5c).
12. Remove the padding from the ulna and transfer it to the inside of the trough.
13. Attach Velcro straps (e and f) to the forearm trough (Fig. 9-2c).

*Stay:*

14. Heat the thermoplastic, fold over the top and bottom long edges 1 in. (2.5 cm) to strengthen the stay.
15. Overlap the short ends of the thermoplastic approximately 2 in. (5 cm) to form a cylinder.

*Bonding the stay to the body shell and forearm trough:*

16. Apply solvent or alcohol to the surfaces of the body shell, trough, and stay that will be bonded.
17. Dry heat the surfaces of the body shell and trough that will be bonded to the stay.
18. Apply the body shell and trough to the trunk and arm.
19. If the stay was heated in water, dry heat the surface with a heat gun to enhance its surface stickiness.
20. While holding the shoulder in the desired position, attach the stay to the body shell and trough.
21. After the stay has cooled, remove the orthosis and check the strength of the bond. If the components can be pulled apart, apply solvent or alcohol and dry heat to create a permanent bond.

*Waist belt:*

22. Follow the steps in Figure 9-4.
23. Apply hook Velcro G (Fig. 9-2b) to the orthosis, corresponding to the loop Velcro F on the inside of the waist belt.

*Shoulder pad (or use a prefabricated Tubular Sling Pad[4]):*

24. Use fabric (H) to sew a cover to enclose the foam (I).
25. Fold lengthwise and sew down long edge, creating a cylinder 3½ × 10 in. (9 × 25 cm).
26. Apply the orthosis to the client, slip the waist belt through the stay, and secure the loop Velcro F to the hook Velcro G on the orthosis.

*Shoulder strap (Fig. 9-2b):*

27. Sew a D-ring to one end of webbing J.
28. Slip the shoulder pad (or prefabricated sling pad) onto the shoulder strap.
29. Pin onto the waist belt, marking the location of the hook and loop Velcro.
30. Remove the waist belt with the attached shoulder strap. Sew the shoulder strap in place on the belt.
31. Sew the hook and loop Velcro closure.

**Application and Removal**

- With the forearm trough supported on a table, the client leans away to ease in or out of the orthosis.

**Wearing Regimen**

- Can be worn over a T-shirt, dressing the affected side first. To facilitate safe dressing, open up the side seam on the affected side and sew Velcro straps along opening.
- Remove only for sponge bathing, and use pillow protection to maintain shoulder position.
- Gradually wean during the last 2 weeks of use.

*Precautions*

- The client may feel faint or nauseated and be in much pain.
- Avoid any restricted joint motions during the fabrication process and the healing period.
- The orthosis is usually fitted 1 day postoperatively; the therapist must carefully remove the pillow dressing, maintaining the safe joint position(s).
- Encourage the client to maintain range of motion of the unaffected joints.

*Options*

- If the client's forearm is particularly long, an additional cylindrical stay, 3 in. (7.5 cm) wide, can be bonded to support the hand portion of the forearm trough.

*Alternatives*

- Prefabricated Rolyan® SCOI Shoulder Brace[5]—for positioning of shoulder and elbow after orthopedic surgery
- Prefabricated Freedom Gunslinger Shoulder Orthosis[1]

---

## Name: **Lateral Trunk-Based Static (or Serial-Static) Shoulder-Abduction (Elbow-Wrist) Orthosis** (Fig. 9-6)

The shoulder is the target joint. Inclusion of the elbow and wrist is optional, depending on the degree of shoulder abduction. If the shoulder is abducted more than 120°, the elbow and wrist joints can be excluded, which is why they are bracketed.

*Common Names*     Axilla/airplane splint/conformer

*SCS Name*     120° shoulder abduction immobilization/mobilization; type 3[4]—i.e., 3 secondary joints (elbow, forearm, and wrist) + shoulder = 4 joints

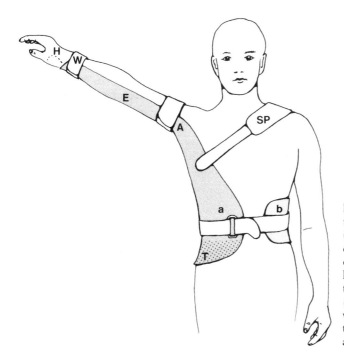

**FIGURE 9-6.** Lateral trunk-based static (or serial-static) shoulder-abduction (elbow-wrist) orthosis. Inclusion of the elbow and wrist is optional if these joints do not require immobilization. Shows landmarks for measurements for the pattern in Figure 9-7. (*a*) Main component. (*b*) Waist conformer. H = hand; W = wrist; E = elbow; A = axilla; T = trochanter; SP = shoulder pad; stippled area = foam/gel lining.

| | |
|---|---|
| *Objectives* | • To elevate the hand to prevent edema<br>• To prevent or reduce an axilla contracture<br>• To maintain or restore shoulder mobility<br>• To immobilize the upper extremity after skin grafting<br>• To apply pressure to prevent or reduce hypertrophic scarring in the axilla |
| *Indications* | • Axilla burns or skin grafting<br>• Shoulder adduction contractures |
| *Materials* | • ⅛ in. (3.2 cm) category A or B thermoplastic; for serial-static correction of contracture, use a thermoplastic with memory<br>• 2 in. (5 cm) wide self-adhesive hook Velcro<br>• 2 in. (5 cm) wide padded Velcro straps<br>• 2 in. (5 cm) wide webbing<br>• 2 in. (5 cm) wide nonadhesive hook and loop Velcro<br>• 2 in. D-ring<br>• Fabric and foam for shoulder pad (see previous orthosis) or use a prefabricated Tubular Sling Pad[4]<br>• Self-adhesive foam or gel padding |
| *Equipment and Tools* | • Heating pan<br>• Elastic bandage, Thera-Band, or Orfiband (for molding category A thermoplastics)<br>• Measuring tape<br>• Scissors |
| *Client's Position* | • Side lying (for gravity-assisted molding), preferably on an elevated plinth at a comfortable work height for the therapist. The shoulder is positioned in the desired amount of shoulder abduction and 10° to 15° horizontal adduction (forward flexion) to prevent stress to anterior shoulder joint capsule.[6] |
| *Therapist's Position* | • Standing beside the plinth.<br>• Assistance from a second person is useful for this large orthosis. |
| *Design Options* | • To minimize pressure on the lower edge of the orthosis, position the shoulder in more abduction and increase the surface area by lengthening the trunk base.<br>• Inclusion of the elbow and hand is optional if these joints do not require immobilization.<br>• If the shoulder is adequately abducted, elbow immobilization is not required. If elbow immobilization is required, determine the optimal elbow position before molding. |
| *Pattern* | • Figure 9-7 |
| *Fabrication* | 1. Heat and cut out the pattern.<br>2. Reheat and check the temperature of the thermoplastic.<br>3. Apply foam or gel padding to inside of the orthosis over the iliac crest (Fig. 9-6).<br>4. Mold the orthosis in its entirety or mold in two stages—one for trunk and one for upper extremity. |

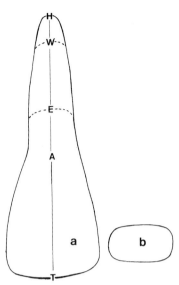

**FIGURE 9-7.** Pattern for lateral trunk-based static (or serial-static) shoulder-abduction (elbow-wrist) orthosis. *(a)* Main component: orthosis can end at elbow (E), wrist (W), or hand (H), depending on the amount of shoulder abduction. Measure the distances between H, W, A (axilla), and T (trochanter) to support entire upper extremity. Alter measurements if the wrist or elbow are excluded. Take half of the circumference of the limb and the trunk at H, W, A, and T. Lay out the pattern with the midline of orthosis as half of measurement T. Divide the measurement on each side of the midline. *(b)* Waist conformer, approximately 8 × 12 in. (20 × 30 cm).

5. Wrapping with elastic bandage, Thera-Band, or Orfiband helps to form the contours, especially for category A materials.
6. For gravity-assisted molding, firmly stroke the thermoplastic into the contours of the limb.
7. Flare the proximal and distal edges.
8. When the material is almost cool, unwrap, mark the trim lines, remove the orthosis, and trim.
9. Mold the waist component ("b" in Figures 9-6 and 9-7).
10. Sew the shoulder pad as described for the previous orthosis, or use a prefabricated Tubular Sling Pad.
11. Attach straps. Note the direction of pull of the D-ring waist belt toward the unaffected hand to facilitate fastening.

*Wearing Regimen*
- As appropriate for the situation.

*Adjustment*
- For serial-static reduction of contracture, reheat and remold every few days as abduction range improves.

*Precautions*
- Be sure to incorporate 10° to 15° of forward flexion to prevent stress to the anterior shoulder joint capsule.
- To control hypertrophic scarring, the orthosis must conform precisely to the contours of the axilla, avoiding compression of neurovascular structures. Educate the client regarding signs of nerve or vascular compression.
- Ensure that the strap does not stress the neck.

*Options*
- Elbow: flexed or extended; included or excluded.
- Hand included or excluded.
- If the shoulder is not abducted at least 120°, the axilla region may need reinforcement with a strip of aluminum or thermoplastic (heated, rolled into a tube, and bonded to orthosis) spanning from the iliac crest to the wrist.

***Alternatives***   • Prefabricated Rolyan® SCOI Shoulder Brace[5]—for positioning of shoulder and elbow after orthopedic surgery; can elevate the hand to control edema; enables static-progressive correction of shoulder contractures. However, this orthosis does not apply pressure to control hypertrophic scarring.

---

**Name:**    **Static Shoulder-Elbow-Wrist Sling** (Fig. 9-8*a*)[7–14]

***Common Names***   Sling; hemi arm sling

***SCS Name***   Not categorized

***Objectives***
- To immobilize the shoulder and elbow
- To support the weight of the upper extremity across the contralateral shoulder, without stress to the back of the neck
- To prevent brachial plexus traction
- To relieve pain and prevent shoulder subluxation

***Indications***
- Shoulder subluxation caused by flaccid hemiplegia—however, it is controversial whether shoulder subluxation is favorably or unfavorably affected by a sling[15,16]
- Brachial plexus injury
- Rotator cuff injury
- Upper extremity trauma (e.g., crush injury)
- Shoulder surgery

***Materials***
- ¼ in. (0.6 cm) wide #1 Plastazote or 4E AliPlast
- 2 in. (5 cm) wide webbing
- 2 in. (5 cm) wide D-ring
- 2 in. (5 cm) wide hook and loop Velcro
- 2 in. (5 cm) self-adhesive hook and loop Velcro
- Fabric and foam for a shoulder pad—see the lateral trunk-based static shoulder-elbow-wrist orthosis—or use a prefabricated Tubular Sling Pad[4]

***Equipment and Tools***
- Sewing machine
- Measuring tape
- Scissors

***Joint Positions***
- This sling positions the shoulder in internal rotation and the elbow in approximately 90° flexion so that forearm is horizontal. If desired, increase

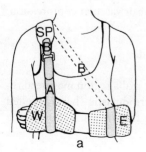

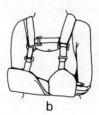

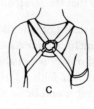

**FIGURE 9-8.** Two types of slings. (*a*) Static shoulder-elbow-wrist sling. (*b, c*) Static shoulder-elbow sling with bilateral suspension from both shoulders (prefabricated Rolyan® Universal Arm Sling[5]). W = wrist cuff; E = elbow cuff; SP = shoulder pad; A = webbing A; B = webbing B.

elbow flexion to position the hand above the elbow to help control hand edema.

| | |
|---|---|
| *Client's Position* | • Seated or standing |
| *Therapist's Position* | • Seated or standing |
| *Pattern* | • Cut wrist and elbow cuffs (W and E) out of Plastazote or AliPlast (Fig. 9-8*a*). |
| *Fabrication* | 1. Use a prefabricated Tubular Sling Pad or sew a shoulder pad as described for the lateral trunk-based static shoulder-elbow-wrist orthosis described previously. |
| | 2. Sew the D-ring to one end of the webbing B, slip B through the shoulder pad, wrap it around the elbow cuff, and then cut it to this length. Sew the end to form a loop around the elbow cuff. |
| | 3. Sew hook and loop Velcro to one end of the webbing A, wrap it around the wrist cuff, and then cut it to this length. Sew the end to form a loop around the wrist cuff. |
| | 4. Attach the cuffs to the webbing by attaching self-adhesive hook Velcro on the cuffs and sewing nonadhesive loop Velcro to the webbing. |
| *Wearing Regimen* | • For shoulder subluxation: when walking or transferring; not appropriate when sitting because hand function is inhibited; instead use a forearm trough or tray on wheelchair to support the limb. |
| | • For shoulder trauma, as appropriate. |
| *Precautions* | • Discourage prolonged use of slings after trauma because immobilization and a dependent position of the hand (i.e., below the heart) promotes edema, joint stiffness, disuse atrophy, and shoulder-hand syndrome.[14] |
| *Alternatives* | • Figures 9-8*b* and *c*. |
| | • Prefabricated versions are relatively inexpensive. |

---

● ● ● ● ● ● ● ● ● ● ● ● ● ● ● ● ● ● ● ● ● ● ● ● ● ● ● ● ● ● ● ● ● ● ● ● ● ● ● ● ● ●

◉ **Name:** **Circumferential Nonarticular Humerus-Stabilizing Orthosis** (Fig. 9-9)[17]

| | |
|---|---|
| *Common Name* | Humeral fracture/functional brace; Sarmiento humeral brace |
| *SCS Name* | Nonarticular splint—humerus |
| *Objectives* | • To stabilize fracture to promote healing without immobilizing any joints. |
| *Indications* | • Fractures of the humeral shaft—usually applied 5 to 10 days after injury, although the time varies with physician and type of fracture. |
| *Rationale* | • Applies circumferential compression to the soft tissues of the upper arm to maintain alignment of the fracture site. |
| | • See Chapter 2, "Fractures of Long Bones." |
| *Materials* | • $\frac{3}{32}$ or $\frac{1}{8}$ in. (2.4 or 3.2 mm) thick slightly perforated thermoplastic—opaque category A, B, or C; translucent category B or C |

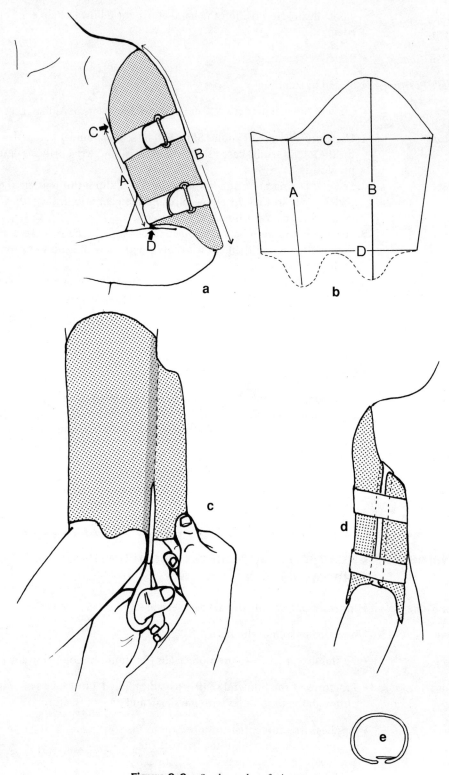

**Figure 9-9.** See legend on facing page.

- For the insert: ¹⁄₁₆ in. (1.6 mm) thick thermoplastic, category B or C—about 2 in. (5 cm) wide and 15 in. (37.5 cm) long—Orfit Classic works well because of its surface stickiness when warm that helps it cling to the skin during molding
- 2 Velcro plastic (radiolucent) D-ring closures, 1 in. (2.5 cm) wide
- Stockinette or Tubigrip
- ⅛ in. (3.2 mm) thick self-adhesive foam or gel padding
- Solvent or alcohol

*Equipment and Tools*
- Heating pan
- Scissors
- For the pattern: measuring tape or flexible clear plastic with permanent marker and straight pins, stapler, or tape

*Client's Position*
- Seated, supporting the injured arm at the wrist with the opposite hand. During molding, the client should lean toward the injured side, allowing the arm to slightly abduct away from the body. Ideally, seated on a height-adjustable stool to bring the humerus to a comfortable work height for the therapist.

*Therapist's Position*
- Seated or standing.
- The assistance of a second person is helpful.

*Pattern*
- Figure 9-9*b*.
- This pattern is designed with a posterior opening; however, the pattern can be modified to position the opening on the lateral or anterior aspect of the limb.

*Fabrication*
1. Decide on the location of the opening—posterior, lateral, or anterior.
2. Measure and lay out the pattern. Heat and cut out the pattern.
3. Apply foam or gel padding over the medial epicondyle.
4. Mold the insert at the location of the opening.
5. Apply a layer of Stockinette or Tubigrip over the molded insert. Use two layers if using a translucent material to compensate for shrinkage.
6. Heat the thermoplastic and align the proximal edge with the acromion process.
7. Use both hands to stretch thermoplastic around the limb from anterior to posterior, and then squeeze together at the location of the insert.
8. Cut off excess material flush with the limb while the material is warm, creating a closed seam (Fig. 9-9*c*).
9. Mark trim lines around the axilla and elbow to ensure unrestricted motion and no irritation.
10. When the material is cold, pop open the edges that were pinched together and remove the orthosis. If it has adhered to the Stockinette, cut

**FIGURE 9-9.** *(a)* Circumferential nonarticular humerus-stabilizing orthosis. *(b)* Pattern. If fracture is proximal, extend proximal edge to the acromion process and distal edge can end above elbow at D. If fracture is distal, extend more distally over the epicondyles but terminate proximal to acromion. A = measurement from the axilla to the tip of the medial epicondyle; B = measurement from the acromion process to the tip of the lateral epicondyle; C = circumference of the upper arm plus 2 in. (5 cm); D = circumference above the elbow plus 2 in. (5 cm). *(c)* To form posterior opening, squeeze thermoplastic together along the upper arm, then cut off excess material flush with limb while thermoplastic is warm, creating a closed seam over the insert (shaded). *(d)* Posterior view of circumferential humeral-stabilizing orthosis showing posterior opening and insert (broken line) to prevent pinching of the skin. *(e)* Superior view showing the insert bonded to one side of the thermoplastic cylinder.

through the Stockinette to remove the orthosis. Once the orthosis is off the arm, the Stockinette can be peeled away.

11. Transfer the epicondyle pad to the inside of the orthosis or discard it to leave a space.

12. Cut along the trim lines and remove about ½ in. (1 cm) from each side of the opening. Adhere the insert to one inside edge using solvent or alcohol and dry heat (Fig. 9-9*d* and *e*).

13. Apply the orthosis and attach two D-ring straps (Fig. 9-9*a*).

14. With the orthosis in place, confirm fracture alignment with an x-ray.

| | |
|---|---|
| ***Wearing Regimen*** | • Worn at all times.<br>• When the fracture is stable, the orthosis can be removed carefully for bathing, as per the physician's recommendations.<br>• Continue with the orthosis until fracture healing is complete. |
| ***Application and Removal*** | • Circumferential orthoses can be difficult to apply and may require assistance from another person to hold the sides open. |
| ***Precautions*** | • If edema develops in the hand because of compression around the arm, apply two layers of Tubigrip over the hand and forearm before applying the orthosis. Institute other edema controls. (See Chapter 3, "Edema.")<br>• Encourage gravity pendulum exercise as soon as the acute symptoms have subsided to prevent adhesive capsulitis.[18]<br>• Encourage range of motion of all the upper extremity joints.<br>• Discourage prolonged use of a sling (i.e., no longer than a few days) because immobilization and a dependent position of the hand promotes edema, joint stiffness, disuse atrophy, and shoulder-hand syndrome.[14] |
| ***Options*** | • If the fracture is proximal, extend the proximal edge to the acromion process; the distal edge can end above elbow at D (Fig. 9-9*b*).<br>• If the fracture is more distal, extend the distal edge over the epicondyles (broken line in Fig. 9-9*b*); proximal edge does not need to cover the deltoid muscle.<br>• Bivalved design with anterior and posterior slabs that overlap at the sides. |
| ***Alternatives*** | • Precut humerus brace kits, including Rolyan® AquaForm Humeral Fracture Brace[5] with zipper closure<br>• Preformed humerus braces |

○ **Names:** **Posterior Static Elbow (Wrist) Orthosis** (Fig. 9-10)
**Posterior Static Elbow Flexion-Blocking Orthosis**

Option: The distal edge can be extended to the MCPs to support the ulnar side of the hand, thus incorporating the wrist.

| | |
|---|---|
| ***Common Name*** | (Posterior) elbow splint |
| ***SCS Name*** | 90° elbow flexion immobilization; type 0[1]—i.e., no secondary joints, just the elbow. If the wrist was included, it would be named 90° elbow flexion immobilization; type 1[1] |

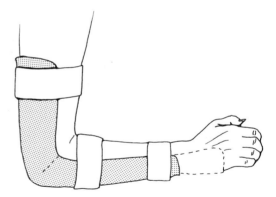

**FIGURE 9-10.** Posterior static elbow orthosis. Broken line shows optional hand support and mitered elbow seam.

| | |
|---|---|
| ***Objectives*** | • To support and rest the elbow to relieve pain<br>• To immobilize the elbow to promote healing<br>• To block elbow extension |
| ***Indications*** | • Rheumatoid arthritis<br>• Elbow surgery<br>  ◦ Ulnar nerve transposition<br>  ◦ Tendon transfers<br>  ◦ Nerve repairs |
| ***Materials*** | • ⅛ in. (3.2 mm) thick thermoplastic<br>  ◦ For gravity-resisted molding, use category B<br>  ◦ For gravity-assisted molding, use category C<br>• 2 in. (5 cm) wide self-adhesive hook Velcro<br>• 2 in. (5 cm) wide loop Velcro or padded alternative |
| ***Equipment and Tools*** | • Heating pan<br>• Scissors<br>• Elastic bandage, Thera-Band, or Orfiband<br>• For the pattern: measuring tape or flexible clear plastic with permanent marker and straight pins, stapler, or tape |
| ***Client's Position*** | • For gravity-assisted molding: prone with the upper arm supported on plinth and forearm hanging vertically and use category C thermoplastic. The thermoplastic can be molded around the flexed elbow without a seam (i.e., seamless). Ideally, lying on a height-adjustable plinth at a comfortable work height for the therapist.<br>• For gravity-resisted molding: seated and use category B thermoplastic and forming a mitered elbow seam. Ideally, on a height-adjustable stool at a comfortable work height for the client.<br>• The elbow is usually flexed about 90° and the forearm is neutral so that the orthosis supports the ulnar side of the forearm (and hand). |
| ***Therapist's Position*** | • Standing beside the plinth or stool.<br>• Assistance from a second person is helpful for gravity-resisted molding. |
| ***Pattern***<br>(Fig. 9-3*a, b,* and *d*) | • Select the method of molding and the elbow design: seamless or mitered seam. |

- Decide where the distal edge should terminate—at the wrist or MCPs (which supports the hand but restricts wrist motion).
- If the elbow can be fully extended, you can make a pattern using flexible clear plastic, or follow the steps in Figure 9-3 and measure the distances between U, E, W, and H while the elbow is positioned in the desired amount of flexion.
- Lay out the pattern.

*Fabrication*

1. Heat and cut out the pattern.
2. Reheat, check the temperature, and then place the warm thermoplastic against the posterior of the upper arm and the ulnar surface of forearm.
3. For gravity-resisted molding, use an elastic bandage. Thera-Band, or Orfiband to spiral wrap the thermoplastic from distal to proximal. Guard against twisting of the material around the limb with this technique.
4. Create a seamless or mitered elbow seam (Fig. 9-5). A seamless elbow is easy to form during gravity-assisted molding. During gravity-resisted molding, it can be achieved by stretching and pinching together the corresponding edges about every 4 in. (10 cm)(see Fig. 7-6*b*).
5. Flare the distal edge.
6. When the material is almost cool, unwrap, mark trim lines, remove the orthosis, and trim. Any thermoplastic that was stretched along the edges is cut off.
7. Attach straps (Fig. 9-10).

*Wearing Regimen*

- As appropriate for the situation.

*Options*

- Delete the straps and secure with either sterile gauze bandage (for acute burns) or elastic bandage (for edema).
- Seamless or mitered elbow seam.
- With or without support to the ulnar side of the hand.
- To convert the orthosis to an extension-blocking design: Add an extra strap above the elbow and delete the forearm and wrist straps, securing the orthosis to the upper arm only, leaving the forearm free to flex out of the orthosis.

*Alternatives*

- Preformed elbow orthosis
- Precuts, including QuickCast[4,19] or Dynacast Rapide Elbow Splint[5]
- See "Anterior Static Elbow Orthosis" or "Bisurfaced Static Elbow Orthosis"

---

## Names:    **Anterior Static Elbow Orthosis** (Fig. 9-11)
**Anterior Serial-Static Elbow Corrective-Extension Orthosis**
**Anterior Static Elbow Flexion-Blocking Orthosis**

*Common Name*    (Anterior) elbow splint

*SCS Name*    Elbow extension immobilization or mobilization; type 0[1]

*Objectives*
- To prevent or correct elbow flexion contractures
- To block elbow flexion

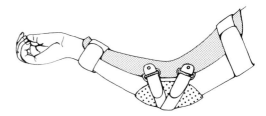

**FIGURE 9-11.** Anterior static elbow orthosis.

| | |
|---|---|
| *Indications* | • Burns     • Elbow injury or surgery |

*Indications*
- Burns
- Ulnar nerve entrapment
- **Capsular tightness**
- Elbow injury or surgery
  - Multiple trauma
  - Intra-articular fractures
  - Triceps rupture
  - Tumor **resection**
  - Total elbow arthroplasty

*Materials*
- ⅛ in. (3.2 mm) thick category B or C thermoplastic; for serial-static correction of contracture, use a thermoplastic with memory
- For the elbow pad:
  - ½ in. (1.2 cm) thick, perforated foam thermoplastic—#1 Plastazote or 4E AliPlast
  - 4 D-rings, 1 in. (2.5 cm) wide
  - 1 in. (2.5 cm) wide self-adhesive hook Velcro
  - 1 in. (2.5 cm) wide loop Velcro
  - 4 Chicago screws/nylon screws/rapid rivets
- For straps:
  - 2 in. (5 cm) wide self-adhesive hook Velcro
  - 2 in. (5 cm) wide loop Velcro or padded alternative

*Equipment and Tools*
- Heating pan • Scissors • Elastic bandage, Thera-Band, or Orfiband

*Client's Position*
- If the objective is to provide gentle, prolonged stretch to reduce a flexion contracture, it is easier to maintain extension during fabrication with the client lying supine on a bed or, ideally, on a height-adjustable plinth at a comfortable height for the therapist.

*Therapist's Position*
- Standing beside the bed or plinth.

*Pattern*
- Measure the distances between U, E, and W (Fig. 9-3*a*, *b*, and *e*).
- Take three fifths of the circumference at U, E, and W so that the trough will extend slightly more than halfway up the sides.
- Lay out the pattern. The midline of the orthosis is three fifths of U, divided in half.
- Cut out a circle of Plastazote or AliPlast to cover the olecranon process (Fig. 9-11).

*Fabrication*
1. Heat and cut out the pattern.
2. Reheat, check the temperature, and then place the warm thermoplastic against the anterior surface of the limb.
3. If desired, use a bandage to help form the contours of a category B material. Spiral wrap the thermoplastic from distal to proximal. Guard against twisting of the material around the limb with this technique. Assistance from a second person may be necessary to control the position of the elbow.

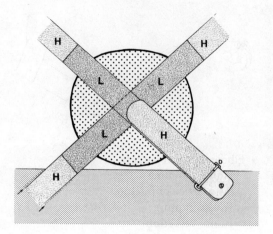

**FIGURE 9-12.** Construction of elbow or knee pad. Heat the Plastazote/AliPlast and mold it over olecranon process (or knee). If the elbow or knee is too painful, mold to the opposite side. Cut two strips of self-stick loop Velcro (L) to criss-cross the pad. Cut four strips of hook Velcro (H) and sew to the ends of the loop Velcro. Heat the adhesive backing of the loop Velcro with a heat gun and attach to the pad, crossing one strap over the other. After the orthosis has been molded, position the pad and mark where the hook straps overlap the orthotic shell (arrows). Attach four D-rings to the orthotic shell with a piece of 1 in. (2.5 cm) loop Velcro (or leather or webbing) and a screw or rivet. In this figure, only one D-ring (D) has been anchored.

4. If no bandage is used, stroke the thermoplastic into contours of the limb.
5. Flare the proximal and distal edges.
6. When the material is almost cool, unwrap, mark the trim lines, remove the orthosis, and trim.
7. Attach the straps.
8. Construct the elbow pad and attach four D-ring anchors to the orthosis (Fig. 9-12).

*Adjustment*

- For a serial-static design, reheat and remold as the contracture is reduced (see Fig. 1-9).

*Precautions*

- Ensure that the natural valgus "carrying angle" of the elbow is accommodated (Fig. 9-13).

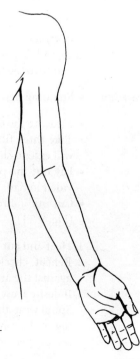

**FIGURE 9-13.** The natural valgus (lateral deviation) carrying angle of the elbow.

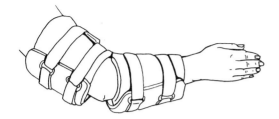

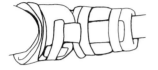

**FIGURE 9-14.** Prefabricated circumferential Rolyan® Progressive™ Elbow Splint[5] (original design courtesy of Lynn Swedberg, MS, OTR), made of soft foam/plush, washable orthosis with remoldable Ezeform insert. Especially good for clients in long-term care environments. (U.S. patent granted).

- When attempting to reduce a flexion contracture and increase elbow extension, avoid excessive extension force. (See Chapter 2, "Promoting Tissue Growth to Reduce Contractures.")
- Elbows are susceptible to developing **heterotopic ossification** in the surrounding soft tissues, especially after a severe burn.[20]
- Encourage motion of all unrestricted upper extremity joints.
- Edema can develop in the hand because of the wrist strap and positioning the hand below the heart; institute measures to control edema. (See Chapter 3, "Edema.")

*Options*

- Delete straps and elbow pad and secure with either sterile gauze bandage (for acute burns) or elastic bandage (for edema).
- To convert the orthosis to a flexion-blocking design: Add another strap above the elbow and delete the elbow pad and wrist strap, securing the orthosis to the upper arm only, leaving the forearm free to extend out of the orthosis.

*Alternatives*

- Posterior static elbow orthosis
- Bisurfaced static elbow orthosis
- Serial plaster casting[21]
- Prefabricated static-progressive elbow hinge
- Figure 9-14
- Dynamic corrective-extension orthoses[22,23]
- Elbow CPM orthosis (see Fig. 1-15*b*)

---

 **Names:** **Bisurfaced Static Elbow Orthosis** (Fig. 9-15)
**Bisurfaced Serial-Static Elbow Corrective-Flexion/ Extension Orthosis**
**Bisurfaced Static Elbow Flexion-Blocking Orthosis**

*Common Name*     Elbow splint

*SCS Name*     Elbow extension immobilization; type 0[1]

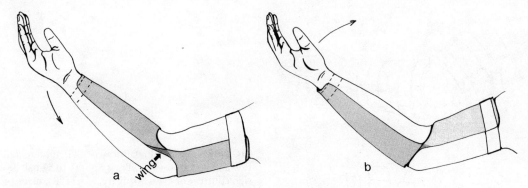

**FIGURE 9-15.**   Bisurfaced static elbow orthoses. *(a)* Posterior-radial style molded to the posterior upper arm and radial aspect of forearm. When the wrist strap (broken line) is omitted, active extension out of the orthosis is permitted while elbow flexion is blocked. When the wrist strap is fastened, the orthosis is static and no elbow motion is permitted. *(b)* Anterior-ulnar style molded to the anterior upper arm and ulnar aspect of forearm to block elbow extension. Wrist strap (broken line) is optional.

| | |
|---|---|
| ***Objectives and Indications*** | • See posterior static elbow orthosis and anterior static elbow orthosis, earlier in this chapter. |
| ***Materials*** | • ⅛ in. (3.2 mm) thick category B or C thermoplastic; for serial-static correction of contracture, use a thermoplastic with memory<br>• 2 in. (5 cm) wide self-adhesive hook Velcro<br>• 2 in. (5 cm) wide loop Velcro or padded alternative |
| ***Equipment and Tools*** | • Heating pan<br>• Measuring tape<br>• Scissors |
| ***Client's Position*** | • Seated, ideally on a height-adjustable stool at a comfortable height for the therapist, with elbow resting on a table. |
| ***Therapist's Position*** | • Standing beside the client. |
| ***Pattern*** | • Figure 9-3*a*, *b*, and *f*<br>• Cut out the cross-hatched area in the pattern to create the elbow hole. |
| ***Fabrication*** | 1. Similar to anterior static elbow orthosis, except that the hand and forearm are slipped through the elbow hole so that the material drapes over the radial border of the forearm and lies against the posterior aspect of the arm.<br>2. While maintaining the elbow in the desired position, fold the "wings" upward along the fold lines (Fig. 9-3*b*).<br>3. Gently flare the proximal and distal edges.<br>4. Mark the trim lines, remove the orthosis, and trim when the material is still partially warm.<br>5. Using a heat gun, seal the folded wings to eliminate any crevices unless using a serial-static design.<br>6. Attach straps. |
| ***Adjustment*** | • For serial-static correction of a flexion contracture, remold and reposition the elbow every few days, as the contracture reduces. |

| | |
|---|---|
| *Precautions* | • See anterior static elbow orthosis |
| *Options* | • Mold to the anterior upper arm and the ulnar side of the forearm to create a static extension-blocking orthosis (Fig. 9-15*b*). The wrist strap is optional. |
| *Alternatives* | • See anterior static elbow orthosis<br>• Other flexion-blocking orthoses[24–26] |

---

 **Name:** **Static-Progressive Elbow-Flexion Harness** (Fig. 9-16*a* through *c*)

Designed by Dorcas Beaton, O.T.(C); Barbara Shankland, O.T.(C); and Shawn O'Driscoll, M.D., Ph.D., FRCSC, at St. Michael's Hospital, Toronto, Ontario

| | |
|---|---|
| *Common Name* | Elbow flexion splint |
| *SCS Names* | Elbow flexion mobilization; type 1[2]<br>Elbow (primary joint) + shoulder = 2 joints |
| *Objectives* | • To increase elbow flexion range of motion (ROM)<br>• To maintain surgically gained flexion ROM |
| *Indications* | • Flexion contractures caused by<br>  ◦ Intra-articular fractures<br>  ◦ Multiple trauma<br>  ◦ Capsular tightness<br>  ◦ Supracondylar fracture<br>  ◦ Radial head fracture<br>• Postoperatively: total elbow arthroplasty |
| *Rationale* | • See Chapter 2, "Promoting Tissue Growth to Reduce Contractures." |
| *Materials* | • Webbing: 1 and 2 in. (2.5 and 5 cm) wide<br>• Hook Velcro: 1 and 2 in. (2.5 and 5 cm) wide<br>• Three 2 in. (5 cm) wide D-rings<br>     • One 1 in. (2.5 cm) wide D-ring<br>     • Padded strapping or self-adhesive foam or gel padding<br>     • Loop Velcro: 1 in (2.5 cm) and 2 in. (5 cm) wide<br>     • Moleskin or microfoam tape |
| *Equipment and Tools* | • Sewing machine     • Scissors     • Straight pins |
| *Client's Position* | • Seated or standing |
| *Therapist's Position* | • Seated or standing |
| *Pattern* | • No specific pattern required |
| *Fabrication*<br>(Fig. 9-16*a* through *e*)<br>The letters in these | *Waist Belt:*<br>A. Measure waist circumference; add 8 to 10 in. (20 to 25 cm). Cut 2 in. (5 cm) wide webbing to this length. |

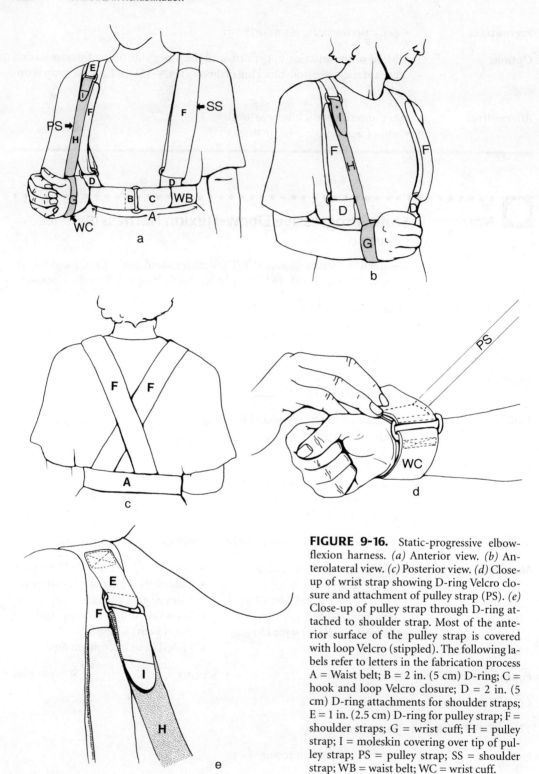

**FIGURE 9-16.** Static-progressive elbow-flexion harness. *(a)* Anterior view. *(b)* Anterolateral view. *(c)* Posterior view. *(d)* Close-up of wrist strap showing D-ring Velcro closure and attachment of pulley strap (PS). *(e)* Close-up of pulley strap through D-ring attached to shoulder strap. Most of the anterior surface of the pulley strap is covered with loop Velcro (stippled). The following labels refer to letters in the fabrication process A = Waist belt; B = 2 in. (5 cm) D-ring; C = hook and loop Velcro closure; D = 2 in. (5 cm) D-ring attachments for shoulder straps; E = 1 in. (2.5 cm) D-ring for pulley strap; F = shoulder straps; G = wrist cuff; H = pulley strap; I = moleskin covering over tip of pulley strap; PS = pulley strap; SS = shoulder strap; WB = waist belt; WC = wrist cuff.

figures refer to the letters in the fabrication process.

B. Sew D-ring to one end of the strap.

C. Sew hook and loop Velcro to the other end. (Loop Velcro should be on the loose end of the strap to avoid snagging hook Velcro on clothes.) Apply the waist belt to the client.

*Shoulder straps:*

D. Sew 2 in. (5 cm) D-ring to a 4 in. (10 cm) length of 2 in. (5 cm) wide webbing. Repeat for other side. Pin to the front of the waist belt.

E. Sew 1 in. (2.5 cm) D-ring to a 4 in. (10 cm) length of 1 in. (2.5 cm) wide webbing.

F  Using 2 in. (5 cm) wide webbing, pin one end of shoulder strap to the waist belt, lateral to the spine (Fig. 9-16*c*). Then bring the loose end of the strap across and over the opposite shoulder to the waist belt in front. Add enough webbing for the hook and loop Velcro closure at the front. Repeat for the other shoulder strap. Pin D-ring webbing (E) to the shoulder strap on the side of the affected arm (Fig. 9-16*e*). Remove and sew the components together.

*Wrist cuff (Fig. 9-16d):*

G. Sew 2 in. (5 cm) D-ring to one end of 2 in. (5 cm) wide webbing. Measure the length of the strap by wrapping it around the client's wrist, feeding the loose end through the D-ring and allowing 3 in. (7.5 cm) extra for overlap. Sew the hook and loop Velcro closure to the other end. Sew padding to the inside of the cuff, or apply self-adhesive foam or gel padding. The wrist cuff should fit loosely and the closure should be positioned toward the contralateral hand for easy fastening of the Velcro.

*Pulley Strap (Fig. 9-16e):*

H. Sew 1 in. (2.5 cm) webbing to the proximal edge of the wrist strap. Feed the loose end of the webbing through the D-ring (E) on the shoulder strap, add 4 in. (10 cm), and then cut off. Sew 4 in. (10 cm) length of 1 in. (2.5 cm) wide hook Velcro over the loose end of the pulley strap and 1 in. (2.5 cm) loop Velcro to the remainder of the pulley strap.

I.  Cover the cut end of the webbing with moleskin or microfoam tape to prevent fraying.

*Application and Adjustment*

• Adjust tension in the pulley strap until the client feels a slight stretch but no pain. After 10 minutes of wear, tighten the strap slightly.

• As the flexion range improves, the moleskin tip will be attached lower on the pulley strap, getting closer to the hand. Use pen marks on the pulley strap to record improvement.

*Wearing Regimen*

• Worn several hours per day to apply gentle, prolonged stretch to promote desired soft tissue growth.

• When using any corrective-flexion orthosis, the extension range can be compromised. Remove frequently to move the elbow into extension.

• If the client lacks range in both flexion and extension, develop a cyclical wearing schedule. During the day, alternate between an anterior or bisurfaced static (or serial-static) elbow orthosis and the elbow flexion harness every 3 to 4 hours, with gentle, active ROM exercises in between. During the night, use either the orthosis or the harness, depending on which range is more limited.

| | |
|---|---|
| *Precautions* | • Caution the client against overtightening the pulley strap. Overzealous stretching will injure contracted soft tissues. The client should feel pull, not pain. |
| | • If tingling occurs because of ulnar nerve traction at the elbow, reduce the tension in the pulley strap. |
| | • Initially, ROM increases quickly, but the rate of improvement slows down and can take months to achieve final results. |
| *Alternatives* | • Prefabricated progressive elbow hinges. |
| | • Elbow CPM (see Fig. 1-15*b*), which is better for maintaining ROM rather than increasing it. |
| | • Replace the webbing of trunk harness and wrist strap with a thermoplastic vest and wrist orthosis, respectively.[27] |

---

● ● ● ● ● ● ● ● ● ● ● ● ● ● ● ● ● ● ● ● ● ● ● ● ● ● ● ● ● ● ● ●

⬤ **Name:**     **Circumferential Nonarticular Proximal Forearm Strap**[28,29]  (Fig. 9-17*a* and *b*)

| | |
|---|---|
| *Common Names* | Tennis elbow strap; counterforce strap |
| *SCS Name* | Nonarticular splint—proximal forearm |
| *Objectives* | • To reduce pain and inflammation by reducing tensile force exerted by wrist extensors or flexors at their origins from the lateral or medial epicondyle, respectively[28,29] |
| *Indications* | • Inflammation of the common tendon origin of |
| | ○ Wrist extensors: lateral epicondylitis (tennis elbow) |
| | ○ Wrist flexors: medial epicondylitis (golfer's elbow) |
| *Materials* | • 2 in. (5 cm) wide webbing |
| | • 2 in. (5 cm) wide loop Velcro—5 in. (12.5 cm) long |
| | • 2 D-rings—1 in. (2.5 cm) wide |
| | • 1 in. (2.5 cm) nonadhesive hook Velcro |
| | • Thin self-adhesive foam or gel padding or microfoam tape |
| | • ½ in. (1 cm) thick gel padding (e.g., Akton) or foam lining (e.g., T-foam) |
| | • For reinforcement: polyethylene or low-temperature thermoplastic: $\frac{1}{32}$ or $\frac{1}{16}$ in. (0.8 or 1.6 mm) thick |
| *Equipment and Tools* | • Sewing machine            • Scissors |
| *Client's Position* | • Seated |
| *Therapist's Position* | • Seated |
| *Pattern* | • Measure the circumference around the proximal forearm, about 1 in. (2.5 cm) below the elbow. Cut the webbing to this length plus 3 in. (7.5 cm). |
| *Fabrication* (Fig. 9-17*c*) | 1. For lateral epicondylitis, position the opening over the medial aspect of the forearm; for medial epicondylitis, position the opening over the lateral aspect of the forearm. |
| | 2. Sew under ½ in. (1 cm) at each end. |

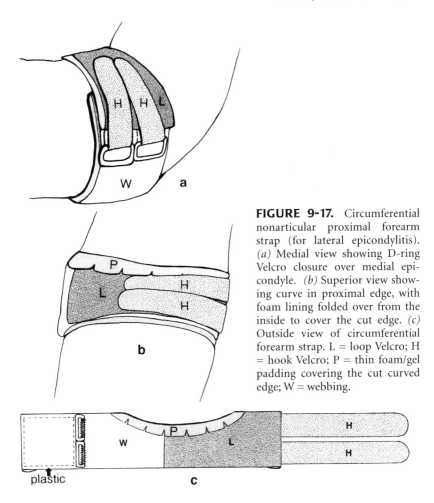

**FIGURE 9-17.** Circumferential nonarticular proximal forearm strap (for lateral epicondylitis). *(a)* Medial view showing D-ring Velcro closure over medial epicondyle. *(b)* Superior view showing curve in proximal edge, with foam lining folded over from the inside to cover the cut edge. *(c)* Outside view of circumferential forearm strap. L = loop Velcro; H = hook Velcro; P = thin foam/gel padding covering the cut curved edge; W = webbing.

3. Sew loop Velcro (L) to the outside surface, two hook (H) Velcro straps to one end, and two D-rings 2 in. (5 cm) in from the other end.
4. Cut a curve out of the proximal anterior edge. Cover the cut edge with the thin foam or gel sheeting or microfoam tape.
5. Cover the inner surface with foam or gel padding. Insert the plastic reinforcement between the webbing and foam.

***Wearing Regimen***

- Strap is worn immediately below the elbow, directly over the inflamed muscles, during activities that cause pain.

***Precautions***

- Strap is to be worn as tight as tolerable without causing swelling, numbness, or tingling in the hand.
- Educate the client about recognizing signs of circulatory restriction. When the arm is inactive, tension must be slackened at least every 3 to 4 hours to restore full blood flow to the hand.
- Do not wear at night.

***Options***

- Adhere a patch of ½ in. (0.5 cm) thick gel padding or foam lining adjacent to inflamed muscle origin to absorb vibration, increase conformity, and increase pressure.

| | |
|---|---|
| *Alternatives* | • Prefabricated designs. |
| | • If after a few days symptom relief is insufficient, provide an immobilizing wrist orthosis to completely rest inflamed wrist muscles (see Chapter 10). |

● ● ● ● ● ● ● ● ● ● ● ● ● ● ● ● ● ● ● ● ● ● ● ● ● ● ● ● ● ● ● ● ● ● ● ● ● ● ● ● ●

⬤ **Name:** **Spiral Dynamic Forearm-Rotation Thumb-Abduction Strap** (Fig. 9-18*a*)

Developed by Christine Casey at Gillette Children's Hospital, 1986[30]

| | |
|---|---|
| *Common Names* | Thumb abduction supination splint[30] |
| | Prefabricated Rolyan® Upper Extremity TAP™ (*Tone and Positioning*) Splint[6] |
| *SCS Name* | Forearm pronation/supination mobilization, thumb abduction mobilization; type 1[3]—i.e., thumb MCP is the secondary joints; primary joints are forearm and thumb CMC; total joints = 3 |
| *Objectives* | • To abduct the thumb and, depending on the direction in which the strap is wrapped, to promote either supination or pronation. The elbow and wrist are free to move. |
| | • To reduce the tone of hypertonic muscles by abducting the thumb and supinating the forearm. |
| | • To assist weak muscles. |
| | • To promote functional use of the hand. |
| | • To increase either supination or pronation range of motion. |
| *Indications* | • **hypertonicity** or **hypotonicity** associated with |
| | ◦ Head injury ◦ **Multiple sclerosis** |
| | ◦ **Cerebral palsy** ◦ **Cerebrovascular accident** |
| | • Forearm stiffness secondary to cast immobilization for a wrist fracture |
| *Materials* | • Neoprene strap—⅛ in. (3.2 mm) thick, 2 in. (5 cm) wide[1,4,6] |
| | • Neoprene sheeting ¹⁄₁₆ in. (1.6 mm) thick[4] |
| | • Hook Velcro—1 in. (2.5 cm) wide |
| *Equipment and Tools* | • Sewing machine • Scissors • Measuring tape |
| *Pattern* | • Measure the length of the neoprene strap—circumference above the elbow and then spiraling around the forearm, wrist, and through the first web space. Cut the neoprene strap to this length. |
| | • Figure 9-18*b* for thumb abduction glove. |
| *Fabrication* | 1. Sew thumb abduction glove (Fig. 9-18*c*). |
| | 2. Sew 2 in. (5 cm) length of hook Velcro to each end of the neoprene strap. |
| *Application* | • To promote supination, wrap the strap around the limb, as shown in Figure 9-18*a*. |
| | • To promote pronation, reverse the direction of the wrapping. |
| *Precautions* | • Adjust tension carefully to avoid excessive rotational force. |

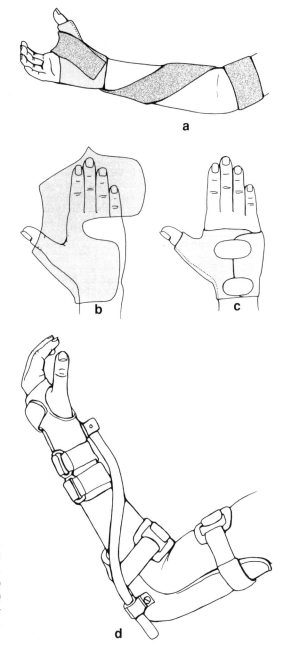

**FIGURE 9-18.** *(a)* Spiral dynamic forearm-rotation thumb-abduction strap (prefabricated Rolyan® TAP™ [Tone and Positioning] Splint[5]). The direction of wrapping promotes forearm supination. *(b)* Pattern for neoprene thumb-abduction glove. *(c)* Completed glove, showing seam along radial border and hook Velcro (H). *(d)* Rolyan® Preformed Dynamic Supination/Pronation Splint.

*Alternatives*

- Prefabricated version: Rolyan® Upper Extremity TAP™ Splint[5]
- To increase supination or pronation, Rolyan® Preformed Dynamic Pronation/Supination Splint (Fig. 9-18*d*)[5]
- Air bag splints[31]
- Dynamic pronation orthoses[32–33]
- Dynamic supination orthoses[34–35]

● **References**

1. AliMed Orthopedic Rehabilitation Products Catalog, 1997.
2. Richards, RR: Soft Tissue Reconstruction in the Upper Extremity. Churchill Livingston, New York, 1995.
3. Tenney, CG, and Lisak, JM: Atlas of Hand Splinting. Little, Brown, Boston, 1986.
4. Sammons Preston Catalog, 1997.
5. Smith & Nephew Inc.: Rehabilitation Division Catalogue, 1997. (Rolyan, TAP, and Progressive are trademarks of Smith & Nephew Inc.)
6. Daugherty, MB, and Carr-Collins, JA: Splinting techniques for the burn patient. In Richard, RL, and Staley, MJ (eds): Burn Care and Rehabilitation: Principles and Practice. FA Davis, Philadelphia, 1994, p 589.
7. Bellefeuille-Reid, D: Arm sling for controlling extensor tonus pattern: a case study. Can J Occup Ther 48:125, 1981.
8. Shea, R: Upper limb sling for use with a Hoffman external fixation device. Can J Ocup Ther 49:137, 1982.
9. Claus, BS, and Godfrey, KJ: A distal support sling for the hemiplegic patient. Am J Occup Ther 39:536, 1985.
10. Walker, J: Modified strapping of roll sling. Am J Occup Ther 37:110, 1983.
11. Neal, MR, and Williamson, J: Collar sling for bilateral shoulder subluxation. Am J Occup Ther 34:400, 1980.
12. Sullivan, BE, and Rogers, SL: Modified Bobath sling with distal support. Am J Occup Ther 43:47, 1989.
13. Smith, RO: Checklist for the prescription of slings for the hemiplegic patient. Am J Occup Ther 35:91, 1981.
14. Sadra, H: New technical designs: Universal arm splint for brachial plexus injuries. Can J Occup Ther 62:216, 1995.
15. Davis, JZ: Neurodevelopmental treatment of adult hemiplegia: The Bobath approach. In Pedretti, LW (ed): Occupational Therapy: Practice Skills for Physical Dysfunction, ed 4. Mosby, St. Louis, 1996, p 449.
16. Linden, CA, and Trombly, CA: Orthoses: Kinds and purposes. In Trombly, CA (ed): Occupational Therapy for Physical Dysfunction, ed 4. Williams & Wilkins, Baltimore, 1995.
17. Davila, S: Upper extremity fracture bracing. J Hand Ther 5:157, 1992.
18. Sarmiento, A, Ross, SDK, and Racette, WL: Functional Fracture Bracing. Orthomerica Products Inc., February 1, 1996.
19. North Coast Medical Hand Therapy Catalog, 1997.
20. Dutcher, K, and Johnson, C: Neuromuscular and musculoskeletal complications. In Richard, RL, and Staley, MJ (eds): Burn Care and Rehabilitation: Principles and Practice. FA Davis, Philadelphia, 1994, p 589.
21. King, TI: Plaster splinting as a means of reducing elbow flexor spasticity: A case study. Am J Occup Ther 36:671, 1982.
22. Parker, BC: A dynamic elbow extension splint. Am J Occup Ther 41:825, 1987.
23. Dellon, AL, Kofkin, J, and Tobing, M: Dynamic elbow splint following tendon transfer to restore triceps. Am J Occup Ther 34:680, 1981.
24. McClure, MK, Holtz-Yotz, M: The effects of sensory stimulatory treatment on an autistic child. Am J Occup Ther 45:1138, 1991.
25. Harper, BD: The drop-out splint: An alternative to the conservative management of ulnar nerve entrapment at the elbow. J Hand Ther 3:199, 1990.
26. Sharpe, PA, and Ottenbacher, KJ: Use of an elbow restraint to improve finger-feeding skills in a child with Rett syndrome. Am J Occup Ther 44:328, 1990.
27. Kamil, NI, and Correia, AL: A dynamic elbow flexion splint for an infant with arthrogryposis. Am J Occup Ther 44:460, 1990.
28. Clements, LG, and Chow, S: Effectiveness of a custom-made below elbow lateral counterforce splint in the treatment of lateral epicondylitis. Can J Occup Ther 60:137, 1993.
29. Nirschl, RP: Symposium on treatment of acute hand injuries. Washington Hand Symposium, Washington, DC, 1990.
30. Casey, CA, and Kratz, EJ: Soft splinting with neoprene: The thumb abduction supinator splint. Am J Occup Ther 42:395, 1988.
31. Barr, K: The use of air bag splints to increase supination and pronation in the arm. Am J Occup Ther 48:746, 1994.
32. Hage, G: Two pronation splints. Am J Occup Ther 39:265, 1985.
33. Hokken, W, et al: A dynamic pronation orthosis for the C6 tetraplegic arm. Arch Phys Med Rehabil 74:104, 1993.
34. Murphy, MS: An adjustable splint for forearm supination. Am J Occup Ther 44:936, 1990.
35. Berger-Feldscher, S: Adaptation of the Murphy supination splint. J Hand Ther 8:270, 1995.

# *Forearm-Based Orthoses*

## *Chapter Outline*

This chapter describes the fabrication process for 21 forearm-based orthoses. With the exception of the circumferential nonarticular forearm-stabilizing orthosis, all the designs influence wrist motion. The orthoses are organized from proximal to distal; as the chapter progresses, the orthoses incorporate more distal joints in the hand.

The illustrated patterns can be enlarged with a photocopier to produce a standard pattern that matches the size of the client's hand. Measure the bird's-eye width across the dorsum of the client's hand from the radial side of the second MC head to the ulnar side of the fifth MC head. Compare this measurement with the MCP width in the illustrated pattern, and determine the amount of enlargement required to match the client's MCP width.

The following acronyms are used:

- SCS—splint classification system
- MC—metacarpal
- MP or MCP—metacarpophalangeal joint
- PIP—proximal interphalangeal joint
- DIP—distal interphalangeal joint
- IP—interphalangeal joints
- CMC—carpometacarpal joint

Other abbreviations are D1 (thumb), D2 (index finger), D3 (middle finger), D4 (ring finger), and D5 (small finger).

An evaluation form for upper extremity orthoses can be found at the end of Chapter 7. It can be used as a guideline for designing, fabricating, and evaluating many of the orthoses in Chapter 10. Refer to the introduction to Chapter 8 for more information.

● ● ● ● ● ● ● ● ● ● ● ● ● ● ● ● ● ● ● ● ● ● ● ● ● ● ● ● ● ● ● ● ● ● ● ● ● ● ● ● ●

## ⬤ Name: Circumferential Nonarticular Ulna-Stabilizing Orthosis[1] (Fig. 10-1)

| | |
|---|---|
| ***Common Name*** | Ulnar fracture/functional brace |
| ***SCS Name*** | Nonarticular splint—ulna |
| ***Objectives*** | • To stabilize an ulnar fracture to promote healing, without immobilizing any joints<br>• To protect fragile bones from fracture |
| ***Indications*** | • Midshaft ulnar fractures |
| ***Rationale*** | • Applies circumferential compression to soft tissues of the forearm to maintain alignment of the fracture site.<br>• See Chapter 2, "Fractures of Long Bones." |
| ***Materials*** | • ³⁄₃₂ or ⅛ in. (2.4 or 3.2 mm) thick slightly perforated thermoplastic—opaque category A, B, or C; translucent category B or C<br>• For the insert: ¹⁄₁₆ in. (1.6 mm) thick thermoplastic, category B or C—about 1½ in. (4 cm) wide and 12 in. (30 cm) long—Orfit Classic works well because of its surface stickiness when warm that helps it cling to the skin during molding<br>• ⅛ in. (3.2 mm) thick self-adhesive foam or gel padding<br>• Stockinette or Tubigrip<br>• Solvent or alcohol<br>• Self-adhesive hook Velcro<br>• Loop Velcro<br>• Two plastic (radiolucent) D-rings (optional) |

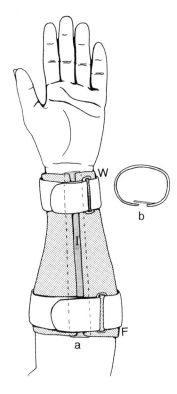

**FIGURE 10-1.** Circumferential nonarticular ulna-stabilizing orthosis. *(a)* Volar view. *(b)* Cross section showing insert strip bonded to one side of the opening. W = wrist; I = insert; F = two thirds up the forearm.

*Equipment and Tools*
- Heating pan
- Scissors
- Heat gun
- For the pattern: paper towel or flexible clear plastic with permanent marker and straight pins, stapler, or tape

*Client's Position*
- Seated with the elbow resting on a table for vertical molding and forearm neutral

*Therapist's Position*
- Seated beside the client

*Pattern*
- Make a circumferential pattern using plastic or paper towel, allowing 1 in. (2.5 cm) extra along each side.
- Alternatively, measure the distances between the wrist (W) and two thirds up the forearm (F). Take circumferences at W and F and add 2 in. (5 cm).
- A precise pattern is not required because of the stretch technique used to mold.

*Fabrication*
1. Decide on the location of the opening—volar, dorsal, radial, or ulnar.
2. Apply padding to the ulnar head.
3. Insert: Heat the material, check the temperature, and mold against the skin at the location of the opening.
4. Apply a layer of Stockinette or Tubigrip over the molded insert. Because of shrinkage, use two layers if using translucent material.
5. Heat material and gently stretch around limb. Pinch excess material together and cut flush with limb while material is warm, creating a closed seam (see Fig. 9-9c).
6. Conform to the contours.
7. Mark the trim lines at the proximal and distal edges to ensure unrestricted motion and no irritation.

8. When cold, pop open the edges that were pinched together and remove the orthosis. If it has adhered to the Stockinette, cut through the Stockinette to remove the orthosis. Once the orthosis is off the forearm, the Stockinette can be peeled away.

9. Transfer the ulnar head pad to the inside of the orthosis or discard it to leave a space.

10. Cut along the trim lines and remove about ½ in. (1 cm) from each side of the opening. Adhere the insert to one inside edge using solvent or alcohol and dry heat (Fig. 10-1*b*).

11. Apply the orthosis and attach two overlap or D-ring straps.

12. With the orthosis in place, confirm fracture alignment with an x-ray.

| | |
|---|---|
| ***Wearing Regimen*** | • Worn at all times except for bathing.<br>• Continue with the orthosis until fracture healing is complete. |
| ***Application*** | • Circumferential orthoses can be difficult to apply and may require assistance from another person to hold the sides open. |
| ***Precautions*** | • If edema develops in the hand because of compression around the arm, apply two layers of Tubigrip over the hand and forearm before applying the orthosis. Institute other edema controls. (See Chapter 3, "Edema.")<br>• Encourage range of motion of all the upper extremity joints.<br>• Discourage prolonged use of a sling (i.e., no longer than a few days) because immobilization and a dependent position of the hand promotes edema, joint stiffness, disuse atrophy, and shoulder-hand syndrome. |
| ***Options*** | • The opening can be volar (as shown), dorsal, radial, or ulnar.<br>• Bivalved—2 overlapping half-shells.<br>• Replace the low-temperature thermoplastic with a combination of polyethylene and Plastazote, and use the technique described later for circumferential forearm-based static wrist orthosis. |
| ***Alternatives*** | • Precut ulnar brace kit[2]<br>• Prefabricated ulnar fracture brace |

---

## ● Half-Shell Wrist Orthoses

**Names:**     **Volar Forearm-Based Static Thumb-Hole Wrist Orthosis** (Fig. 10-2*a* and *b*)
**Dorsal Forearm-Based Static Wrist Orthosis** (Fig. 10-3*a* and *b*)
**Ulnar Forearm-Based Static Wrist Orthosis**[3,4] (Fig. 10-4*a*)
**Radial Forearm-Based Static Thumb-Hole Wrist Orthosis**[4] (Fig. 10-5*a*)

***Common Names***

• Volar/palmar wrist splint
• Volar wrist cock-up splint
• Wrist immobilization splint
• Carpal tunnel splint
• Drop wrist splint

• Wrist extension immobilization splint
• Work splint
• Working splint
• Ulnar gutter splint
• Radial gutter splint

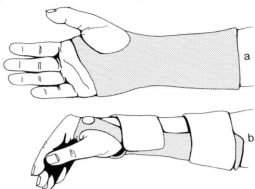
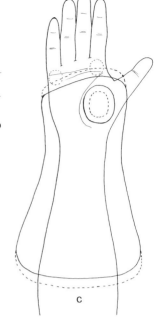

**FIGURE 10-2.** Volar forearm-based static thumb-hole wrist orthosis. *(a)* Volar view shown without straps. *(b)* Radial view. *(c)* Pattern. When using ³⁄₃₂ or ⅛ in. (2.4 or 3.2 mm) thermoplastic, cut out the pattern along solid line. When using ¹⁄₁₆ in. (1.6 mm) thick thermoplastic, extend the proximal and distal borders to the broken line and allow an extra ½ in. (1 cm) around the thumb hole (broken line); when molding, fold back distal and proximal edges and roll back thumb hole ½ in. (1 cm). These folds strengthen the orthosis when thin thermoplastic is used and create smooth edges. After molding, the distal edge terminates just proximal to second metacarpal head and ¼ in. (½ cm) proximal to fifth metacarpal head.

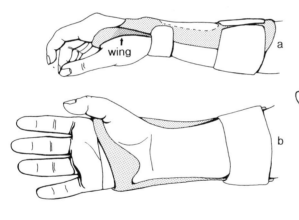
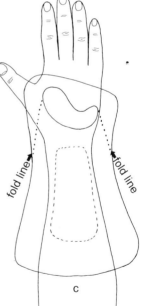

**FIGURE 10-3.** Dorsal forearm-based static wrist orthosis. *(a)* Radial view. *(b)* Volar view. *(c)* Pattern. The hole over the dorsal forearm (broken line), a design innovation by Paul Van Lede, OTR, of Orfit Industries, is optional. The hole makes the orthosis lighter by removing unnecessary thermoplastic. The dotted lines are fold lines. This design has an integrated palmar bar.

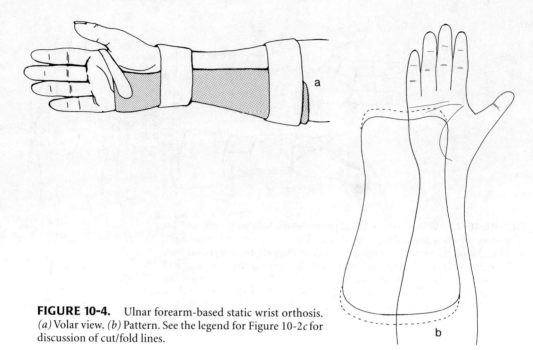

**FIGURE 10-4.** Ulnar forearm-based static wrist orthosis. *(a)* Volar view. *(b)* Pattern. See the legend for Figure 10-2*c* for discussion of cut/fold lines.

| | |
|---|---|
| *SCS Name* | • Wrist extension immobilization; type 0[1] |
| *Design Considerations* | • *Volar:* provides optimal support to the carpal bones; recommended for joint inflammation or instability; the volar surface of the hand is naturally well padded and tolerates the palmar base well; can be used to mount flexion outriggers |

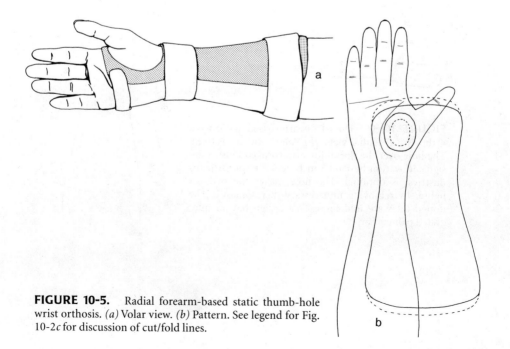

**FIGURE 10-5.** Radial forearm-based static thumb-hole wrist orthosis. *(a)* Volar view. *(b)* Pattern. See legend for Fig. 10-2*c* for discussion of cut/fold lines.

- *Dorsal:* less coverage of the volar surface than other designs, thus blocking sensation less than other designs; ulnar head requires padding; can be used to mount extension outriggers; has integrated palmar bar
- *Ulnar:* easiest to make; ulnar head requires padding; can be used to mount flexion or extension outriggers
- *Radial:* restricts wrist motion less than other designs, permitting wrist ulnar deviation and some flexion; the palmar strap is important to compensate for lack of ulnar support from the thermoplastic; can be used to mount flexion or extension outriggers

| *Objectives* | *Indications* | |
|---|---|---|
| • To reduce pain and inflammation | • Tendinitis/tenosynovitis of wrist tendons | |
| | • Joint inflammation, such as rheumatoid arthritis (RA) | |
| • To protect against joint damage | • Joint inflammation (e.g., RA) | |
| • To immobilize to promote healing | • Skin graft | • **Synovectomy** |
| | • Unstable wrist joint | • Wrist fracture—once callus has |
| | • Wrist sprain | formed |
| • To promote hand function | • Unstable wrist joint | |
| | • Weak/paralyzed wrist extensors (e.g., radial nerve palsy) | |
| • To prevent or correct contractures | • Congenital hand deformities (e.g., radial club hand) | |
| | • Weak/paralyzed wrist extensors | |
| • To provide base for outriggers | • Volar style for flexion outriggers | |
| | • Dorsal style for extension outrigger | |
| | • Radial or ulnar style for either flexion or extension outriggers | |
| • To optimally position | | |
| ○ To correct radial deviation and prevent/reduce MCP ulnar drift | • Joint inflammation (e.g., RA) | |
| ○ To reduce carpal tunnel pressure[5–9] | • Carpal tunnel syndrome | |

| *Materials* | • Opaque/translucent category C or translucent category B thermoplastic—$\frac{1}{16}$ or $\frac{3}{32}$ in. (1.6 or 2.4 mm) thick—use $\frac{1}{8}$ in. (3.2 mm) thickness for dorsal design and to mount wire outrigger, although spring wire is thin enough to mount onto $\frac{1}{16}$ or $\frac{3}{32}$ in. (1.6 or 2.4 mm) |
|---|---|
| | • For a more flexible (but bulkier) support, use Kushionsplint |
| | • $\frac{1}{8}$ in. (3.2 mm) thick self-adhesive foam or gel padding |
| | • Self-adhesive hook Velcro |
| | • Loop Velcro or padded alternative |

| *Equipment and Tools* | • Heating pan      • Scissors      • Heat gun |
|---|---|
| | • For the pattern: paper towel or flexible clear plastic with permanent marker and straight pins, stapler, or tape |
| | • Oven for Kushionsplint |

| *Wrist Position* | • See Chapter 2, "Joint Mechanics and Considerations for Positioning Hand Joints." |
|---|---|

| *Client's Position* | • Seated with forearm positioned to promote gravity-assisted molding: volar—supination (see Fig. 7-4*a*); dorsal—pronation (see Fig. 7-4*b*); ulnar—fore- |
|---|---|

arm neutral and elbow flexed; radial—forearm neutral with elbow extended

**Therapist's Position**
- Seated across from the client who is seated on a chair or standing beside the client who is seated on a height-adjustable stool.

**Pattern**
- From the proximal palmar crease to two thirds up the forearm.
- Figures 10-2*c*, 10-3*c*, 10-4*b*, 10-5*b*.
- When using ¹⁄₁₆ in. (1.6 mm) thick thermoplastic, extend the patterns in Figures 10-2*c*, 10-4*b*, and 10-5*b* to the broken lines and fold the distal and proximal edges over about ½ in. (1 cm) during molding to strengthen the orthosis. Similarly, use the broken line for the thumb hole to allow an extra ½ in. (1 cm) to fold back the thermoplastic around the thumb hole.

**Fabrication**
1. For ulnar or dorsal designs, apply padding to the ulnar head.
2. For the volar design, slip the thumb through hole and then stretch the material ulnarly to uncover the thenar eminence. See Chapter 7 for more in-depth directions for the volar design.
3. For the dorsal design, position yourself behind the client's affected shoulder.
   - Slip the hand through the hole, positioning the distal edge at the proximal edge of the second MC head and ¼ in. (½ cm) proximal to the fifth MC head.
   - Drape the material over the dorsum of the forearm.
   - Fold the "wings" upward along the fold lines and hold them in place with the thenar eminence of your hands (see Fig. 7-4*b*).
   - Use the index or middle finger of one hand to conform the material to the transverse arch. At the same time, control wrist flexion/extension and deviation to achieve the desired wrist positioning.
4. For all designs, mark the trim lines, remove the orthosis when the material is set but still warm, and trim.
5. Ensure that MCP flexion and thumb and elbow motion are unrestricted.
6. Gently flare the proximal volar edge.
7. Apply the straps.

**Wearing Regimen**
- As appropriate for the situation.

**Precautions**
- Avoid pressure points, especially over the ulnar head/styloid and radial styloid.
- Ensure full range of motion of the MCPs, thumb (clear the thenar eminence), and elbow.
- During molding, control wrist flexion/extension and deviation.
- With joint inflammation, immobilizing the wrist increases stress on the MCPs.
- Ensure that the straps are easy to manage for arthritic fingers (see Fig. 3-16).
- Some wrist orthoses have a negative impact on grip strength.[10–12]

**Options**
- Fold over the distal edge once to clear the MC heads during molding.
- Apply gel padding over an incision or hypertrophic scar before molding and transfer the padding to the inside of the orthosis when the material has set.
- The hand strap can be omitted from the volar design to allow active wrist extension out of the orthosis.
- Add a magnet to assist with object retrieval if the client has little or no finger dexterity.[13]

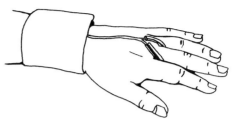

**FIGURE 10-6.** Prefabricated Daytimer Carpal Tunnel Support—blocks flexion via tension through the nonelastic finger loop but permits extension and ulnar and radial deviation. The finger loop is anchored to a fabric wrist cuff.

| *Alternatives* | • Precuts for thumb-hole styles—cut the thumb hole to enlarge it to 1½ in. (3 cm) before molding (see Fig. 7-7*a*).<br>• Dorsal forearm-based dynamic joint-aligned coil-spring wrist-assistive extension orthosis (Fig. 10-8) (described later in this chapter)<br>• Prefabricated Daytimer Carpal Tunnel Support[14] (Fig. 10-6) |
|---|---|

 **Names:** **Circumferential Forearm-Based Static Wrist Orthosis (With Ulnar Opening)** (Fig. 10-7*a*)
**Circumferential Forearm-Based Polyethylene/ Plastazote Static Wrist Orthosis[15]**

This design can be directly molded to the client using either low-temperature thermoplastic or polyethylene lined with Plastazote. Polyethylene is a high-temperature plastic that can be directly molded to the client when there is a Plastazote interface and the client's limb is protected with a double layer of Stockinette or Tubigrip or a splint liner.

| *Common Name* | • Circumferential work(ing) splint; gauntlet immobilization splint |
|---|---|
| *SCS Name* | • Wrist extension immobilization; type 0[1] |
| *Objectives and Indications* | • As for half-shell orthoses, but the circumferential design provides greater wrist stability<br>• As an evaluation tool before wrist arthrodesis (fusion) to determine the optimal wrist position and the impact of fusion on hand function<br>• To immobilize and stabilize a fracture of the radius or base of an MC |

| *Materials* | *Low-temperature thermoplastic* | *Polyethylene/Plastazote* |
|---|---|---|
| | • Category B or C thermoplastic:<br> ○ ⅟₁₆ or ³⁄₃₂ in. (1.6 or 2.4 mm) thick<br> ○ For the insert: ⅟₃₂ or ⅟₁₆ (0.8 or 1.6 mm) thick—1¼ in. (4 cm) wide<br>• For a more flexible but bulkier orthosis, use Kushionsplint[16]<br>• ⅛ in. (3.2 mm) thick self-adhesive foam or gel padding<br>• Velcro straps<br>• Three D-rings (optional) | • ⅟₁₆ in. (1.6 mm) thick low-density polyethylene—10 × 10 in. (25 × 25 cm)<br>• ⅟₁₆ in. (1.6 mm) #1 perforated Plastazote<br>• 2 in. (5 cm) wide Stockinette or Tubigrip<br>• Coban tape or self-adhesive padding to protect the thumb during molding |

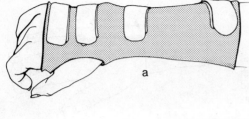

**FIGURE 10-7.**    Circumferential forearm-based static wrist orthosis (with ulnar opening). *(a)* Radiodorsal view. *(b)* Pattern. See the legend for Figure 10-2c for discussion of cut/fold lines when using ¹⁄₁₆ in. (1.6 mm) thermoplastic. Use solid lines as cut lines for polyethylene. Cut Plastazote to extend about ¼ in. (½ cm) beyond the edges of the polyethylene.

| | Low-temperature thermoplastic | Polyethylene/Plastazote |
|---|---|---|
| | • Six rivets (optional) | • ⅛ in. (3.2 mm) thick self-adhesive foam or gel padding<br>• Velcro straps<br>• Three D-rings (optional)<br>• Six rivets (optional) |
| *Equipment and Tools* | • Heating pan | • Oven<br>• Heavy cotton gloves<br>• Awl<br>• Hammer (if rivets used)<br>• Metal tray lined with release paper, cornstarch, or talcum powder<br>• Wrist-thumb splint liner or Stockinette or Tubigrip |
| | • Scissors<br>• For the pattern: paper towel or flexible clear plastic with permanent marker and straight pins, stapler, or tape | • Scissors |
| *Wrist Position* | • See Chapter 2, "Joint Mechanics and Considerations for Positioning Hand Joints." | |
| *Client's Position* | • Seated (near oven) with elbow resting on the table for vertical molding. The forearm is neutral. | |
| *Therapist's Position* | • Seated beside the client. The assistance of a second person is helpful because of the short working time of the polyethylene/Plastazote (about 30 seconds). | |

***Pattern***
(Fig. 10-7*b*)

- Make a circumferential pattern using plastic or paper towel, allowing 1 in. (2.5 cm) extra along each side.
- Unlike half-shell forearm-based orthoses, circumferential designs need to extend only halfway up the forearm from the waist.
- A precise pattern is not required because of the stretch technique used during molding.
- When using ¹⁄₁₆ in. (1.6 mm) thick thermoplastic, extend the pattern in Figure 10-7*b* to the broken lines and fold the distal and proximal edges over about ½ in. (1 cm) during molding to strengthen the orthosis. Similarly, use the broken line for the thumb hole to allow an extra ½ in. (1 cm) to fold back the thermoplastic around the thumb hole.
- Design it with either a dorsal or ulnar opening.
- Polyethylene shrinks in one direction and stretches in the perpendicular direction. Lay out the pattern, allowing for shrinkage and stretch. The Plastazote should extend ½ in. (1 cm) beyond the edges of polyethylene when both are heated to protect the client's skin from burns.

***Thermoplastic Fabrication***

1. Apply padding to the ulnar head.
2. Heat, check the temperature, and then mold the insert against the skin at the location of the opening.
3. Apply a splint liner or layer of Stockinette or Tubigrip over the molded insert. Because of shrinkage, use two layers if using translucent material.
4. Heat the material and slip the thumb through the hole.
5. Gently stretch the material around the limb and pinch the excess material together. While the material is warm, cut it flush with the limb, creating a closed seam (see Fig. 9-9*c*).
6. If using ¹⁄₁₆ in. (1.6 mm) thickness, roll back once at the thumb hole and fold over ½ in. (1 cm) at the proximal and distal edges.
7. Conform the material to the contours.
8. Mark the trim lines to ensure unrestricted MCP, thumb, and elbow motion.
9. When cold, pop open the edges that were pinched together and remove the orthosis. If it has adhered to the Stockinette, cut through the Stockinette to remove the orthosis. Once the orthosis is off the forearm, the Stockinette can be peeled away.
10. Transfer the ulnar head pad to the inside of the orthosis or discard it to leave a space.
11. Cut along the trim lines and remove about ½ in. (1 cm) from each side of the opening. Adhere the insert to one inside edge using solvent or alcohol and dry heat (Fig. 10-1*b*).
12. Gently flare the proximal volar edge.
13. Attach three or four overlap or D-ring Velcro straps.

***Polyethylene-Plastazote Fabrication***

1. Preheat oven to 250°F (140°C).
2. To protect the client's skin from burns, apply a double-layer wrist-thumb splint liner to two layers of Stockinette or Tubigrip. Protect the thumb by wrapping it with cohesive tape or self-adhesive padding. Therapist must wear heavy gloves when handling hot polyethylene.
3. If the Plastazote is unperforated, punch holes in it with an awl or a nail to prevent air bubbles from being trapped between Plastazote and polyethylene during heating.

4. Place the polyethylene, outer surface down, on the metal sheet and heat until it begins to turn transparent. Then set the Plastazote on top and continue to heat both layers together until the polyethylene is transparent. Plastazote and polyethylene autobond when heated together.

5. Remove from the oven. With Plastazote on the inside, work quickly to mold the material into the transverse arch while pulling it around to the dorsum of the hand; ensure a snug fit at the wrist. Because the working time is short (30 seconds), another person may help by simultaneously molding the forearm portion.

6. Trim to clear the MC heads, thenar eminence, and elbow, and then attach three or four overlap or D-ring Velcro straps.

| | |
|---|---|
| ***Wearing Regimen*** | • As appropriate for the application |
| ***Precautions*** | • See "Half-Shell Wrist Orthoses." |
| | • The opening should not pinch. |
| | • Do not mold polyethylene/Plastazote to a client with inadequate protective sensation. |
| | • Circumferential orthoses can be difficult to apply and may require assistance from another person to hold the sides open. |
| | • Ensure that straps are easy to manage for arthritic fingers (see Fig. 3-16). |
| ***Options*** | • Add a circumferential thumb piece to the thermoplastic design. |
| | • The opening can be dorsal or ulnar. |
| ***Alternatives*** | • Circumferential prefabricated wrist orthoses |
| | • Circumferential precuts such as Dynacast Rapide[16] or QuickCast[17,18] or Wrist Splints; Orfizip[2] or Aquaform[16] Zippered Wrist Splint (see Fig. 7-7c) |
| | • Other custom thermoplastic designs[19] |
| | • Custom Fabric Circumferential Wrist Orthosis[20] |

---

● ● ● ● ● ● ● ● ● ● ● ● ● ● ● ● ● ● ● ● ● ● ● ● ● ● ● ● ● ● ● ● ● ● ● ● ● ●

## ◖ Name: Dorsal Forearm-Based Dynamic Joint-Aligned Coil-Spring Wrist Assistive-Extension Orthosis[21]
(Fig. 10-8 *a, b,* and *c*)

| | |
|---|---|
| ***Common Name*** | Dynamic wrist extension splint |
| ***SCS Name*** | Wrist extension mobilization; type 0[1] |
| ***Objectives*** | • To passively extend the wrist while allowing active wrist flexion |
| | • To prevent contracture of unopposed, innervated wrist flexors |
| ***Indications*** | • Weak or paralyzed wrist extensors (e.g., radial nerve palsy) |
| ***Materials*** | • Category B or C (Aquaplast Resilient is not recommended because it resists imbedding of wires) • Self-adhesive hook Velcro • Loop Velcro or padded equivalent • Thin self-adhesive gel padding • Two prefabricated wrist extension coil springs[2] (see Fig. 4-4c) or 1.5 mm gauge spring wire • Solvent or alcohol |

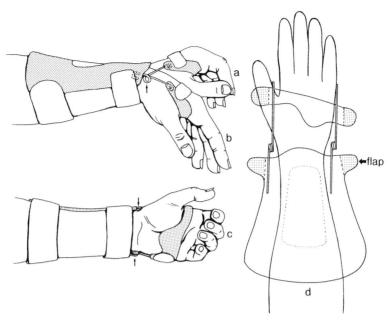

**FIGURE 10-8.** Dorsal forearm-based dynamic-joint-aligned coil-spring wrist assistive-extension orthosis. *(a)* A pair of coil springs, which are aligned with the wrist joint axis, passively extend wrist to about 20° extension. When the wrist is extended, metacarpophalangeals (MCPs) flex. Because of paralysis of the extensor digitorum, active MCP extension is absent. *(b)* The wrist can flex against the resistance of the coil springs. Wrist flexion promotes extension at MCPs despite paralysis of extensor digitorum because of tenodesis action. *(c)* Palmar view. Coil springs (arrows) are aligned with wrist joint axis. The integrated palmar bar is positioned and trimmed to permit full finger MCP and thumb mobility. *(d)* Pattern. The forearm hole (dotted line) is optional. Broken lines represent fold lines. Stippled areas are the flaps that are folded over the bent ends of the coil spring wire. Use the forearm component of the pattern without the flaps and hole for the dorsal forearm-based dynamic arching spring-wire wrist and D1-5 MCP assistive-extension orthosis and the dorsal slab of the bivalved forearm-based dynamic MCP-IP protective-extension and flexion-blocking orthosis.

| | |
|---|---|
| ***Equipment and Tools*** | • Heating pan       • Wire cutter |
| | • Heat gun       • Wire-bending jig to make custom coil springs |
| | • Two pairs of pliers       from spring wire |
| ***Pattern*** | • Figure 10-8*d* |
| ***Fabrication*** | |

1. Cut a strip of gel padding 1¼ in. (3 cm) wide. Apply across the distal forearm to pad the ulnar head and prevent migration.
2. Heat the forearm component; check the temperature and mold.
3. Attach the proximal forearm strap.
4. Heat the palmar component; check the temperature and mold.
5. Align the center of one coil spring over the wrist joint axis medially. Bend the ends of the wire and cut off the excess wire. Mark the location of wire bends on forearm and palmar components. Repeat for the other coil spring on the lateral side.
6. Heat the ends of the wire over the heat gun nozzle and embed them into the thermoplastic.
7. Apply solvent or alcohol, dry heat the flaps, and fold them over the bent ends of the wires. Blend in all edges for a firm bond and for elimination of dirt-collecting crevices.
8. Attach the remaining straps.

| | |
|---|---|
| ***Wearing Regimen*** | • Daytime use to promote function. |
| | • At night use a static wrist orthosis if desired. |
| ***Precaution*** | • Spring wires are easily deformed. |
| | • To prevent injury from a piece of flying wire, cut the wire under a towel, pillowcase, or sheet. |
| ***Alternatives*** | • See Table 7-2. |
| | • Prefabricated static or dynamic orthoses. |

 **Name:** **Dorsal-Volar Forearm-Based Static Wrist Writing/Painting Orthosis** (Fig. 10-9*a* through *d*)

Developed by Matthew Fleet and Brenlee Mogul-Rotman, O.T.(C.) at Lyndhurst Spinal Cord Centre, Toronto, Ontario.

| | |
|---|---|
| ***Common Name*** | Writing splint |
| ***SCS Name*** | Wrist extension immobilization; type 0[1] |
| ***Objectives*** | • To enable writing, drawing, or painting by positioning the wrist in functional extension and providing an attachment for a pen, pencil, or paintbrush. |
| | • To enable erasing of pencil marks or turning of pages with the mounted eraser. |
| ***Indications*** | • **Spinal cord injury** at level C5 or above (wrist extensors are paralyzed) |
| ***Materials*** | • Category B or C—⅛ in. (3.2 mm) thick —Orfit Classic works well because its surface stickiness when warm helps it cling to the client's skin to facilitate molding <ul><li>Self-adhesive hook Velcro</li><li>Loop Velcro</li><li>Solvent or alcohol</li></ul> |
| | • Double nylon roller catch (for cupboard door—available from hardware store) <ul><li>Pen, pencil, paintbrush, and pencil-style eraser (optional)</li></ul> |
| ***Equipment and Tools*** | • Heating pan   • Heat gun   • Scissors |
| ***Pattern*** | • 1 in. (2.5 cm) wide strips of thermoplastic (Fig. 10-9*e*) |
| ***Fabrication*** (Fig. 10-9*e*) | 1. Heat the hand strip, check the temperature, and mold it around the radial side of the hand, leaving the ulnar side of the hand open. |
| | 2. Apply solvent or alcohol, dry heat, bond the volar forearm strip to the hand strip, and then mold it to the client's hand and forearm with the wrist in the desired position. |
| | 3. Heat and bond the J-shaped dorsal piece to the hand strip, mold it over the dorsum of the hand and wrist, around the radial side of the forearm, and then bond it to the volar strip. Attach a Velcro strap that spans the volar strip and the J-shaped piece and a second strap around the ulnar opening of the hand strip. |
| | 4. Heat and attach the two thermoplastic mounting strips to the roller catch. Bond the mounting strips to the handpiece with one strip attached to the inside surface and one to the outside surface. Ensure that the |

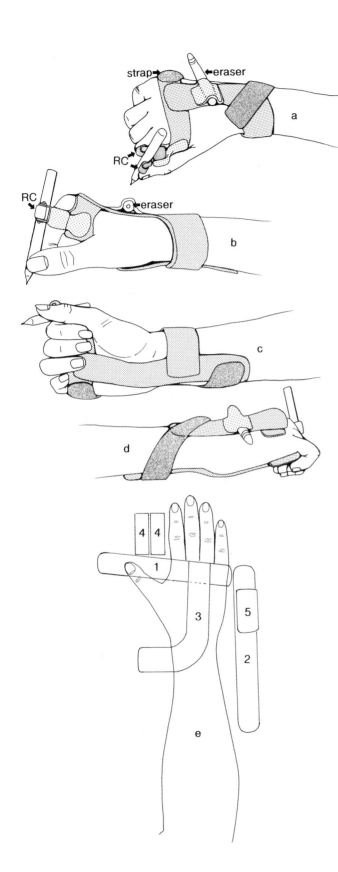

**FIGURE 10-9.** Dorsal-volar forearm-based static wrist-writing/painting orthosis. *(a)* Dorsal view showing the roller catch (RC) gripping a pen and an eraser bonded to the "J"-shaped dorsal piece. *(b)* Radial view. *(c)* Palmar view. *(d)* Ulnar view. The hand strap has been excluded to show the ulnar opening in the hand-piece. *(e)* Pattern. These numbers also refer to the steps in the fabrication process. 1 = hand strip; 2 = volar forearm strip; 3 = J-shaped dorsal piece; 4 = two strips of thermoplastic to mount the roller catch onto the hand strip; 5 = strip of thermoplastic to mount the eraser to the J-shaped dorsal piece.

roller catch is optimally positioned to orient a pen, pencil, or paintbrush toward a working surface. Slip a pen, pencil, or paintbrush between the rollers.

5. Attach the eraser to the J-shaped piece with the piece of thermoplastic.

| | |
|---|---|
| *Wearing Regimen* | • For writing, drawing, or painting activities. |
| *Precautions* | • Extra caution is required when checking the temperature of the warm thermoplastic because the client lacks full sensation in the forearm and hand. |
| | • Ensure that the client can apply and remove the orthosis independently. |
| *Options* | • Mount a second roller catch for the eraser. |
| | • Delete the eraser. |
| | • Incorporate the thumb and index into the design for increased support. |
| *Alternatives* | • Prefabricated forearm- or hand-based writing orthoses[22,23] |

---

**Name:**     **Radial Forearm-Based Static Wrist-Thumb Orthosis[24]**
(Fig. 10-10*a* and *b*)

| | |
|---|---|
| *Common Names* | • De Quervain's static splint |
| | • Wrist and thumb static splint |
| | • Long thumb CMC immobilization splint |
| | • Long opponens splint |
| | • Radial thumb gutter splint |
| | • Wrist-thumb orthosis for de Quervain's tenosynovitis |
| *SCS Name* | • Thumb MP extension immobilization; type 2[3]<br>(The secondary joints are the thumb CMC and the wrist.) |
| *Objectives* | • To immobilize the wrist, thumb CMC and MCP joints, which are crossed by the inflamed tendons (the IP is generally left free because the inflamed tendons do not cross it) |
| | • To rest and reduce inflammation |
| *Indications* | • De Quervain's tenosynovitis (stenosing tenosynovitis)—inflammation of the tendons of abductor pollicis longus and extensor pollicis brevis in their synovial sheaths in extensor tunnel 1 (Fig. 10-10*c*) |
| *Advantage of This Design* | • Compared with the volar version described later, the radial design allows more mobility of the distal transverse arch and the ulnar side of wrist. |
| *Materials* | • Category C or D thermoplastic—¹⁄₁₆ or ³⁄₃₂ in. (1.6 or 2.4 mm) thick |
| | • For a more flexible but bulkier support, use Kushionsplint[16] |
| | • Self-adhesive hook Velcro |
| | • Loop Velcro or padded alternative |
| | • ¹⁄₁₆ in. (1.6 mm) self-adhesive foam padding or hand cream |

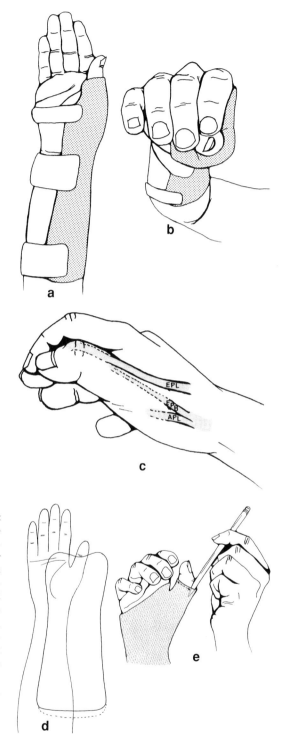

**FIGURE 10-10.** Radial forearm-based static wrist-thumb orthosis. *(a)* Volar view. *(b)* Fingertip view. *(c)* Tendons of the anatomical snuffbox affected by de Quervain's tenosynovitis. The abductor pollicus longus (APL) and extensor pollicus brevis (EPB) in the first tunnel under the extensor retinaculum are inflamed. The APL acts on the first CMC while EPB acts on the first MCP. As a result, these two joints, as well as the wrist, must be immobilized to reduce tendon inflammation. The extensor pollicus longus (EPL), acting on the interphalangeal joint (IP), is usually not involved; as a result, the IP can be left free to move. *(d)* Pattern. See the legend for Figure 10-2*c* for discussion of cut/fold lines at proximal edge. *(e)* Flaring around thumb edge with a pencil, shown on the volar forearm-based static wrist-thumb orthosis.

| | |
|---|---|
| ***Equipment and Tools*** | • Heating pan    • Scissors    • Heat gun    • Oven for Kushionsplint<br>• For the pattern: paper towel or flexible clear plastic with permanent marker and straight pins, stapler, or tape |
| ***Client's Position*** | • Seated with the forearm neutral and resting on the ulnar border for gravity-assisted molding |
| ***Therapist's Position*** | • Seated beside or across from the client |
| ***Joint Positions*** | • Wrist: as appropriate for most functional activities<br>• Thumb: positioned to promote easy opposition |
| ***Pattern*** | • Figure 10-10*d* |
| ***Fabrication*** | 1. When using translucent thermoplastics with memory, wrap the thumb with ⅟₁₆ in. (1.6 mm) self-adhesive foam to prevent excessive shrinkage as the thermoplastic cools, or apply hand cream to the client's thumb.<br>2. Heat, check the temperature, and drape the material over the radial side of the forearm and thumb, overlapping the material in the first web space.<br>3. Place the thumb in opposition with the index and middle fingers (see Fig. 2-25*b*).<br>4. Gently flare the distal thumb edge by running a pencil or pen under it (Fig. 10-10*e*).<br>5. Smooth out any creases at the base of the thumb by stretching the thumb piece upward.<br>6. Mark the trim lines to allow full finger MCP and thumb IP flexion, remove the orthosis, and trim.<br>7. Gently flare the proximal edge and smooth all edges.<br>8. Apply three Velcro straps around the forearm, wrist, and hand. |
| ***Wearing Regimen*** | • All the time to rest inflamed tendons |
| ***Precautions*** | • Ensure easy thumb opposition. If wrist and MCPs need to radially deviate for the middle finger to oppose the thumb, insufficient opposition was achieved. Remold to correct thumb position.<br>• Ensure that wrist position is a good compromise to facilitate most activities.<br>• The finger MCPs and thumb IP should be unrestricted.<br>• Avoid pressure over the radial styloid.<br>• Provides minimal support for an inflamed or unstable wrist joint—use the volar design described next. |
| ***Options*** | • Extend the thumb piece distally to immobilize the IP circumferentially, or provide a dorsal IP extension block.<br>• Volar forearm-based static wrist-thumb orthosis described next.<br>• Build up a pen with self-adhesive foam or Rubazote to relieve some irritation to inflamed tendons when writing. |
| ***Alternatives*** | • Zipper precuts—Orfizip Wrist and Thumb Splint[2]; Rolyan® Aquaform Zippered Wrist and Thumb Splint[16]<br>• Precuts—Dynacast Rapide[16] or QuickCast[17,18] Thumb Spica Forearm Splint<br>• Prefabricated soft radial or circumferential designs |

**Name:** **Volar Forearm-Based Static Wrist-Thumb Orthosis**[25,26]
(Fig. 10-11*a*)

| | |
|---|---|
| ***Common Names*** | • See previous orthosis<br>• Scaphoid fracture splint |
| ***SCS Name*** | • Thumb MC extension immobilization; type 2[3] |
| ***Objectives*** | • To immobilize the wrist and thumb CMC and MCP joints<br>• To rest the hand to reduce inflammation<br>• To stabilize the wrist and thumb |
| ***Indications*** | • De Quervain's tenosynovitis (stenosing tenosynovitis) (Fig. 10-10*c*)<br>• Quadriplegia[27–29]<br>• Instability or joint inflammation of the wrist and thumb CMC/MCP (e.g., rheumatoid arthritis)[30]<br>• Scaphoid fracture<br>• Bennett's fracture-dislocation—at the base of the first MC |
| ***Advantage of This Design*** | • Provides better volar support for the carpal bones than the radial design |
| ***Materials*** | • Category C thermoplastic— $\frac{1}{16}$ or $\frac{3}{32}$ in. (1.6 or 2.4 mm) thick<br>• For a more flexible but bulkier support, use Kushionsplint[16]    • Self-adhesive hook Velcro<br>• Loop Velcro or padded alternative<br>• $\frac{1}{16}$ in. (1.6 mm) self-adhesive foam padding or hand cream |

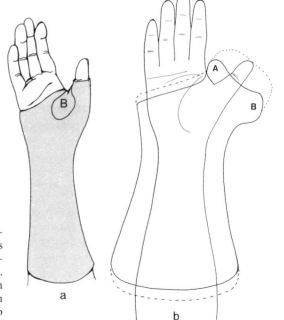

**FIGURE 10-11.** Volar forearm-based static wrist-thumb orthosis. *(a)* Volar view. Dotted line shows optional IP extension block. *(b)* Pattern. See the legend for Figure 10-2*c* for discussion of cut/fold lines. If IP immobilization is necessary, extend the pattern distally around the thumb to the dotted line. When molding, flap A is pulled dorsally through the thumb web space and flap B is pulled volarly.

| | |
|---|---|
| ***Equipment and Tools*** | • Heating pan      • Scissors      • Heat gun<br>• Oven for Kushionsplint<br>• For the pattern: paper towel or flexible clear plastic with permanent marker and straight pins, stapler, or tape |
| ***Client's Position*** | • Seated with forearm supinated for gravity-assisted molding |
| ***Joint Position*** | • Wrist: as appropriate for the condition<br>• Thumb: positioned to promote easy opposition (see Fig. 2-25*b*) |
| ***Pattern*** | • Figure 10-11*b*<br>• Extend the pattern to the broken line when using ¹⁄₁₆ in. (1.6 mm) thick thermoplastic, and fold the distal and proximal edges over about ¼ in. (½ cm) during molding to strengthen the orthosis. |
| ***Fabrication*** | 1. See the radial design described previously.<br>2. Stretch A through the web space of the thumb from volar to dorsal.<br>3. Stretch B around the dorsum of the thumb and through the web space from dorsal to volar.<br>4. Smooth out any creases at the base of the thumb by stretching the thumb piece upward.<br>5. Gently flare the proximal edge.<br>6. Apply three straps over the proximal forearm and wrist and optionally across the hand. |
| ***Wearing Regimen*** | • As appropriate for the condition. |
| ***Precautions*** | • See radial design described previously. |
| ***Options*** | • See radial design described previously.<br>• Extend the thumb portion distally (to the dotted line) to immobilize the thumb IP (Fig. 10-11*b*). |
| ***Alternatives*** | • See radial design. |

**Name:** **Volar Forearm-Based Static Wrist and D2-5 MCP-Stabilizing Orthosis**[30] (Fig. 10-12*a* and *b*)

| | |
|---|---|
| ***Common Name*** | Wrist MCP splint |
| ***SCS Name*** | Wrist and index through small finger MP extension immobilization; type 0[5] |
| ***Objectives*** | • To immobilize the wrist and finger MCPs<br>• To relieve pain and inflammation<br>• To prevent or correct joint deformity (e.g., wrist radial deviation and volar subluxation; MCP ulnar drift and volar subluxation)<br>• To unload lax joint capsules and ligaments or promote resorption and correct joint instability |
| ***Indications*** | • Joint inflammation (e.g., rheumatoid arthritis with or without carpal tunnel syndrome) |

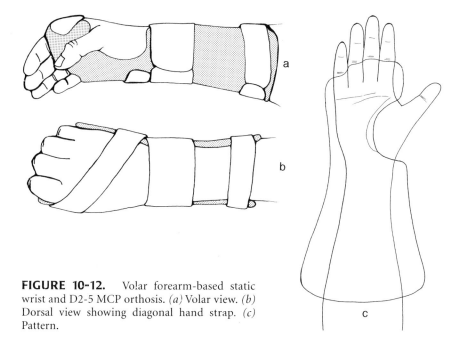

**FIGURE 10-12.** Volar forearm-based static wrist and D2-5 MCP orthosis. *(a)* Volar view. *(b)* Dorsal view showing diagonal hand strap. *(c)* Pattern.

| | |
|---|---|
| *Rationale* | • See Chapter 2. |
| *Advantages of This Design* | • In contrast to a full hand orthosis, the finger IPs and thumb are left free for opposition, allowing enough dexterity to apply the contralateral orthosis and manipulate light switches, bed covers, and other items.<br>• The IPs and thumb naturally fall into their loose-packed positions. |
| *Materials* | • Category C thermoplastic—3/32 in. (2.4 mm) thick, perforated, or use Hexcelite for ventilation and light weight<br>• Self-adhesive hook Velcro<br>• Padded Velcro strap |
| *Equipment and Tools* | • Heating pan          • Scissors          • Heat gun |
| *Joint Positions* | • Wrist neutral to slight extension, no deviation; MCPs in slight flexion so that opposition with thumb is possible; thumb unrestricted.<br>• See Chapter 2, "Joint Mechanics and Considerations for Positioning Hand Joints." |
| *Client's Position* | • Seated with forearm supinated for gravity-assisted molding. If supination is difficult, gravity-resisted molding with the forearm in pronation is possible, using category B thermoplastic and bandage wrapping. |
| *Therapist's Position* | • Seated across from the client. |
| *Pattern* | • Figure 10-12*c* |
| *Fabrication* | 1. Heat the pattern and cut out.<br>2. Reheat, check temperature, and mold, positioning the joints as described previously and conforming to the contours, especially the transverse arch. |

3. Gently flare the proximal and distal edges.

4. Attach the straps. Note the diagonal orientation of the strap across the hand to avoid volar forces over the proximal phalanges, which would promote MCP volar subluxation (Fig. 10-11*b*).

*Wearing Regimen*

• Worn at night.
• When joints are inflamed, use also during daytime rest periods.

*Precautions*

• A strap across the proximal phalanges is contraindicated because it promotes MCP volar subluxation.
• Ensure that the straps are easy to manage for arthritic fingers (see Fig. 3-16).
• Finger IPs and thumb should be unrestricted.
• Immobilization of MCPs puts more stress on distal joints, which could aggravate inflammation in susceptible arthritic joints.

*Alternatives*

• Volar or circumferential forearm-based static wrist orthosis (Figs. 10-2*a* and 10-7*a*)
• Circumferential prefabricated wrist orthoses/splints
• Volar (or circumferential) hand-based static D2-5 MCP-stabilizing orthosis (see Fig. 11-2)
• Circumferential hand-based dynamic traction D2-5 MCP corrective-radial-deviation orthosis (see Fig. 11-3)
• Prefabricated hand-based MCP orthoses/splints

---

● **● ● ● ● ● ● ● ● ● ● ● ● ● ● ● ● ● ● ● ● ● ● ● ● ● ● ● ● ● ● ● ● ● ● ● ● ● ● ● ●**

**Name:** **Dorsal Forearm-Based Dynamic Arching Spring-Wire D1-5 MCP Assistive-Extension Orthosis**[21,31]
(Fig. 10-13*a* through *d*)

The wrist is immobilized but not named because it is not a target joint. However, identifying the forearm base implies the inclusion of the wrist.

*Common Name*

Radial nerve splint; MCP extension-assist splint; MCP arthroplasty splint

*SCS Name*

Index through small finger MP extension mobilization; type 1[5](The wrist is the secondary joint.)

*Objectives*

• To immobilize the wrist in a functional position and passively extend the MCPs to 0° while permitting full active MCP flexion and unrestricted IP motion
• To prevent contractures

*Indications*

• When the extensors of the wrist, finger MCPs, and thumb are paralyzed or weak.[32] (For a radial nerve lesion, IP extensors, i.e., lumbricals and interossei, are unaffected because they are innervated by the median and ulnar nerves.)
• MCP arthroplasty—angle the wires to pull the MCPs radially.

*Advantages of This Design*

• When the client makes a fist, the wires are pulled in close and the hand can be slipped into a pocket.
• The hand can be slipped through a loose sleeve with the orthosis on.

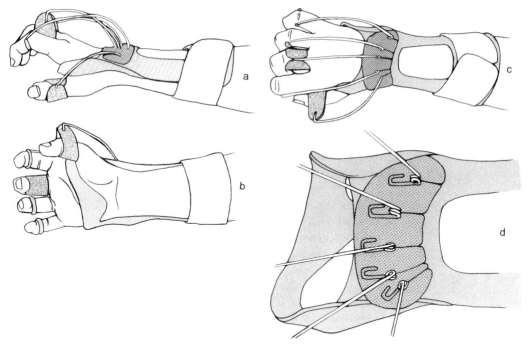

**FIGURE 10-13.** Dorsal forearm-based dynamic arching spring-wire D1-5 MCP assistive-extension orthosis. *(a)* and *(b)* This orthosis demonstrates finger loops for the thumb and middle fingers. The index, ring, and little fingers have finger hooks formed from the coil spring wire, covered with thin thermoplastic. The finger hooks create a lower profile than the finger loops; however, loops are easier to fabricate. Use either all loops or all hooks for consistency. *(c)* Dorsal view. *(d)* Close-up of embedded coil spring bases covered with a reinforcement strip of thermoplastic (stippled). Note the orientation of the bases or the coil springs and the more proximal location of the bases for the ring and little fingers.

| | |
|---|---|
| *Materials* | • Category C thermoplastic—⅛ in. (3.2 mm) for the orthosis; 1/16 in. (1.6 mm) to cover finger hooks<br>• Thin self-adhesive foam or gel padding<br>• Self-adhesive foam or gel padding<br>• Self-adhesive hook Velcro<br>• Loop Velcro or padded alternative<br>• Prefabricated finger extension-assist coil springs (0.9 mm gauge)[2]<br>• Finger loops (alternative to finger hooks)<br>• Solvent or alcohol |

*Equipment and Tools*

• Heating pan
• Heat gun
• Scissors
• Permanent marker

• Two pairs of pliers—ideally, one is round nosed to form the finger hooks
• Wire cutter

*Wrist Position*

• Position the wrist in the desired amount of extension and deviation. (See Chapter 2, "Joint Mechanics and Considerations for Positioning Hand Joints.")

*Client's Position*

• Seated with the forearm pronated for gravity-assisted molding on a height-adjustable stool at a comfortable work height for the therapist

*Therapist's Position*  • Standing behind the client's shoulder to mold the thermoplastic base (see Fig. 7-4*b*)

*Pattern*  • Use Figure 10-3*c*.

*Fabrication*

1. Apply padding to the ulnar head.
2. Mold the thermoplastic base as for the dorsal forearm-based static wrist orthosis described earlier in this chapter.
3. Attach the forearm strap. A wrist strap is optional.
4. Apply the orthosis and mark the location for each coil spring base, near the wrist, aligned with the radial side of each finger (midway between the MC heads) and the ulnar side of thumb. Position the base for the small finger as close to the wrist as possible (Fig. 10-13*d*). Note that the fifth PIP is about 1 in. (2.5 cm) closer to the wrist than the third PIP. If the base is anchored too distal, the arching wire will be too short and cause MCP hyperextension.
5. For MCP arthroplasty, increase the radial orientation of the wire to each finger to apply force in the radial direction to the MCP joint capsule.
6. With the orthosis on the client's hand to stabilize it, heat the base of each coil spring in turn over the heat gun nozzle and embed the coil springs at the marked locations, using pliers to push the hot wire into the thermoplastic. *Be careful not to injure the eyes with the sharp ends of the coil springs.*
7. Apply solvent or alcohol around the embedded wires and a reinforcement strip of thermoplastic, 1 × 4 in. (2.5 × 10 cm). Use the heat gun to slightly warm the recipient area of the orthosis and to fully heat the reinforcement strip. Bond the reinforcement over the top of the coil spring bases (Fig. 10-13*d*). Blend in all the edges for a firm bond and to eliminate dirt-collecting crevices. *Do not stress the wires before the reinforcement has fully cooled.*
8. Forming the finger hooks:
   a. While the client makes a fist, bend the coil spring down until it intersects the volar side of the PIP, and mark this location with a permanent marker.
   b. Remove the orthosis and use pliers to bend the wire 90° at the mark, down toward the palm.
   c. Use round-nose pliers to form a U-shaped hook that matches the contour of volar side of the PIP.
   d. When the finger flexors are relaxed, the wires will passively extend the MCPs to 0°, and each hook should be positioned at, or just proximal to, the PIP.
   e. Ask the client to make a fist and check that the arching wire passes between the MC heads without impinging on the web space. If impingement occurs, adjust the shape of the arch. If this does not relieve the impingement, the hook was formed too proximally and the wire will need to be unbent and the hook re-formed more distally. If a wire hits an MC head, bend it to pass between MC heads.
   f. Cut off the extra wire.
   g. Remove the orthosis. Heat a piece of the thin thermoplastic, about ½ × 1½ in. (1 × 3 cm) and cover each hook, blending in any crevices.
9. Alternate method—finger loops:

a. One finger at a time, hold the MCP in extension with the wire parallel to the finger. Mark the midpoint of the proximal phalanx and bend the wire 90° at the mark, down toward the palm.

b. Use a prefabricated finger loop, or use loop Velcro to make a custom sling to slip over the proximal phalanx.

c. Using pliers, bend the wire through the holes of the finger loop and cut off the excess wire.

*Wearing Regimen*
- During functional activities.
- At night, or for social situations, use a static wrist orthosis—custom (described earlier) or prefabricated.

*Precautions*
- Spring wires are easily bent and thus not appropriate for some clients.
- Ensure that the wires do not impinge on the web spaces or the MC heads when the fingers are flexed.
- Ensure that the MCPs are not hyperextended.
- To prevent injury from a piece of flying wire, cut the wire under a towel, pillowcase, or sheet.

*Options*
- Thermoplastic-covered wire hooks or finger loops.
- Delete the thumb wire for MCP arthroplasty.

*Alternatives*
- Static half-shell or circumferential wrist orthoses (described earlier in this chapter).
- See Figures 1-11*b*, 3-10*a* and*b*.
- See Table 7-2.
- For MCP arthroplasty.[33,34]
- Other outrigger designs.[35]

---

**Name:** **Dorsal Forearm-Based Dynamic Arching Spring-Wire Wrist and D1-5 MCP Assistive-Extension Orthosis** (Fig. 10-14)

*Common Name*     Radial nerve splint; wrist-MCP extension-assist splint

*SCS Name*     Wrist and MP extension mobilization; type 0[5]

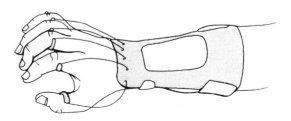

**FIGURE 10-14.** Dorsal forearm-based dynamic arching spring-wire wrist and D1-5 MCP assistive-extension orthosis.

| | |
|---|---|
| *Objectives* | • To passively extend the wrist to about 20° and the MCPs to 0°, while permitting passive wrist and MCP flexion and unrestricted IP motion. |
| *Indications* | • See previous orthosis.<br>• Not suitable for MCP arthroplasty because of the lack of wrist support. |
| *Advantages of This Design* | • See previous orthosis.<br>• Applies dynamic forces to the wrist and MCPs. |
| *Materials* | • See previous orthosis.<br>• Very thin self-adhesive gel padding. |
| *Equipment and Tools* | • Heating pan       • Scissors<br>• Heat gun          • Two pairs of pliers—ideally, one is round nosed<br>• Elastic bandage roll    to form finger hooks |
| *Client's Position* | • Seated with forearm pronated for gravity-assisted molding, on a height-adjustable stool at a comfortable height for the client |
| *Therapist's Position* | • Standing behind the client's shoulder to mold the thermoplastic base (see Fig. 7-4*b*) |
| *Pattern* | • Use the forearm piece in Figure 10-8*d*, deleting the flaps.<br>• The forearm base begins at the wrist, extends two thirds up the forearm from the wrist and two thirds down the sides of the forearm. The hole over the forearm is optional. |
| *Fabrication* | 1. Heat the thermoplastic and apply gel padding to the entire inner surface of the thermoplastic, and then mold it to the forearm. Alternatively, apply a 2 in. (5 cm) wide strip to the thermoplastic at the distal end of the forearm.<br>2. Mold the material.<br>3. Attach the wrist and forearm straps. The location of the embedded coil springs at the wrist necessitates side patches for the wrist strap.<br>4. To prop up the wrist in the desired amount of extension, place a bandage roll in the palm of the hand.<br>5. Attach the wires to the distal end of the forearm as per the previous orthosis.<br>6. Either form thermoplastic-covered hooks or use finger loops (Fig. 10-13*a* through *c*). |
| *Wearing Regimen* | • See dorsal forearm-based dynamic arching spring-wire MCP assistive-extension orthosis |
| *Precautions* | • See dorsal forearm-based dynamic arching spring-wire MCP assistive-extension orthosis |
| *Options* | • Thermoplastic-covered hooks or use finger loops |
| *Alternatives* | • See Table 7-2<br>• See dorsal forearm-based dynamic arching spring-wire MCP assistive-extension orthosis<br>• Dorsal forearm-based dynamic low profile wrist and D2-5 MCP assistive-extension orthosis[36] (Fig. 10-15) |

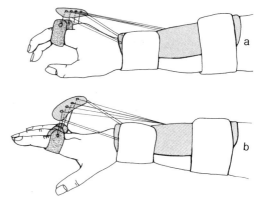

**FIGURE 10-15.** Dorsal forearm-based dynamic low-profile wrist and D2-5 MCP assistive-extension orthosis. This design uses a low-profile outrigger formed from outrigger wire. Thermoplastic has been bonded over the end and holes have been punched through to act as pulleys. *(a)* When the muscles are relaxed, the elastics pull the wrist into extension and the MCPs are somewhat flexed. *(b)* When the wrist flexes, the elastics pull the MCPs into extension.

 **Name:** **Volar Forearm-Based Dynamic D2-5 MCP Corrective-Flexion Orthosis**[37] (Fig. 10-16)

The wrist is immobilized but not named because it is not a target joint. However, identifying the forearm base implies the inclusion of the wrist.

| | |
|---|---|
| *Common Name* | Dynamic MCP flexion splint |
| *SCS Name* | Index through small finger MP flexion mobilization; type 1[5] |
| *Objectives* | • To gently stress the MCP collateral ligaments to promote desired growth and increase flexion range |
| *Indications* | • Extension contracture of the MCPs caused by shortened collateral ligaments |
| *Rationale* | • See Chapter 2, "Promoting Tissue Growth to Reduce Contractures." |
| *Advantages of This Design* | • The maxi-perforated thermoplastic pulley enables a 90° angle of pull on the proximal phalanx. (See "Adjustment" following.) |
| *Materials* | • For the static base: category C thermoplastic—³⁄₃₂ in. (2.4 mm) thick |
| | • For the pulley: maxi-perforated translucent category B or C thermoplastic—⅛ in. (3.2 mm) thick |
| | • ¹⁄₁₆ in. (1.6 mm) self-adhesive gel lining to prevent distal migration |
| | • Solvent or alcohol |
| | • Self-adhesive hook Velcro |
| | • Loop Velcro or padded alternative |
| | • Finger slings |
| | • Long elastic bands, elastic thread, or wrapped elastic cord |
| *Equipment and Tools* | • Heating pan   • Heat gun   • Scissors |
| *Client's Position* | • Seated with the forearm supinated for gravity-assisted molding (Fig. 7-4*a*) |

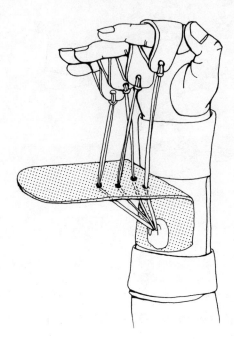

**FIGURE 10-16.** Volar forearm-based dynamic MCP corrective-flexion orthosis. Maxi-perforated thermoplastic projecting from the forearm base acts as a pulley to ensure that the line of pull of the elastic band traction is 90° to the axis of the proximal phalanx and toward the scaphoid bone. The elastics are anchored proximally to a hook molded from thermoplastic.

| | |
|---|---|
| *Therapist's Position* | • Seated across from the client |
| *Pattern* | • Use Figure 10-2*c*. |
| *Fabrication* | 1. Heat, check the temperature, and mold the forearm base as for the volar forearm-based static thumb-hole wrist orthosis described earlier in this chapter. |
| | 2. Gently flare the proximal and distal edges. |
| | 3. Attach the proximal forearm and hand straps. |
| | 4. Apply solvent or alcohol, dry heat, and bond the thermoplastic pulley to the forearm base. |
| | 5. Form a thermoplastic hook and bond it to the base, proximal to the pulley. |
| | 6. Slip the finger loop over the proximal phalanx. |
| | 7. Tie an elastic to each finger sling. |
| | 8. Flex each MCP until the client feels slight stretch, ensuring that the elastic pulls 90° to the long axis of the phalanx and generally toward the scaphoid bone. |
| | 9. Thread each elastic through an appropriate hole in the maxi-perforated thermoplastic pulley, and attach the proximal end of each elastic to the thermoplastic hook. |
| *Adjustment* | • When MCP flexion is limited, the elastics will pass through holes near the tip of the pulley. As flexion range improves, rethread the elastic through holes progressively closer to the forearm base. |
| *Wearing Regimen* | • Several hours per day to provide gentle, prolonged stretch. |
| *Precaution* | • Avoid excessive flexion force. |

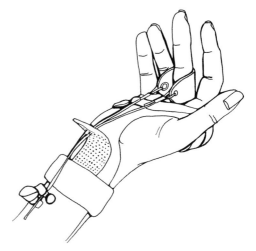

**FIGURE 10-17.** Volar forearm-based static-progressive MERiT™-screw MCP-flexion orthosis. The prefabricated MERiT component has a thumb screw to tighten the nylon lines attached to the finger slings in small increments as MCP flexion improves. (MERiT™ is a trademark of Upper Extremity Technology [UE Tech]).

| | |
|---|---|
| *Options* | • Replace the thermoplastic pulley with a static progressive outrigger (MERiT screw) (Fig. 10-17).<br>• Apply corrective force to the specific affected digit(s). |
| *Alternatives* | • Prefabricated flexion glove |

 **Name:** **Volar Forearm-Based Static (or Serial-Static) C-Bar Wrist-Hand Orthosis** (Fig. 10-18*a* through *c*)

| | |
|---|---|
| *Common Name* | Resting hand splint |
| *SCS Name* | Wrist extension, index through small finger MCP and IP extension, thumb CMC palmar abduction immobilization/mobilization; type 0[16] |
| *Objectives* | • To immobilize the wrist, MCPs, and IPs of fingers and thumb<br>• To prevent or reduce contractures<br>• To reduce pain and inflammation |

| *Indications* | | |
|---|---|---|
| | • Skin graft | • Burns[40] |
| | • Scleroderma[38] | • Inflammatory joint disease[41,42] |
| | • **Dupuytren's** release[39] | • Crush injury |
| | • Boxer's fracture (neck of fifth MC) | • **Replantation** |
| | | • **Flaccid** paralysis[43] |

| | |
|---|---|
| *Materials* | • Category A, B, or C thermoplastic—$\frac{3}{32}$ or $\frac{1}{8}$ in. (2.4 or 3.2 mm) thick<br>• Self-adhesive hook Velcro<br>• Loop Velcro or padded alternative |

| *Equipment* | | |
|---|---|---|
| | • Heating pan | • For the pattern: paper towel or flexible clear plastic with permanent marker and straight pins, stapler, or tape |
| | • Heat gun | |
| | • Scissors | • Elastic bandage, Thera-Band, or Orfiband for gravity-resisted molding |

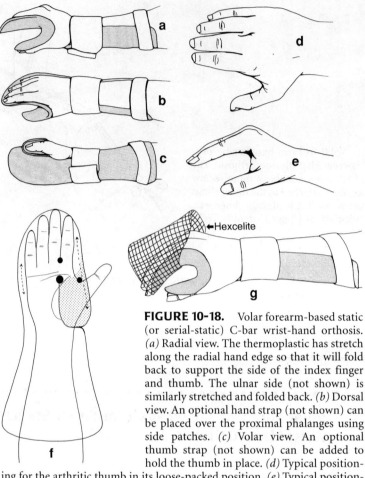

←Hexcelite

**FIGURE 10-18.** Volar forearm-based static (or serial-static) C-bar wrist-hand orthosis. *(a)* Radial view. The thermoplastic has stretch along the radial hand edge so that it will fold back to support the side of the index finger and thumb. The ulnar side (not shown) is similarly stretched and folded back. *(b)* Dorsal view. An optional hand strap (not shown) can be placed over the proximal phalanges using side patches. *(c)* Volar view. An optional thumb strap (not shown) can be added to hold the thumb in place. *(d)* Typical positioning for the arthritic thumb in its loose-packed position. *(e)* Typical positioning for the burned hand. The thumb web space is well rounded. When the dorsum of the fingers has been burned, the IPs must be completely extended. *(f)* Pattern. Mark the base of the first and second web spaces (small dots) to landmark the end of the cut line for the thumb piece (large dot). The thumb piece (stippled) can be deleted if thumb support is not required. The arrows (broken lines) indicate where the thermoplastic should be prestretched when using category A or B, so that thermoplastic will fold back to support sides of hand. *(g)* Hexcelite (open weave thermoplastic) has been bonded to the orthosis to create a protective hood, for example after replantation.

*Joint Positions*

- For inflammatory joint disease: wrist neutral to slight extension; MCPs and IPs slightly flexed; thumb neutral with well-rounded web space (Fig. 10-18*d*).
- For hand trauma: MCPs flexed about 60°, IPs extended (for dorsal burns) or slightly flexed; well-rounded first web space (Fig. 10-18*e*). For boxer's fracture, delete the thumb support.
- For Dupuytren's release, position the joints to maintain surgically gained extension of the MCPs and IPs.
- See Chapter 2, "Joint Mechanics and Considerations for Positioning Hand Joints."

orearm supinated for gravity-assisted molding. If
ult, gravity-resisted molding with the forearm in
le, using category A or B thermoplastic and bandage
-5).

| | |
|---|---|
| ***Pattern*** | • Figure 10-18*f* |
| ***Fabrication*** | 1. Heat and cut out the pattern.<br>2. Reheat. If using category A or B, prestretch the thermoplastic along the edge that borders the first web space and beside the fifth MC head before molding on client (Fig. 10-18*f* ).<br>3. Mold to the volar surface of the hand, controlling positions of all the incorporated joints.<br>4. Mark trim lines, remove the orthosis when the material is set but still warm, and trim.<br>5. Gently flare the proximal edge.<br>6. Apply straps (Fig. 10-18*a* through *c*). |
| ***Wearing Regimen*** | • For inflamed joints, during night and daytime rest periods<br>• For acute burns or other trauma, all the time |
| ***Precautions*** | • Thumb abduction occurs at the CMC joint. Do not stress the ulnar collateral ligament of the first MCP when attempting to abduct the thumb, especially if the CMC is contracted or the MCP is lax.<br>• Check carefully for pressure points, especially if the client lacks full sensation and may not feel discomfort. |
| ***Options*** | • The hand strap is optional, depending on the situation. It can be placed across the proximal phalanges or diagonally as in Figure 10-12*b*.<br>• Delete straps and use either sterile gauze bandage (for acute burns) or elastic bandage (for edema).<br>• For Dupuytren's release, not all the fingers need to be immobilized.<br>• Leave the IPs free (Fig. 10-12*a* and *b*).<br>• Omit the thumb piece and use it as the volar component of the bivalved forearm-based dynamic MCP-IP protective-extension flexion-blocking orthosis for extensor tendon repair (described later).<br>• Attach a Hexcelite protective hood (Fig. 10-18*g*)<br>• For inflamed joints, leave the thumb and finger IPs free as in volar forearm-based static wrist-MCP orthosis described earlier.<br>• Mold the orthosis from Hexcelite for a lightweight well-ventilated orthosis.<br>• Delete the forearm base and convert it into a hand-based orthosis, especially for Dupuytren's release. |
| ***Alternatives*** | • Precuts<br>• Preformed splints<br>• Bisurfaced forearm-based static wrist-hand orthosis (following) |

● ● ● ● ● ● ● ● ● ● ● ● ● ● ● ● ● ● ● ● ● ● ● ● ● ● ● ● ● ● ● ● ● ● ● ● ● ● ● ● ● ● ● ● ● ● ● ● ●

## ◐ Name: Bisurfaced Forearm-Based Static (or Serial-Static) Wrist-Hand Orthosis[21,31] (Fig. 10-19*a* and *b*)

| | |
|---|---|
| ***Common Names*** | Antispasticity splint; dorsal volar hand splint |
| ***SCS Name*** | Wrist extension, index through small finger MCP and IP extension, thumb CMC palmar abduction immobilization/mobilization; type 0[16] |
| ***Objectives*** | • To immobilize the wrist, MCPs, and IPs of fingers and thumb<br>• To prevent or reduce contractures<br>• To reduce tone of hypertonic muscles[44–47] |

***Indications***

- Hand trauma or surgery (see previous orthosis) when it is desirable for the proximal palm or volar surface of the forearm to be uncovered

- High tone associated with
  - Head injury
  - Cerebral palsy
  - Multiple sclerosis
  - Cerebrovascular accident

***Materials***

- Category B or C thermoplastic —³⁄₃₂ or ⅛ in. (2.4 or 3.2 mm) thick
- Loop Velcro or padded alternative

- Self-adhesive hook Velcro
- Thin self-adhesive foam or gel padding
- Solvent or alcohol

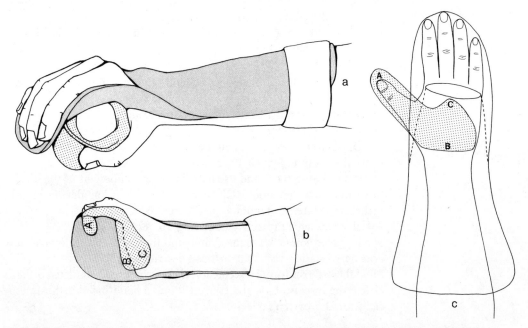

**FIGURE 10-19.**   Bisurfaced forearm-based static (or serial static) wrist-hand orthosis. *(a)* Radial view. *(b)* Volar view. A, B, and C correspond to labels on the pattern. *(c)* Pattern. When the thumb piece (stippled) is bonded to the base, B is attached under the MC heads, A is attached under the index fingertip, and C is oriented toward the wrist.

| | |
|---|---|
| *Equipment and Tools* | • Heating pan    • Scissors    • Heat gun<br>• For the pattern: paper towel or flexible clear plastic with permanent marker and straight pins, stapler, or tape |
| *Joint Positions* | • For hand trauma: MCPs flexed about 60°; IPs extended or slightly flexed; wrist extended 20° to 30° to balance tension in long finger flexors and extensors (see Fig. 2-9*b*)<br>• For high tone: wrist and IPs in submaximal extension (rationale: see Chapter 2, "Spasticity") |
| *Client's Position* | • Seated with forearm pronated for gravity-assisted molding on a height-adjustable stool at a comfortable height for the therapist. |
| *Therapist's Position* | • Standing behind the client's shoulder to mold the thermoplastic base (see Fig. 7-4*b*). The assistance of a second person may be helpful if tone is high. |
| *Pattern* | • Figure 10-19*c*.<br>• Use the contralateral hand for the pattern if necessary. |
| *Fabrication* | 1. Before molding, use tone-inhibiting techniques to suppress flexor tone, if appropriate.<br>2. Apply padding to the ulnar head. When using thermoplastics with memory, adhere a 1 in. (2.5 cm) wide strip of thin padding around the MC heads to avoid excess shrinkage.<br>3. Heat the thermoplastic, check the temperature, and slip the hand through the hole, draping the material over the forearm and the volar material against the MC heads and fingers.<br>4. Fold the "wings" upward along the fold lines and hold them in place with the thenar eminence of each hand (see Fig. 7-4*b*).<br>5. Use the index or middle finger of one hand to conform the material to the transverse arch. At the same time, control wrist flexion/extension and deviation to achieve the desired wrist positioning.<br>6. Position the MCPs and IPs. If it is difficult to control all joints simultaneously, heat and mold in two stages—forearm and then hand.<br>7. Mark the trim lines, remove the orthosis when the material is set but still warm, and trim.<br>8. Discard the padding around the MC heads and transfer the padding from the ulnar head to the inside of the orthosis, or discard to leave a space.<br>9. Attach a forearm strap; a wrist strap is optional.<br>10. Thumb piece attachment (Fig. 10-19*b*): Apply solvent or alcohol to the attachment sites on the base and thumb pieces; use the heat gun to warm the recipient areas and fully heat the thumb piece. Invert the thumb piece from its orientation in Figure 10-19*c*, attach B at the MC heads, and reflect A back to attach at the tip of the index finger. C is molded to the palm of the hand. As the material cools, position the thumb as desired. |
| *Wearing Regimen* | • As appropriate for the condition. |
| *Precautions* | • Avoid pressure points around the MC heads where the wings begin distally.<br>• Check carefully for pressure points, especially if the client lacks full sensation and may not feel discomfort. |

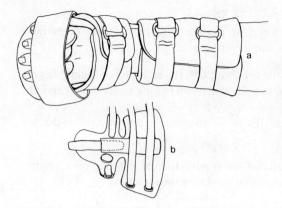

**FIGURE 10-20.** Alternative for custom wrist-hand orthosis: Prefabricated Rolyan® Progressive™ Palm Protector Splint[16] (original design courtesy of Lynn Swedberg, MS, OTR). This soft foam/plush washable orthosis is especially good for long-term care. *(a)* Dorsal view. *(b)* Volar view showing a strip of Ezeform (partly inserted into pocket) that can be remolded to adjust the position of the wrist as extension improves.

- Ensure that the thumb piece will not break off and that all crevices are sealed shut.

*Options*
- Expand the area for finger support and position the MCPs in abduction.
- Optional straps can be attached at the wrist, over the proximal phalanges, and around the thumb.
- Adhere gel padding under the fingers.

*Alternatives*
- Ulnar forearm-based static wrist-hand cone-style tone-reducing orthosis (following)
- Soft prefabricated (e.g., Rolyan's® Progressive Hand Splint,[16] Fig. 10-20)
- Preformed ball splints (see Fig. 7-7*d*)

---

⬤ • • • • • • • • • • • • • • • • • • • • • • • • • • • • • • • • • • • •

**Name:**  **Ulnar Forearm-Based Static Wrist-Hand Cone-Style Tone-Reducing Orthosis** (Fig. 10-21*a*)

*Common Name*  Antispasticity cone splint

*SCS Name*  Wrist extension, index through small finger MCP and IP extension, thumb CMC palmar abduction immobilization/mobilization; type 0[16]

*Objectives*
- To prevent flexion contractures
- To reduce tone of hypertonic muscles[44–47]

*Rationale*
- See Chapter 2, "Spasticity."

*Indications*
- High tone associated with
  ○ Head injury
  ○ Cerebral palsy
  ○ Multiple sclerosis
  ○ Cerebrovascular accident (CVA)

*Materials*
- Category B or C thermoplastic— ⅛ in. (3.2 mm) thick
- Self-adhesive hook Velcro
- Loop Velcro or padded alternative

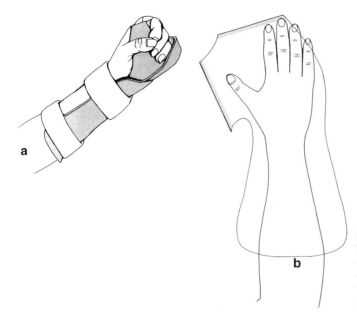

**FIGURE 10-21.** Ulnar forearm-based static wrist-hand cone-style tone-reducing orthosis. *(a)* Radial view. *(b)* Pattern. When molding, bond the stippled edges together to form the cone shape.

|  |  |
|---|---|
| | • ⅛ in. (3.2 mm) thick foam or gel padding for the ulnar head    • Solvent or alcohol |
| **Equipment and Tools** | • Heating pan    • Heat gun    • Scissors    • Cone |
| **Joint Positions** | • Submaximal extension (see Chapter 2, "Spasticity"). |
| **Pattern** | • Figure 10-21*b*.<br>• Use the contralateral hand for the pattern. |
| **Fabrication** | 1. Before molding, use tone-inhibiting techniques to suppress flexor tone.<br>2. Apply padding to the ulnar head.<br>3. Heat the distal half, apply solvent or alcohol to the stippled areas in the pattern, and then overlap them.<br>4. Mold it over a cone, rolling the edges up around the ulnar side of the hand of the client or a model.<br>5. Heat the forearm component, check temperature, and mold it to the client's forearm in submaximal wrist extension.<br>6. Transfer the ulnar head padding to the inside of the orthosis or discard it to leave a space.<br>7. Apply straps.<br>8. If desired, apply self-adhesive padding to the surface of the cone. |
| **Wearing Regimen** | • At night and during periods of inactivity during the day |
| **Precautions** | • Check for pressure points because the client lacks full sensation and may not feel discomfort. |
| **Alternatives** | • Preformed version |

- Bisurfaced forearm-based static wrist-hand orthosis
- Preformed ball splint (see Fig. 7-7*d*)

---

 **Name:** **Volar Forearm-Based Tenodesis Wrist-Hand Orthosis**[48] (Fig. 10-22*a* through *c*)

| | |
|---|---|
| *Common Name* | Rehabilitation Institute of Chicago (RIC) tenodesis (training) splint |
| *SCS Name* | Not classified |
| *Objectives* | • To train a tenodesis grasp<br>• To promote a strong tripod pinch with wrist extension and finger opening with wrist flexion (see Fig. 2-19)<br>• To promote functional contracture of the long finger flexors |
| *Indication* | • Quadriplegia at the level of C6 with at least a grade 3 strength of the wrist extensors |
| *Rationale* | • See Chapter 2, "Impact of Joint Position on Tissue Tension in the Hand." |
| *Materials* | • Category C thermoplastic—³⁄₃₂ in. (2.4 mm) thick for thumb and forearm components, ¹⁄₁₆ in. (1.6 mm) thick for finger component<br>• Solvent or alcohol<br>• Nonelastic cord<br>• ¹⁄₁₆ in. (1.6 mm) self-adhesive foam or gel padding<br>• Self-adhesive hook Velcro<br>• Loop Velcro<br>• ½ in. (1.3 cm) wide R-Thin or Extra-Thin loop Velcro |
| *Equipment and Tools* | • Heating pan   • Heat gun   • Scissors   • Hole punch |
| *Joint Positions* | • Slight flexion of the finger IPs.<br>• The thumb is aligned to oppose the index and middle fingers, with a well-rounded web space.<br>• Tension in the cord controls the degree of active wrist extension. Wrist flexion occurs when the wrist extensors relax. |
| *Pattern* | • Figure 10-22*d* |
| *Fabrication* | 1. Heat the forearm component, apply self-adhesive gel (to prevent distal migration), check the temperature, and mold it to the forearm. Gently flare the edges.<br>2. Mold the finger and thumb components.<br>3. Apply straps. Use R-Thin or Extra-Thin loop over the fingers.<br>4. Punch a hole in the finger component between the index and middle fingers, centered on the middle phalanx.<br>5. Secure the proximal end of the cord to the forearm piece by bonding a disk of thermoplastic with solvent or alcohol and dry heat.<br>6. Thread the cord through the hole. Determine the length of cord that will create a strong tripod grasp when the wrist extends, and then tie it off against the outside of the finger component. |

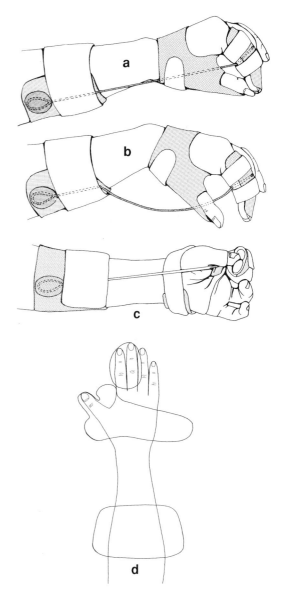

**FIGURE 10-22.** Volar forearm-based tenodesis wrist-hand orthosis. *(a)* Radial view. As the wrist extends, tension in the cord pulls the fingers against the thumb that is stabilized by the hand portion. *(b)* Radial view. When the wrist extensors relax, the wrist flexes, creating tension through the extensor tendons, causing the MCPs to extend. *(c)* Palmar view. *(d)* Pattern consists of three components: finger component for index and middle fingers, hand component to position the thumb in opposition, and forearm component to anchor the cord.

| | |
|---|---|
| ***Wearing Regimen*** | • Used for activities requiring finger prehension.<br>• Often used temporarily while the client learns a tenodesis grasp and the long finger flexors develop functional contractures to promote a strong tripod pinch. Discontinue when the functional tenodesis grasp has been established without the need for an orthosis.<br>• Difficult to apply independently. |
| ***Precautions*** | • Hand component should not restrict wrist motion.<br>• The cord should not contact the palm when the wrist is extended.<br>• Check carefully for pressure points because the client lacks full sensation and may not feel discomfort. |

| *Options* | • Forearm component can be circumferential.<br>• Slip the cord under the hand strap. |
|---|---|
| *Alternatives* | • Custom wrist-driven prehension orthoses fabricated from high-temperature thermoplastics or metal[49–52] |

---

**Name:** **Dorsal Forearm-Based Dynamic MCP-IP Protective-Flexion and MCP Extension-Blocking Orthosis[53]**
(Fig. 10-23*a* through *c*)

Dynamic component designed by Stancie Trueman, OT(C), Toronto, Ontario. The wrist is immobilized but not named because it is not a target joint. However, identifying the forearm base implies the inclusion of the wrist. In this figure, D4 is the target finger.

| *Common Name* | Flexor tendon repair splint; modified Kleinert splint |
|---|---|
| *SCS Name* | Not classified |
| *Objectives* | • To position the wrist in static flexion and passively flex the MCP and IPs while permitting limited active extension of the MCPs and full IP extension<br>• To promote early protected motion and tendon excursion for optimal tendon healing with minimal range-restricting adhesions or risk of rupture[54] |
| *Indications* | • Flexor tendon lacerations (flexor digitorum superficialis and profundus) in zone II[55] |
| *Rationale* | • See Chapter 2, "Tendon Injuries." |
| *Advantages of This Design* | • Incorporates a palmar pulley to promote composite flexion of the MCP, PIP, and DIP<br>• No need to glue a dressing hook to the fingernail |
| *Materials* | • Category C thermoplastic—⅛ in. (3.2 mm) thick<br>• ¹⁄₁₆ in. (1.6 mm) thick self-adhesive foam or gel padding<br>• ⅛ in. (3.2 mm) self-adhesive foam padding<br>• Velfoam or alternative for finger wraps<br><br>• Self-adhesive hook Velcro<br>• Loop Velcro<br>• Solvent or alcohol<br>• Nylon line<br>• Rubber band<br>• Two large plastic-coated paper clips<br>• Nonadhesive hook Velcro |
| *Equipment and Tools* | • Heating pan<br>• Pliers<br><br>• Heat gun<br>• Scissors<br><br>• Hole punch<br>• Wire cutter |
| *Joint Positions* | • Wrist: flexed (e.g., 30°) and MCPs flexed (e.g., 45° to 70°) according to the protocol of the surgeon.<br>• The IPs are molded in extension; traction brings them into almost full flexion. |
| *Client's Position* | • Seated with the elbow resting on the table, allowing wrist and fingers to fall into flexion |

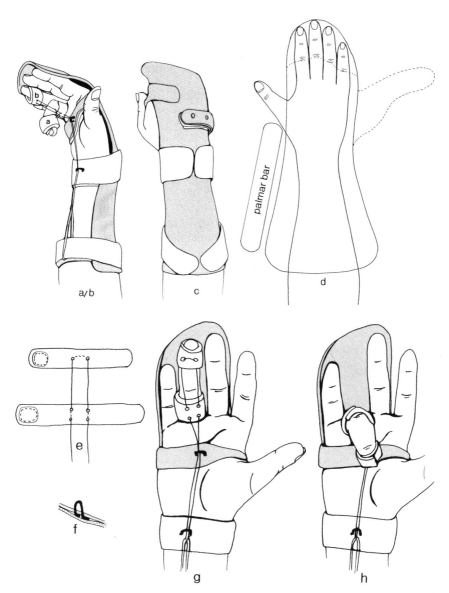

**FIGURE 10-23.** Dorsal forearm-based dynamic MCP-IP protective-flexion and extension-blocking orthosis. *(a)* When the finger extensors are relaxed, the rubber band pulls the IPs into flexion. *(b)* Muscle contraction pulls the IPs into full extension while the dorsal block limits MCP extension. At night, the rubber band traction is disconnected and the fingers are strapped to the dorsal block with the IPs extended. *(c)* Dorsal view. The radial side of the palmar bar has been bonded to the back of the orthosis; the ulnar side has loop Velcro riveted to the underside to attach to hook Velcro adhered to the back of the orthosis. *(d)* Pattern. Solid lines show the pattern for the illustrated orthosis. Dotted line at the PIPs shows alternate distal edge, leaving middle and distal phalanges uncovered. Broken line shows an alternate, integrated palmar bar that extends from ulnar border and attaches with Velcro closure to back of the orthosis on the radial side. *(e)* Finger cuffs for distal (shorter) and proximal phalanges. Each has a patch of hook Velcro sewn to one end. The distal cuff has one pair of holes for the nylon line while the proximal cuff has two pairs of holes. *(f)* Paper clip forming a line guide for the nylon line. *(g)* Volar view showing the ring finger extended to the limit of the dorsal block. The nylon lines pass through two paper clip line guides, one on the palmar bar and one on the wrist cuff. *(h)* When the finger extensors are relaxed, the rubber band pulls the IPs into flexion. Notice the orientation of the flexed ring finger toward the scaphoid.

| | |
|---|---|
| ***Therapist's Position*** | • Seated beside the client |
| ***Pattern*** | • Figure 10-23*d*.<br>• Use the contralateral hand for the pattern. |

***Fabrication***
(Fig. 10-23*e*
through *h*)

1. Apply padding to the dorsum of the hand and wrist, from the MC heads to the ulnar head, to protect bony prominences and prevent migration.
2. Heat the material and check the temperature.
3. While positioning the wrist and MCPs in the desired amount of flexion and IPs in full extension, drape the warm thermoplastic over the dorsum of the hand and forearm. Conform it to the contours of the MC heads and the individual fingers. If you use the pattern with the integrated palmar bar, mold it to the contours of the palm.
4. Attach the forearm and wrist straps.
5. If you use the pattern with the detached palmar bar, heat it and bond it to the radial side of the orthosis and mold across the palm proximal to the MC heads, gently flaring edges. Attach Velcro closure to the ulnar side of the palmar bar.
6. Attach a center patch of hook Velcro over the IP extension block and attach two straps to keep the IPs extended against the extension block at night.
7. For each affected finger, cut two strips of Velfoam—one to wrap around the proximal phalanx and one around the distal phalanx and long enough to overlap dorsally. Sew hook Velcro to one end of each strip. Punch small holes where marked—one pair for the distal phalanx and two pairs for the proximal phalanx. Thread nylon line through the holes (Fig. 10-23*e*).
8. With the orthosis on the client, apply Velfoam cuffs to the distal and proximal phalanges. Flex the finger(s) into the palm, converging toward the scaphoid, and place two horizontal marks on the palmar bar. Punch two holes where marked.
9. Unfold the paper clip once and cut in half, creating a U-shaped hook. Insert the two ends of the hook into the holes, creating a line guide on the front of the palmar bar. Bend the two ends back under the palmar bar and cover the back of the palmar bar with padding (Fig. 10-23*f*).
10. Thread the nylon lines through the paper clip hook.
11. Determine where the nylon lines cross the wrist strap: mark and punch two horizontal holes in the wrist strap.
12. Create another paper clip line guide, insert it into the holes, bend back the ends, and line the wrist strap with padding.
13. Thread the nylon lines through the paper clip hook on the wrist strap.
14. Unfasten one side of the forearm strap and slip a rubber band over it. Attach the nylon lines to the rubber band. Line the forearm strap with padding to keep the rubber band in place (Fig. 10-23*a* and *b*).

***Wearing Regimen***

• Worn continuously. At 3 weeks, if the client is compliant, the orthosis can be removed to wash the hand.
• Keep the traction applied during waking hours. Release tension in the rubber band to permit active extension to the limit of the extension block several times daily according to the protocol of the surgeon.
• At night, disconnect the traction and strap the IPs to the dorsal extension block.

- Generally worn for 6 weeks; if range-limiting adhesions are forming, the orthosis is discontinued sooner; if adhesions are not forming, the orthosis is used longer.

*Precautions*
- The client must not actively flex the involved digit(s) for several weeks.
- Ensure easy application and removal.
- Educate the client for signs of median nerve compression caused by wrist flexion.
- Control edema with elevation; discourage use of a sling beyond a few days.
- Check for PIP flexion contractures and flexor muscle shortening.

*Options*
- Terminate the extension block at the PIPs.[56]
- The number of fingers in addition to the injured finger(s) with attached traction varies from none to all. The number of fingers included in the dorsal block also varies (Fig. 10-23*g* and *h*)
- With the same approach, the orthosis can be designed for the thumb when the flexor pollicus longus is lacerated.
- Alternate traction:
  - Dressing hook or contoured fingernail hook glued to nail (see Fig. 1-12)
  - Rolyan® Wrap-On Finger Hooks[16] if the nails are injured
  - Silicone finger caps[2]
- When using a fingernail hook or finger cap, the combination of nylon line and rubber band can be replaced with elastic thread or wrapped elastic cord.

*Alternatives*
- Prefabricated version of the Velfoam finger cuffs—Rolyan® Biodynamic Flexion/Extension System[16]
- Precut flexor tendon repair kit complete with straps and traction[16]
- Rolyan® Tenodesis Flexor Tendon Repair PreCut[16] and Incremental Wrist Hinge
- Synergistic splint[57]
- Duran static orthosis with passive ROM[58]

---

**Name:** **Bivalved Forearm-Based Dynamic MCP-IP Protective-Extension and Flexion-Blocking Orthosis**
(Fig. 10-24*a* and *b*)

The wrist is immobilized but not named because it is not a target joint. However, identifying the forearm base implies the inclusion of the wrist.

*Common Name*
Extensor tendon repair splint

*SCS Name*
Not classified

*Objectives*
- To position the wrist in static extension and passively extend the MCP and IPs of the affected finger(s) while permitting limited active MCP flexion
- To promote early protected motion and tendon excursion for optimal tendon healing with minimal range-restricting adhesions or risk of rupture[59–60]

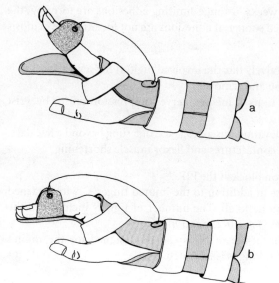

**FIGURE 10-24.** Bivalved forearm-based dynamic MCP-IP protective-extension and flexion-blocking orthosis. This orthosis has two slabs. The coil springs are mounted on the dorsal slab. The finger slings are wide enough to support both the PIP and DIP in extension. If desired, thin thermoplastic can be used to mold individual volar finger troughs to ensure PIP and DIP extension. *(a)* When the finger flexors are relaxed, the coil spring pulls the MCPs into extension. *(b)* Muscle contraction flexes the MCPs to the limit of the volar flexion block.

| | |
|---|---|
| *Indications* | • Extensor tendon lacerations (extensor digitorum, extensor indicis, extensor digiti minimi) in zones 5, 6, and 7 and thumb 4 and 5[59–63] |
| *Rationale* | • See Chapter 2, "Tendon Injuries." |
| *Materials* | • Category C thermoplastic—³⁄₂ or ⅛ in. (2.4 or 3.2 mm) thick <br> • ¹⁄₁₆ in. (1.6 mm) thick self-adhesive foam or gel padding <br> • Prefabricated finger extension-assist coil spring[2] (0.9 mm gauge) <br><br> • Finger loops <br> • Solvent or alcohol <br> • Self-adhesive hook Velcro <br> • Loop Velcro <br> • Padded Velcro strap |
| *Equipment and Tools* | • Heating pan    • Scissors    • Heat gun    • Pliers |
| *Joint Positions for Molding the Static Volar Base* | • Wrist extended (about 30° to 40°), MCPs flexed (about 30° to 40°), IPs extended, according to the protocol of the surgeon. <br> • Traction brings the MCPs into full extension. |
| *Client's Position* | • Seated with the forearm supinated for the volar slab, and pronated for the dorsal slab |
| *Therapist's Position* | • Seated beside or across from the client |
| *Pattern* | • For the volar slab, use Fig. 10-18*f*, excluding the thumb piece. <br> • For the dorsal slab, use Fig. 10-8*d*, deleting the flaps and forearm hole and extending it distally over the hand. <br> • Use the contralateral hand for the pattern. |
| *Fabrication* | 1. Heat, check the temperature, and mold the static volar slab as described earlier for volar forearm-based static C-bar wrist-hand orthosis. <br> 2. Attach a center patch of hook Velcro under the IP flexion block and attach two straps to keep the MCPs flexed and the IPs extended against the flexion block at night. |

3. Heat, check the temperature, and mold the dorsal slab.

4. Attach straps as shown in Figure 10-24*a*.

5. Mount coil springs to dorsal slab, as described earlier for dorsal forearm-based dynamic arching spring-wire wrist-MCP assistive-extension orthosis.

6. Use a wide finger loop to extend the MCP and IPs simultaneously.

7. If desired, use ¹⁄₁₆ in. (1.6 mm) thick thermoplastic and mold a volar slab to each individual finger to support the IPs in extension (not shown).

*Wearing Regimen*

• Actively flex the MCPs to the limit of the flexion block several times daily, according to protocol.

• Both components are worn continuously for 3 weeks (or according to the surgeon's protocol), after which daytime use of the volar slab is discontinued. The dynamic dorsal component is worn alone for 2 to 3 more weeks.[61]

• At night, the dynamic dorsal slab is removed and the IPs are strapped down to the volar flexion block.

*Precautions*

• Do not hyperextend the MCPs.

• MCP extension contractures might develop.

*Options*

• Different extension outrigger designs[62] (see Fig. 10-15).

• With the same approach, the orthosis can be designed for the thumb when extensor pollicus longus is lacerated.

*Alternatives*

• Prefabricated MCP extension orthosis (see Fig. 3-10*a* and *b*)

• Static immobilization (wrist extended 30° to 45°, MCPs and IPs at 0°) until 3 weeks when gentle, active mobilization is introduced[63]

## ● References

1. Schultz, KH: Hand-based metacarpal fracture brace and forearm ulnar or radius fracture brace. J Hand Ther 5:158, 1992.

2. Orfit Industries: Orthotic Products Catalogue. Wijnegem, Belgium, 1997.

3. Kruger, VL, Veer, L, and Nicholls, LA: A modified ulnar gutter wrist splint for the treatment of carpal tunnel syndrome. Can J Occup Ther 59:159, 1992.

4. Johnson, C: Splinting the injured musician. J Hand Ther 5:107, 1992.

5. Gelberman, RH, et al: The carpal tunnel syndrome: A study of carpal canal pressures. J Bone Joint Surg 63A:380, 1981.

6. Kruger, VL, et al: Carpal tunnel syndrome: Objective measure and splint use. Arch Phys Med Rehabil 72:517, 1991.

7. Weiss, ND, et al: Position of the wrist associated with the lowest carpal-tunnel pressure: Implications for splint design. J Bone Joint Surg 77A:1695, 1995.

8. Burke, DT, et al: Splinting for carpal tunnel syndrome: In search of the optimal angle. Arch Phys Med Rehabil 75:1241, 1994.

9. Dolhanty, D: Effectiveness of splinting of carpal tunnel syndrome. Can J Occup Ther 53:275, 1985.

10. Stern, E: Wrist extensor orthoses: Dexterity and grip strength across four styles. Am J Occup Ther 45:42, 1991.

11. Stern, E, Sines, B, and Teague, T: Commercial wrist ex-

12. Stern, EB: Grip strength and finger dexterity across five styles of commercial wrist orthoses. Am J Occup Ther 50:32, 1996.

13. Mildenberger, LA: Magnetic splint for object retrieval. Am J Occup Ther 38:195, 1984.

14. AliMed, Inc.: Orthopedic Rehabilitation Products Catalog, 1996–97.

15. Bielawski, T, and Lehman, JB: A gauntlet work splint. Am J Occup Ther 40:199, 1986.

16. Smith & Nephew, Inc.: Rehabilitation Division Catalogue, 1997. (Rolyan® and Progressive™ are trademarks of Smith & Nephew, Inc.)

17. North Coast Medical: Hand Therapy Catalog, 1997.

18. Sammons Preston Catalog, 1997.

19. Henshaw, JL, Satren, JW, and Wrightsman, JA: The semi-flexible support: An alternative for the hand-injured worker. J Hand Ther 2:35, 1989.

20. Backman, C: Spandex wrist splint: an alternative for the client with arthritis. Can J Occup Ther 55:89, 1988.

21. North Coast Medical, Inc.: Orfit Splinting Material Instruction Manual. North Coast Medical, Inc., San Jose, CA, 1995.

22. Ford, JR, and Duckworth, B: Physical Management for the Quadriplegic Patient, ed 2. FA Davis, Philadelphia, 1987, p 333.

23. Linden, CA, and Trombly, CA: Orthoses: Kinds and purposes. In Trombly, CA (ed): Occupational Therapy for Physical Dysfunction, ed 4. Williams & Wilkins, Baltimore, 1995, p 551.

tensor orthoses: Hand function, comfort, and interference across 5 styles. J Hand Ther 7:237, 1994.

24. Johnson, C: Splinting the injured musician. J Hand Ther 5:107, 1992.
25. Eaton, R: Entrapment syndrome in musicians. J Hand Ther 5:91, 1992.
26. Tenney, CG, and Lisak, JM: Atlas of Hand Splinting. Little, Brown, Boston, 1986.
27. Fishwick, G, and Sellers, JN, Jr: Occupational therapy for patients with cervical cord injury. In Pierce, DS, and Nickel, VH (eds): The Total Care of Spinal Cord Injuries. Little, Brown, Boston, 1977, p 205.
28. Linden, CA, and Trombly, CA: Orthoses: Kinds and purposes. In Trombly, CA (ed): Occupational Therapy for Physical Dysfunction, ed 4. Williams & Wilkins, Baltimore, 1995, p 551.
29. Malick, MH, and Meyer, CMH: Manual on the Management of the Quadriplegic Upper Extremity. Maude H Malick, Pittsburgh, 1978, p 54.
30. Melvin, JL: Rheumatic Disease in the Adult and Child, Occupational Therapy and Rehabilitation, ed 3. FA Davis, Philadelphia, 1989.
31. Orfit Industries: Orfit Splinting Guide, Antwerp, 1990.
32. Dillingham, T, et al: Nerve injuries after a humeral fracture. J Hand Ther 5:212, 1992.
33. Fairleigh, A, and Hacking, S: Post-operative metacarpophalangeal arthroplasty dynamic splint for patients with rheumatoid arthritis. Can J Occup Ther 55:141, 1988.
34. Steadman, AK, and Netscher, DT: A detachable thumb spica combined with an outrigger brace simplifies postoperative management of the rheumatoid hand. J Hand Ther 3:205, 1990.
35. May, EJ, and Silfverskiold, KL: A new power source in dynamic splinting: Experimental studies. J Hand Ther 2:164, 1989.
36. Colditz, CJ: Splinting for radial nerve palsy. J Hand Ther 1:18, 1987.
37. Tenney, CG, and Lisak, JM: Atlas of Hand Splinting. Little, Brown, Boston, 1986.
38. Furst, DE, and Seeger, MW: Effects of splinting in the treatment of hand contracture in progressive systemic sclerosis. Am J Occup Ther 41:118, 1987.
39. Prosser, R, and Conolly, WB: Complications following surgical treatment for Dupuytren's contracture. J Hand Ther 9:344, 1996.
40. Willis, B: The use of Orthoplast Isoprene splints in the treatment of the acutely burned child: Preliminary report. Am J Occup Ther 23:57, 1969.
41. Brandt, KD, and Feinberg, J: Use of resting splints by patients with rheumatoid arthritis. Am J Occup Ther 35:173, 1981.
42. Callinan, NJ, and Mathiowetz, V: Soft versus hard resting hand splints in rheumatoid arthritis: Pain relief, preference, and compliance. Am J Occup Ther 50:347, 1996.
43. Krajnik, SR, and Bridle, MJ: Hand splinting in quadriplegia: Current practice. Am J Occup Ther 46:149, 1992.
44. Aalderks, M, et al: A comparison of dorsal and volar resting hand splints in the reduction of hyper tonus. Am J Occup Ther 36:664, 1982.
45. Kinghorn, J, and Roberts, G: The effect of an inhibitive weight-bearing splint on tone and function: a single-case study. Am J Occup Ther 50:807, 1996.
46. Scherling, E, and Johnson, H: A tone-reducing wrist-hand orthosis. Am J Occup Ther 43:609, 1989.
47. McPherson, JJ: Objective evaluation of a splint designed to reduce hypertonicity. Am J Occup Ther 35:189, 1981.
48. Fess, EF, and Philips, CA: Hand Splinting: Principles and Methods, ed 2. Mosby, St. Louis, 1987, p 355.
49. Bedbrook, GM: The Care and Management of Spinal Cord Injuries. Springer-Verlag, New York, 1981, p 189.
50. Ford, JR, and Duckworth, B: Physical Management for the Quadriplegic Patient, ed 2. FA Davis, Philadelphia, 1987, p 333.
51. Malick, MH, and Meyer, CMH: Manual on the Management of the Quadriplegic Upper Extremity. Maude H Malick, Harmarville Rehabilitation Center, Pittsburgh, 1978, p 54.
52. Shepherd, CC, and Ruzicka, SH: Tenodesis brace use by persons with spinal cord injuries. Am J Occup Ther 45:81, 1991.
53. Clark, EN, and Saldana, MJ: Kleinert traction: Rubber loop to nail fixative method. J Hand Ther 3:161, 1990.
54. Strickland, JW: Biologic rationale, clinical application, and results of early motion following flexor tendon repair. J Hand Ther 2:71, 1989.
55. Peck, FH, et al: An audit of flexor tendon injuries in zone II and its influence on management. J Hand Ther 9:306, 1996.
56. May, EJ, and Silfverskiold, KL: A new power source in dynamic splinting: Experimental studies. J Hand Ther 2:164, 1989.
57. Horii, E, et al: Comparative flexor tendon excursion after passive mobilization: an in vitro study. J Hand Surg (Am) 16:1145, 1991.
58. Gratten, P: Early active mobilization after flexor tendon repairs. J Hand Ther 6:285, 1990.
59. Evans, R: Clinical application of controlled stress to the healing extensor tendon: a review of 112 cases. Phys Ther 69:1041, 1989.
60. Dovelle et al: Rehabilitation of extensor tendon injury of the hand by means of early controlled motion. Am J Occup Ther 43:115, 1989.
61. Steward, KM: Tendon injuries. In Stanley, BG, and Tribuzi, SM (eds): Concepts in Hand Rehabilitation. FA Davis, Philadelphia, 1992.
62. Thomas, D, Moutet, F, and Guinard, D: Post-operative management of extensor tendon repairs in zones V, VI and VII. J Hand Ther 9:309, 1996.
63. Walsh, M, et al: Early controlled motion with dynamic splinting versus static splinting for zones III and IV extensor tendon lacerations. J Hand Ther 7:232, 1994.

CHAPTER **11**

# Hand-, Finger-, Thumb-Based Orthoses

This chapter describes the fabrication process for 21 hand-, finger-, and thumb-based orthoses, all of which exclude the wrist joint. The orthoses are organized from proximal to distal; as the chapter progresses, the orthoses incorporate more distal joints in the hand.

The illustrated patterns can be adjusted with a photocopier to produce a standard pattern that matches the size of the client's hand. Measure the bird's-eye width across the dorsum of the client's hand from the radial side of the second MC head to the ulnar side of the fifth MC head. Compare this measurement with the MCP width in the illustrated pattern, and determine the amount of adjustment required to match the client's MCP width.

The following acronyms are used:

- SCS—splint classification system
- MC—metacarpal
- MP or MCP—metacarpophalangeal joint
- PIP—proximal interphalangeal joint
- DIP—distal interphalangeal joint
- IP—interphalangeal joints
- CMC—carpometacarpal joint

Other abbreviations are D1 (thumb), D2 (index finger), D3 (middle finger), D4 (ring finger), and D5 (small finger).

An evaluation form for upper extremity orthoses can be found at the end of Chapter 7. It can be used as a guideline for designing, fabricating, and evaluating many of the orthoses in Chapter 11. Refer to the introduction to Chapter 8 for more information.

| **Names:** | **Circumferential Nonarticular Metacarpal-Stabilizing Orthosis**[1] **(without the extension)** (Fig. 11-1*a* and *b*) **Circumferential Hand-Based Static MCP-Stabilizing Orthosis** (Fig. 11-1*a* and *b*) |
|---|---|

The extension stabilizes the MCPs of D4 and 5, converting the nonarticular design to a static design. The extension can include any or all MCPs.

| | |
|---|---|
| *Common Name* | Metacarpal (fracture) brace |
| *SCS Name* | Nonarticular splint—metacarpal |
| *Objectives* | • To stabilize an MC fracture to promote healing |
| *Indications* | • Midshaft fracture of the third, fourth, or fifth MC |
| *Rationale* | • Applies circumferential compression to maintain fracture alignment.<br>• See Chapter 2, "Fractures of Long Bones." |
| *Materials* | • Category C thermoplastic—$\frac{1}{16}$ or $\frac{3}{32}$ in. (1.6 or 2.4 mm) thick<br>• $\frac{1}{32}$, $\frac{1}{16}$, or $\frac{1}{8}$ in. (0.8, 1.6, or 3.2 mm) thick self-adhesive foam or gel padding (optional)<br>• 1 in. (2.5 cm) wide self-adhesive hook Velcro<br>• 1 in. (2.5 cm) wide loop Velcro |
| *Equipment and Tools* | • Heating pan    • Sewing machine for optional buddy strap(s)<br>• Heat gun    • For the pattern: paper towel or flexible clear plastic with<br>• Scissors      permanent marker and straight pins, stapler, or tape |
| *Pattern* | • Figure 11-1*c* |

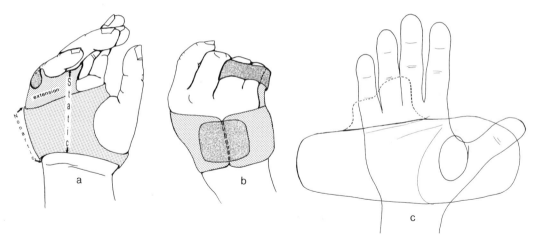

**FIGURE 11-1.** Circumferential nonarticular metacarpal-stabilizing orthosis. *(a)* Volar view. If the fracture is midshaft, the orthosis can terminate at the metacarpal (MC) heads. If the MC head is fractured, extend the orthosis to support the proximal phalanx, immobilizing the MCP in flexion. If the extension is included, the orthosis is called a circumferential hand-based static (D4-5) MCP-stabilizing orthosis. *(b)* Dorsal view showing the dorsal opening and the optional proximal phalanx extension. The opening can also be ulnar or radial, depending on which MC is fractured. *(c)* Pattern. The broken line represents the optional extension to support the proximal phalanges.

- Opening can be ulnar, dorsal, or radial
- May be necessary to restrict MCP flexion slightly to ensure better fixation of fracture[1]

*Fabrication*

1. If desired, apply padding to the dorsum of the MCs.
2. Cut the thermoplastic, heat, and check the temperature of the thermoplastic.
3. Mold circumferentially around the hand.
4. Remove the padding and transfer to the inside of the orthosis or discard.
5. Attach Velcro straps.

*Wearing Regimen*

- Worn at all times.
- When the fracture is stable, the orthosis can be removed carefully for bathing, as per the physician's recommendations.
- Continue with the orthosis until fracture healing is complete.

*Application and Removal*

- Circumferential orthoses can be difficult to apply and may require the assistance of another person to hold the sides open.

*Precaution*

- Ensure full clearance of the thenar eminence and MC heads to prevent any restriction of the thumb or MCP mobility.

*Options*

- Use the nonarticular orthosis in combination with circumferential finger-based PIP-stabilizing buddy straps to provide additional fracture stabilization (see Fig. 11-16).
- If the MC head is fractured, extend the orthosis distally to immobilize the affected MCPs in flexion (Fig. 11-1*a* and *b*).
- Use as a base for dynamic orthoses (see Figs. 11-4, 11-5, 11-8, and 11-12).

| | |
|---|---|
| *Alternative* | • If the base of the MC is fractured, provide a circumferential forearm-based static wrist orthosis (see Fig. 10-7) |

⬤ ● ● ● ● ● ● ● ● ● ● ● ● ● ● ● ● ● ● ● ● ● ● ● ● ● ● ● ● ● ● ● ● ● ● ● ● ● ● ● ● ● ● ● ●

| | |
|---|---|
| **Name:** | **Volar (or Circumferential) Hand-Based Static D2-5 MCP-Stabilizing Orthosis**[2–4] (Fig. 11-2*a* and *b*) |
| *Common Names* | MCP protection splint; static ulnar drift/deviation splint; metacarpal ulnar deviation orthosis; antiulnar deviation splint; trigger finger splint; blocking splint |
| *SCS Name* | Index through small finger MP extension immobilization; type 0[4] |

| *Indications* | *Objectives* |
|---|---|
| • Joint inflammation (e.g., rheumatoid arthritis) | • To promote restabilization of the tendon restraints at MCPs (see Fig. 2-10 and Chapter 2, "Promoting Tissue Resorption")<br>• To prevent or correct MCP volar subluxation (see Fig. 2-11*a*)<br>• To prevent or correct MCP ulnar drift (see Fig. 2-11*b*) |
| • Trigger finger | • To block MCP flexion and limit excursion of the long finger flexors. This prevents tendon triggering at the A1 pulley, which occurs when the affected finger extends from a position of full composite flexion; by eliminating irritation caused by the tendon nodule catching on the A1 pulley, inflammation and triggering subsides.[6] |
| • Surgical release of Dupuytren's contracture | • To maintain surgically gained extension |
| • Extension contractures of the IPs<br>• Intrinsic muscle tightness | • To block the MCP joints so that the flexor digitorum superficialis and profundus can actively stretch the IP joints or intrinsic muscles |
| • MC head fracture | • To stabilize the MC head |

| | |
|---|---|
| *Materials* | • Category C thermoplastic—1⁄16 in. (1.6 mm) thick<br>• 1 in. (2.5 cm) wide self-adhesive hook Velcro<br>• 1 in. (2.5 cm) wide loop Velcro |
| *Equipment and Tools* | • Heating pan<br>• Heat gun<br>• Scissors<br>• For the pattern: paper towel or flexible clear plastic with permanent marker and straight pins, stapler, or tape |
| *Joint Positions* | • Position the MCPs in slight flexion so that the thumb can easily oppose the tips of the index and middle fingers. If triggering is not eliminated, position the MCPs in 0° of flexion.<br>• For intrinsic tightness, position the MCPs in 0° to stretch the intrinsic muscles.<br>• Mold the thermoplastic to support the volar aspect of the proximal phalanges to correct volar subluxation (if appropriate).<br>• Mold the thermoplastic around the ulnar side of the fifth proximal phalanx to correct ulnar drift (if appropriate).<br>• The PIPs and thumb are unrestricted. |

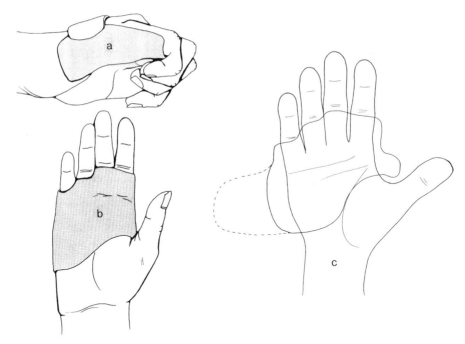

**FIGURE 11-2.** Volar (or circumferential) hand-based static D2-5 MCP-stabilizing orthosis. *(a)* Ulnar view. *(b)* Volar view showing support for all finger MCPs. Alternately, only the affected MCPs can be immobilized. *(c)* Solid line: volar pattern. Broken line: circumferential pattern.

| | |
|---|---|
| ***Pattern*** | • Figure 11-2*c* |
| ***Fabrication*** | 1. Cut the thermoplastic.<br>2. Heat and check the temperature of the thermoplastic.<br>3. Mold to the volar aspect of the hand, controlling the position of the MCP joints.<br>4. Attach strap. |
| ***Wearing Regimen*** | • All the time to prevent or correct deformity and reduce inflammation. Continuous use for several weeks or months can permanently correct mild subluxation or finger triggering. |
| ***Precautions*** | • Ensure full clearance of the PIPs, thenar eminence, and uninvolved MCPs.<br>• Ensure that the straps are easy to manage for arthritic fingers (see Fig. 3-16).<br>• Immobilization of the MCPs puts more stress on the PIPs and DIPs, which could aggravate inflammation in susceptible arthritic joints. |
| ***Options*** | • Instead of a volar design, mold more circumferentially, with a dorsal opening.<br>• Limit flexion only at the MCPs demonstrating inflammation, deformity, or triggering.<br>• Extend distally for individual fingers up to the DIP crease to support/immobilize PIP (see Fig. 11-11*a*).<br>• Convert pattern into a thumb-hole design similar to Figure 11-11*b*. |
| ***Alternatives*** | • For joint inflammation:<br>  ○ Volar forearm-based static wrist and D2-5 MCP orthosis (see Fig. 10-12) |

- Any custom or prefabricated volar or circumferential forearm-based static wrist orthosis to correct wrist radial deviation, which often leads to MCP ulnar drift (see Chapter 10)
- Circumferential hand-based dynamic traction D2-5 MCP corrective radial deviation orthosis
- Prefabricated hand-based orthoses
- For trigger finger:
  - spiral finger-based static PIP extension-blocking orthosis (see Fig. 11-17)—described later in this chapter
- For correction of IP extension contractures:
  - Circumferential hand-based static-progressive MERiT-screw MCP-IP flexion orthosis (see Fig. 11-12a)
  - Circumferential hand-based static-progressive tube-outrigger MCP-IP flexion orthosis (see Fig. 11-12b)

**Name:** **Circumferential Hand-Based Dynamic Traction D2-5 MCP Corrective Radial Deviation Orthosis** (Fig. 11-3a through c)

*Common Name*    Ulnar drift splint; ulnar deviation splint; soft metacarpal ulnar deviation orthosis; antiulnar deviation working splint

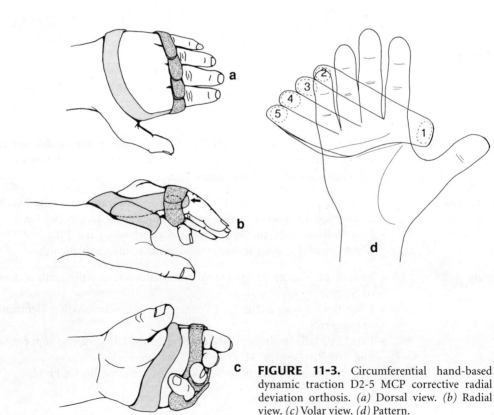

**FIGURE 11-3.** Circumferential hand-based dynamic traction D2-5 MCP corrective radial deviation orthosis. *(a)* Dorsal view. *(b)* Radial view. *(c)* Volar view. *(d)* Pattern.

| | |
|---|---|
| *SCS Name* | Index through small finger MP ulnar deviation restriction; type 0[4] |
| *Objectives* | • To prevent or correct MCP ulnar drift (see Fig. 2-12)<br>• To promote restabilization of the tendon restraints at the MCPs (see Fig. 2-11)<br>• To improve hand function |
| *Indications* | • Joint inflammation (e.g., rheumatoid arthritis) |
| *Rationale* | • See Chapter 2, "Promoting Tissue Resorption." |
| *Materials* | • Category C thermoplastic—$\frac{3}{32}$ or $\frac{1}{8}$ in. (2.4 or 3.2 mm) thick—1 in. (2.5 cm) wide; the length required is about 1½ times the circumference of the hand<br>• Thin self-adhesive foam or gel padding (optional)<br>• Nonadhesive hook Velcro<br>• Self-adhesive loop Velcro<br>• Velfoam or alternative<br>• Solvent or alcohol |
| *Equipment and Tools* | • Heating pan • Heat gun • Scissors • Sewing machine |
| *Joint Positions* | • Second MCP slightly flexed<br>• MCP ulnar deviation reduced to 0° or as tolerated |
| *Pattern* | • Figure 11-3*d* |
| *Fabrication* | 1. Heat and cut the thermoplastic strip.<br>2. Reheat and check the temperature.<br>3. Mold circumferentially around the hand, beginning at the radial side of the proximal phalanx of D2 (arrow in Fig. 11-3*b*), with the D2 MCP slightly flexed and ulnar deviation corrected. Mold across the dorsum with the padding underneath, then across the palm proximal to the MC heads, conforming to the transverse arch. Complete the circle, using solvent or alcohol and dry heat to create a secure bond beside the second MCP. Cut off excess material.<br>4. Apply a self-adhesive loop Velcro tab to the extension beside the second proximal phalanx using a heat gun to ensure a permanent attachment.<br>5. Sew five hook Velcro tabs to the Velfoam (Fig. 11-3*d*).<br>6. Secure hook tab 1 (Fig. 11-3*d*) to the loop Velcro tab on the thermoplastic base.<br>7. Lay the Velfoam against the volar side of the MCPs, wrap strap 2 around the D2 proximal phalanx, and secure with the hook Velcro tab to correct ulnar deviation.<br>8. Continue to wrap one strap around each proximal phalanx of D3, D4, and D5 in turn, securing with sufficient tension to correct ulnar deviation. |
| *Wearing Regimen* | • Worn all the time to prevent or correct deformity or only during strenuous hand activities.<br>• Continuous use for several weeks or months may permanently correct mild, flexible ulnar deviation. |

**Precautions**
- This orthosis does not provide stabilization to rest inflamed MCP joints or prevent volar subluxation.
- MCP flexion is not blocked sufficiently to limit stress to the A1 pulley.

**Options**
- When the MCPs are inflamed or when MCP immobilization can be tolerated, substitute the volar (or circumferential) hand-based static D2-5 MCP-stabilizing orthosis.

**Alternatives**
- Orfit precut kit—ulnar drift splint[7]
- Prefabricated designs
- Soft custom designs[8]

---

## Name: Circumferential Hand-Based Dynamic Arching Spring-Wire MCP Assistive-Extension Orthosis
(Fig. 11-4*a* and *b*)

The orthosis depicted provides spring-wire assistive extension to the middle, ring, and small fingers. However, any or all digits can have a spring-wire extension assist.

**Common Name**
Dynamic MCP extension splint

**SCS Name**
Long through small finger MP extension mobilization; type 0[3]

**Objective**
- To passively extend the MCPs to 0° while permitting full active MCP flexion and unrestricted IP motion

**Indications**
- Weak MCP extensors caused by
  - Radial nerve injury when reinnervation has progressed to the level of the wrist extensors
  - Repair of extensor tendon ruptures associated with rheumatoid arthritis
- Adherent tendons at a fracture site

**Advantages of This Design**
- When the client makes a fist, the wires are pulled in close to the hand permitting it to slip into a loose pocket.
- The hand can be slipped through a loose sleeve with the orthosis on.

**Materials**
- Category C thermoplastic—$\frac{1}{16}$ to $\frac{3}{32}$ in. (1.6 or 2.4 mm) thick
- Thin self-adhesive foam or gel padding
- Self-adhesive hook Velcro
- Loop Velcro
- Prefabricated finger extension-assist coil springs (0.9 mm gauge)[7] (see Fig. 4-4*d*)
- Finger slings (alternative for wire-formed finger hooks)
- Solvent or alcohol

**Equipment and Tools**
- Heating pan
- Heat gun
- Scissors
- Two pairs of pliers—ideally one is round nosed to form the finger hooks
- Wire cutter

**Joint Positions**
- Spring wire extends the MCPs to 0°.

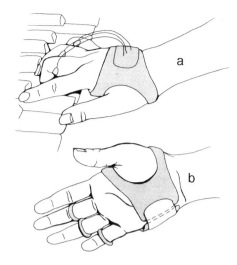

**FIGURE 11-4.** Circumferential hand-based dynamic arching spring-wire D3-5 MCP-assistive extension orthosis. *(a)* Radial view. Orthosis assists client with MCP extension lag to play the piano. Only the three affected fingers have extension assists. *(b)* Volar view showing hooks at the PIPs and the ulnar opening. For pattern, use Figure 11-1*c*.

*Pattern*

- Use Figure 11-1*c*—modify the pattern to incorporate an ulnar opening.

*Fabrication*

1. Heat the thermoplastic of the hand base, apply gel padding to the material against the dorsum, and mold as for the circumferential nonarticular metacarpal-stabilizing orthosis (Fig. 11-1*a*).
2. Attach a strap over the ulnar opening.
3. Mount a coil spring for each affected finger according to fabrication instructions for the dorsal forearm-based dynamic arching spring-wire D1-5 MCP-assistive extension orthosis (see Fig. 10-13).
4. Forming the finger hooks:
   a. While the client makes a fist, bend the wire down until it intersects the volar side of PIP and mark this location with a permanent marker.
   b. Remove the orthosis and bend the wire 90° at the mark, down toward the palm.
   c. Use round-nose pliers to form a ∪-shaped hook that matches the contour of the volar side of the PIP.
   d. While finger flexors are relaxed, the wires will passively extend the MCPs to 0°, and each hook should be positioned at or just proximal to the PIP.
   e. Ask the client to make a fist and ensure that the arching wires pass between MC heads without impinging on the web space. If impingement occurs, the hook was formed too proximal and the wire will need to be unbent and the hook re-formed more distally. If the wire hits an MC head, bend it to run between the MC heads.
   f. Cut off extra wire.
   g. Remove the orthosis. Heat a piece of thin thermoplastic, about ½ × 1½ in. (1 × 3 cm) and cover the hook, blending out any crevices.

*Wearing Regimen*

- For functional activities requiring MCP extension

*Precautions*

- To prevent injury from a piece of flying wire, cut the wire under a towel, pillowcase, or sheet.
- Spring wires are easily bent and thus are not appropriate for some clients.

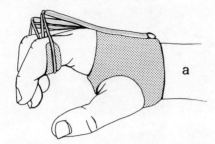

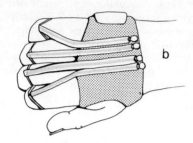

**FIGURE 11-5.** Alternate design for MCP assistive-extension—circumferential hand-based dynamic tube-outrigger MCP assistive-extension orthosis. This design uses Orfitubes, Aquatubes, or ThermoTubes with wrapped elastic cord and thermoplastic finger slings. *(a)* Radial view. *(b)* Dorsal view showing tubes attached to the orthosis. For the pattern, use Figure 11-1*c*.

- Ensure that the wires do not impinge on the web spaces or MC heads when the fingers are fully flexed.
- Ensure that the MCPs are not hyperextended.

*Option*
- Substitute finger loops for the finger hooks (see Fig. 10-13*a* and *b*)

*Alternatives*
- Circumferential hand-based dynamic tube-outrigger D2-5 MCP assistive-extension orthosis (Fig. 11-5)
- Dorsal forearm-based dynamic arching spring-wire D2-5 MCP assistive-extension orthosis (see Fig. 10-13)—this design immobilizes the wrist
- Prefabricated orthoses

---

● **Name:**    **Figure-Eight Hand-Based Static D4-5 MCP Extension-Blocking Orthosis**[2] (Fig. 11-6*a* and *b*)

*Common Name*    Static anticlaw deformity splint; static ulnar nerve splint

*SCS Name*    Ring through small finger MP extension restriction; type 0[2]

*Objectives*
- To stabilize the fourth and fifth MCPs in flexion:
  - To correct hyperextension of fourth and fifth MCPs
  - To prevent shortening of MCP collateral ligaments
  - To promote active IP extension
- To promote hand function

*Indications*
- Ulnar nerve lesion

*Rationale*
- When an ulnar nerve lesion causes paralysis of the lumbricals and interossei of D4 and D5, active MCP flexion and IP extension are lost, caus-

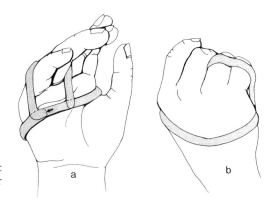

**FIGURE 11-6.** Figure-eight hand-based static D4-5 MCP extension-blocking orthosis. *(a)* Volar view. *(b)* Dorsal view.

ing a partial clawhand deformity (see Fig. 2-17*d*) because the extensor digitorum (extensor of the MCPs) is unopposed. Active IP flexion is unimpaired. By blocking MCP extension of D4 and D5, the force exerted by the extensor digitorum is transferred distally through the extensor expansion to extend the IPs.

| | |
|---|---|
| *Materials* | • Category C or D thermoplastic—³⁄₃₂ or ⅛ in. (2.4 or 3.2 mm) thick—preferably opaque or ³⁄₁₆ or ¼ in. (4.8 or 6.4 mm) thick Aquatubes[12] or ThermoTubes[10]<br>• Solvent or alcohol |
| *Equipment and Tools* | • Heating pan<br>• Heat gun<br>• Scissors |
| *Joint Positions* | • The finger component positions the MCPs in approximately 75° flexion. |
| *Pattern* | • Strip of thermoplastic, ⅜ in. (1 cm) wide and about 12 in. (30 cm) long or a 12 in. (30 cm) length of Aquatube or ThermoTube |
| *Fabrication* | 1. If using an opaque thermoplastic, heat, cut the strip, and then roll to round the edges.<br>2. Reheat (if necessary) and check temperature. When using a tube, squeeze it flat to obliterate the lumen.<br>3. Wrap the strip or tube circumferentially around the hand, beginning at the ulnar aspect of the hand (arrow in Figure 11-6*a*), crossing the dorsum of the hand conforming to the transverse arch in the palm and through the thumb web space. Using solvent or alcohol and dry heat, bond securely to the beginning of the strip to complete the circle.<br>4. While holding the MCPs in about 75° flexion, continue with the strip/tube, molding across the proximal phalanges of D5 and D4, conforming to each phalanx.<br>5. Pass the strip/tube between D3 and D4 and bond securely with solvent or alcohol and dry heat to the palmar strip.<br>6. Cut off the excess thermoplastic.<br>7. Seal all crevices. |
| *Wearing Regimen* | • Worn at all times to prevent contracture of the MCP collateral ligaments |

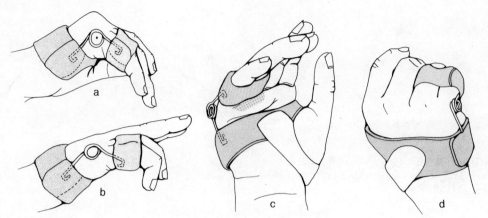

**FIGURE 11-7.** Circumferential hand-based dynamic joint-aligned coil-spring D4-5 MCP assistive-flexion orthosis. *(a)* When extensor digitorum is relaxed, the coil spring (centered over the MCP axis) pushes the MCPs into flexion. *(b)* Contraction of extensor digitorum is able to overcome the resistance of the coil spring to permit MCP extension. Notice how the IPs flex when the MCPs extend because extensor digitorum cannot extend the MCPs and IPs at the same time. *(c)* Volar view shows optional strap around the base of the thumb to prevent distal migration. The stippled area identifies soft tissue susceptible to being pinched if the finger or hand components are too wide. *(d)* Dorsal view.

| *Alternatives* | • Circumferential hand-based dynamic joint-aligned coil-spring, D4-5 MCP assistive-flexion orthosis (Fig. 11-7) |
|---|---|

⬤ • • • • • • • • • • • • • • • • • • • • • • • • • • • • • • • • • • • • • •

| **Name:** | **Circumferential Hand-Based Dynamic Joint-Aligned Coil-Spring D4-5 MCP Assistive-Flexion Orthosis**[9,10] (Fig. 11-7*a* through *d*) |
|---|---|
| *Common Names* | Dynamic anticlaw deformity splint; dynamic ulnar nerve splint; Wynn Perry splint |
| *SCS Name* | Ring through small finger MP flexion mobilization; type 0[2] |
| *Objectives* | • To passively flex the fourth and fifth MCPs while allowing active MCP extension<br> ○ To correct hyperextension of the fourth and fifth MCPs<br> ○ To prevent shortening of MCP collateral ligaments<br> ○ To promote active IP extension |
| *Indications* | • Ulnar nerve lesion |
| *Rationale* | • See figure-eight hand-based static D4-5 MCP extension-blocking orthosis |
| *Materials* | • For the hand base: ³⁄₃₂ or ⅛ in. (2.4 or 3.2 mm) thick category B or C thermoplastic<br>• For the finger piece: ¹⁄₁₆ in. (1.6 mm) thick thermoplastic<br>• Thin self-adhesive gel padding<br><br>• Solvent or alcohol<br>• Self-adhesive hook Velcro<br>• Elasticized loop Velcro<br>• One prefabricated knuckle bender coil spring[7,10] (see Fig. 4-4*b*) or 0.9 mm gauge spring wire |

| | |
|---|---|
| ***Equipment and Tools*** | • Heating pan<br>• Heat gun<br>• Two pairs of pliers—<br>  flat or needle nose<br>• Wire cutter | • Wire-bending jig (or round-nose pliers)<br>  to make custom coil spring from spring<br>  wire if prefabricated coil springs are un-<br>  available |

***Joint Positions***

• At rest, the coil spring will push the MCPs into about 75° flexion.

***Pattern***

• For the hand base: strip of thermoplastic ⅝ in. (15 mm) wide and length equaling the hand circumference plus ¾ in. (2 cm)
• For finger piece: a strip of thermoplastic ⅝ in. (15 cm) wide

***Fabrication***

1. Heat the hand-base strip and apply gel padding to line the thermoplastic over the dorsum of the MCs to prevent distal migration.
2. Beginning at the ulnar side, mold circumferentially around the hand, proximal to the MC heads in the palm and wrapping across the bases of the MCs over the dorsum. Overlap ¾ in. (2 cm) at the ulnar side and cut off excess thermoplastic. Do *not* create a permanent bond.
3. Heat the strip for the fingers and mold circumferentially around the proximal phalanges of D4 and D5, beginning and ending at the ulnar side, overlapping about ¾ in. (2 cm). Do *not* create a permanent bond.
4. Either use a prefabricated coil spring or form a coil spring with a wire-bending jig (see Fig. 7-25) or round-nose pliers.
5. Align the coil spring with the axis of the D5 MCP (Fig. 11-7*a*).
6. Bend the ends of the wire and cut off. Mark the location of the wire bends on the hand and finger strips.
7. Heat the ends of the bent wire over the heat gun nozzle and embed them into the thermoplastic.
8. Apply solvent or alcohol, dry heat the overlaps, and seal. Blend in all edges for a firm bond and to eliminate dirt-collecting crevices.
9. If the orthosis migrates distally with MCP extension, attach a strap around the base of the thumb (Fig. 11-7*c* and *d*).
10. Trim the hand piece and finger piece to prevent pinching of the volar soft tissue (Fig. 11-7*c*).

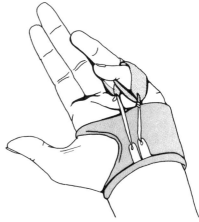

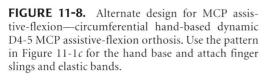

**FIGURE 11-8.** Alternate design for MCP assistive-flexion—circumferential hand-based dynamic D4-5 MCP assistive-flexion orthosis. Use the pattern in Figure 11-1*c* for the hand base and attach finger slings and elastic bands.

| | |
|---|---|
| ***Wearing Regimen*** | • Worn all the time or may be alternated with the figure-eight hand-based static D4-5 MCP extension-blocking orthosis at night. |
| ***Precaution*** | • Spring wire is easily deformed. |
| ***Alternatives*** | • Figure-eight hand-based static D4-5 MCP extension-blocking orthosis<br>• Circumferential hand-based dynamic D4-5 MCP assistive-flexion orthosis, which uses rubber bands attached to finger loops to flex the MCPs[11] (Fig. 11-8)<br>• Prefabricated designs |

- - -

■ **Name:**    **Circumferential Hand-Based Dynamic Joint-Aligned Coil-Spring D2-5 MCP Assistive-Flexion and Thumb Assistive-Opposition Orthosis** (Fig. 11-9*a* and *b*)

| | |
|---|---|
| ***Common Names*** | Dynamic anticlaw deformity splint; dynamic median/ulnar nerve splint; spring wire knuckle bender |
| ***SCS Name*** | Index through small finger MP flexion mobilization and thumb CMC opposition mobilization; type 0[5] |
| ***Objectives*** | • To passively flex finger MCPs while allowing active MCP extension<br>  ○ To correct hyperextension of the MCPs<br>  ○ To prevent shortening of the MCP collateral ligaments<br>  ○ To promote active IP extension<br>• To passively position the thumb in palmar abduction to promote opposition and prevent web space contracture |

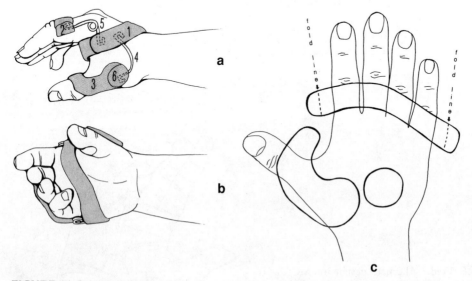

**FIGURE 11-9.**    Circumferential hand-based dynamic joint-aligned coil-spring D2-5 MCP assistive-flexion and thumb assistive-opposition orthosis. *(a)* Radial view. The numbers refer to the steps in the fabrication process. *(b)* Volar view. *(c)* Pattern.

*Indication*   • Combined median and ulnar nerve lesions at the level of the wrist

*Rationale*   • Combined lesions of the median and ulnar nerves at the wrist causes paralysis of all the intrinsic muscles, causing a clawhand deformity (see Fig. 2-17*a* and *b*). Active finger MCP flexion and IP extension are lost, along with the ability to oppose the thumb. Active IP flexion is unimpaired. When the orthosis pushes the MCPs into flexion, forces exerted by the extensor digitorum are transferred distally through the extensor expansion to extend the IPs. The dynamic design also allows active MCP extension against the resistance of the coil springs. The orthosis also positions the thumb in opposition and allows active extension and radial abduction against the resistance of the spring-wire.

*Materials*   
• For the hand base: $\frac{3}{32}$ or $\frac{1}{8}$ in. (2.4 or 3.2 mm) thick category B or C thermoplastic
• For the thumb and finger pieces: $\frac{1}{16}$ in. (1.6 mm) thick thermoplastic
• Thin self-adhesive gel padding
• Solvent or alcohol
• Two prefabricated knuckle bender coil springs[7,10] (Fig. 4-4*b*)
• 0.9 mm gauge spring wire[7]

*Equipment and Tools*   
• Heating pan
• Heat gun
• Two pairs of pliers
• Self-adhesive hook Velcro
• Wire cutter
• Wire-bending jig (or round-nose pliers) to make custom coil spring from spring wire if prefabricated coil springs are unavailable

*Joint Positions*   
• At rest, the coil spring pushes the MCPs into about 75° flexion.
• Thumb is positioned for easy opposition to the tips of D2 and D3.

*Pattern*   • Figure 11-9*c*

*Fabrication*   
1. Heat the hand-base strip and apply gel padding to line the thermoplastic over the dorsum of the MCs to prevent distal migration. Beginning at the ulnar side, mold circumferentially around the hand, wrapping across the bases of the MCs over the dorsum, proximal to the MC heads in the palm, and then across the dorsum again, ending at the radial side of the second MC. Cut off excess thermoplastic. Do *not* create a permanent bond.
2. Heat the finger piece and mold across the dorsum of the proximal phalanges.
3. Heat the thumb piece and mold to the dorsum of the thumb.
4. Using the 0.9 mm wire, create a gentle curve in the thumb-abduction wire, bend the ends, and cut off extra wire. Mark the location of the wire bends on the hand and thumb components.
5. Align the coil springs with the MCP axes of D2 and D5. Bend the ends of the wire and cut off the extra wire. Mark the location of the wire bends on the hand, finger, and thumb components.
6. Heat the thumb end of the curved wire over a heat gun and embed into the thumb piece. Bond a disk of thermoplastic over the embedded wire with solvent or alcohol and dry heat.
7. Open the overlapped thermoplastic across the dorsum of the hand and sandwich the MCP coil springs and the thumb-abduction wire between the layers. Using solvent and dry heat, seal the overlap.
8. Heat the free ends of the MCP coil springs over the heat gun nozzle and embed them into the finger piece.

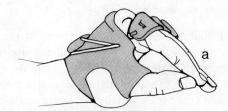

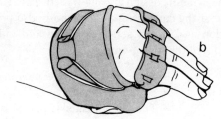

**FIGURE 11-10.** Alternate design to correct claw-hand deformity: circumferential hand-based dynamic MCP assistive-flexion static thumb-MCP orthosis. To fabricate this orthosis, mold a circumferential hand-based static thumb-CMC-MCP orthosis (see Fig. 11-22) with a volar opening to immobilize the thumb in opposition. The assistive flexion component uses rubber bands. *(a)* Radial view. *(b)* Dorsal view.

9. To secure the MCP coil springs to finger piece, apply solvent, dry heat the overlaps, and fold over at the fold lines.

10. Blend in all the edges for a firm bond and to eliminate dirt-collecting crevices.

11. If the orthosis migrates distally during active MCP extension, attach a strap around the base of the thumb as in Figures 11-7*c* and *d*.

| | |
|---|---|
| ***Wearing Regimen*** | • Worn at all times or switch to a static design at night. |
| ***Precaution*** | • Spring wire is easily deformed. |
| ***Option*** | • Delete the thumb piece. |
| ***Alternatives*** | • Circumferential hand-based dynamic D2-5 MCP assistive-flexion static thumb-opposition orthosis uses rubber bands to apply assistive flexion force to the finger MCPs while positioning the thumb in static opposition (Fig. 11-10). |
| | • Modify the figure-eight hand-based static D4-5 MCP extension-blocking orthosis to include all the finger MCPs. |
| | • Prefabricated designs. |

---

 **Name:** **Circumferential Hand-Based Static MCP-PIP Flexion-Blocking Orthosis** (Fig. 11-11*a*)

The orthosis depicted restricts flexion of the index finger. However, any or all digits can be included.

| | |
|---|---|
| ***Common Name*** | Blocking splint |
| ***SCS Name*** | Index finger MCP and PIP extension immobilization; type 0[2] |
| ***Objective*** | • To block MCP and PIP so that the flexor digitorum profundus can actively stretch the DIP to increase the flexion range of motion |

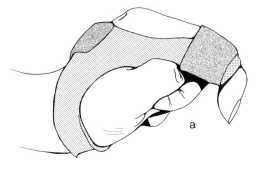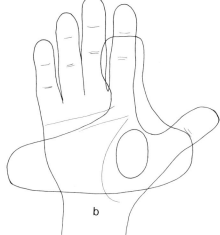

**FIGURE 11-11.** Circumferential hand-based static D2 MCP-PIP flexion-blocking orthosis. (*a*) Radial view. (*b*) Pattern.

| | |
|---|---|
| ***Indication*** | • Extension contracture of the DIP joint |
| ***Rationale*** | • See Chapter 3, "No Unnecessary Restriction of Function" |
| ***Materials*** | • Category C thermoplastic—$\frac{1}{16}$ in. (1.6 mm) thick<br>• 1 in. (2.5 cm) wide self-adhesive hook Velcro<br>• 1 in. (2.5 cm) wide loop Velcro |
| ***Equipment and Tools*** | • Heating pan  • For the pattern: paper towel or flexible clear<br>• Heat gun      plastic with permanent marker and straight pins,<br>• Scissors     stapler, or tape |
| ***Joint Positions*** | • Positions the MCP and PIP of the affected finger in functional flexion so that the thumb can easily oppose the tip of the affected finger.<br>• Thumb and unaffected fingers are unrestricted. |
| ***Pattern*** | • Figure 11-11*b* |
| ***Fabrication*** | 1. Cut the thermoplastic.<br>2. Heat and check the temperature of the thermoplastic.<br>3. Mold to the volar aspect of the hand, controlling the position of the MCP and PIP.<br>4. Attach the straps. |
| ***Wearing Regimen*** | • As tolerated during the waking hours. |
| ***Options*** | • Terminate at the PIP crease to block only MCP flexion.<br>• Include any or all fingers. |
| ***Alternative*** | • Exclude the MCP block and mold a circumferential finger-based orthosis to block PIP motion while leaving the DIP free. |

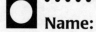

**Name:**    **Circumferential Hand-Based Static-Progressive MERiT-Screw MCP-IP Flexion Orthosis** (Fig. 11-12*a*)
**Circumferential Hand-Based Static-Progressive Tube-Outrigger MCP-IP Flexion Orthosis** (Fig. 11-12*b*)

In both Figures 11-12*a* and *b*, the orthosis depicted is applying corrective force to the middle finger (D3). However, the MERiT screw or tube outrigger can be mounted for any digit.

*Common Name*    Final flexion splint

*SCS Name*    Middle finger MP and IP flexion mobilization; type 0[3]

*Objective*    • To progressively position the MCPs and IPs in composite flexion, applying gentle, prolonged stretch to contracted tissues to reduce extension contractures

*Indications*    • Contracture of the extrinsic extensor tendons with or without contracture of the MCP collateral ligaments
    • IP extension contracture

*Rationale*    • See Chapter 2, "Promoting Tissue Growth to Reduce Contractures."

*Materials*    • For the hand base and finger slings: category C or D thermoplastic—¹⁄₁₆ in. (1.6 mm) thick
    • For mounting the thumb screw—a small piece of ⅛ in. (3.2 mm) thick thermoplastic
    • MERiT Static Progressive Component[12,13] (Fig. 11-12*a*) (The screw is similar to the machine head of a string instrument. When the thumb screw is turned, the nylon line is wrapped around the projecting cylinder, creating tension in the line. The screw allows easy tension adjustment, but it is bulky.)
    • Alternatively, use Orfitube[7] or ⅜ in. (9.5 mm) wide Aquatube[12] or Thermo-Tube[10] (Fig. 11-12*b*)
    • Thin self-adhesive gel padding    • Nylon line

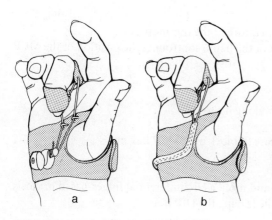

**FIGURE 11-12.**    *(a)* Circumferential hand-based static-progressive MERiT-screw D3 MCP-IP flexion orthosis. *(b)* Circumferential hand-based static-progressive tube-outrigger D3 MCP-IP flexion orthosis.

- Self-adhesive hook Velcro
- Loop Velcro
- Solvent or alcohol
- Two plastic-coated paper clips

***Equipment and Tools***

- Heating pan  • Heat gun  • Scissors  • Hole punch  • Wire cutter
- For the pattern: paper towel or flexible clear plastic with permanent marker and straight pins, stapler, or tape

***Pattern***

- For the hand base, use Figure 11-1*c*, terminating it at the base of the MC heads.
- Finger slings—two pieces: 1 × 1½ in. (2.5 × 4 cm) with rounded corners.

***Fabrication***

1. Mold the hand base as for the circumferential nonarticular metacarpal-stabilizing orthosis and attach a strap over the dorsal opening.
2. Mold the finger slings, ideally with gel padding, over the dorsum of the proximal and distal phalanges of affected digit.
3. Punch small holes in finger slings.

*For the MERiT screw design:*

4. To determine the location of paper clip line guides, estimate where the fingertip would contact the hand base if the finger could fully flex. Punch a pair of small holes in the hand base for each line guide.
5. Unfold each paper clip once and cut in half, creating a U-shaped hook. Insert the two ends of the hook into the holes, creating a line guide on the front of the hand base. Bend the two ends back under the hand base. Repeat for the other line guide and cover the hook ends with gel padding (see Fig. 10-23*f* ).
6. Mount the MERiT screw onto the hand base near the wrist, using solvent or alcohol, the heat gun, and ⅛ in. (3.2 mm) thick thermoplastic.
7. Cut two lengths of nylon line and tie one to each hole in the distal phalanx sling. Thread the lines through the holes in the proximal phalanx sling, through the line guides, and tie them onto the MERiT screw.
8. Turn the thumb screw to adjust the tension in the nylon lines until the client feels a slight stretch.

*For the tube outrigger:*

9. Shape the tube outrigger to conform to the contours of the hand base. The tube must open distally in line with the tip of the affected finger. Aquatubes and ThermoTubes must be moist heated to shape; Orfitubes can be bent without heating.
10. Bond the Aquatube or ThermoTube to the hand base with solvent or alcohol and dry heat. To attach an Orfitube, cut two strips of thermoplastic and secure the tube to the hand base with solvent and dry heat as shown in Figure 11-13*a*.
11. Cut two lengths of nylon line and secure one to each hole in the distal phalanx sling. Thread the lines through the holes in the proximal phalanx sling, through the tube outrigger, and out the proximal end.
12. Adjust the tension in the nylon line until the client feels a gentle stretch that can be tolerated for several hours.
13. Heat a scrap of thermoplastic or a ¼ in. (½ cm) length of Aquatube/ThermoTube and adhere to the proximal end of the nylon line, creating a bead stop as in Figure 11-13*a*.

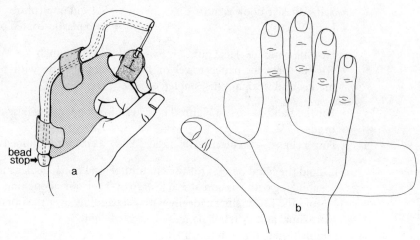

**FIGURE 11-13.** Circumferential hand-based dynamic tube-outrigger D2 PIP corrective-extension orthosis. *(a)* Radial view showing 90° angle of pull of the finger loop on the middle phalanx. Volar opening is not visible. *(b)* Pattern.

| | |
|---|---|
| *Adjustment* | • As the flexion range improves, either<br>  ○ Turn the MERiT screw to maintain the gentle stretch, adjusting tension in small increments, or<br>  ○ Take up the slack in the nylon line and move the bead stop to shorten the line |
| *Wearing Regimen* | • At night and a few hours during the day as tolerated without undue interference with hand function. |
| *Precautions* | • Monitor the extension range of motion and encourage extension exercises when the orthosis is off. |
| *Options* | • Replace the paired thermoplastic finger slings with one thermoplastic cuff.[14]<br>• Replace the thermoplastic finger slings with Velfoam finger cuffs (see Fig. 10-23).<br>• Replace the nylon line with wrapped elastic cord, converting the static-progressive orthosis into a dynamic design. |
| *Alternatives* | • Prefabricated flexion glove<br>• Prefabricated joint cinch<br>• Other custom thermoplastic designs[14–19] |

● **Name:** **Circumferential Hand-Based Dynamic Tube-Outrigger PIP Corrective-Extension Orthosis** (Fig. 11-13*a*)

| | |
|---|---|
| *Common Names* | Low profile dynamic PIP extension splint; short dorsal outrigger |
| *SCS Name* | Index finger extension mobilization; type 1[2] |

| | |
|---|---|
| *Objectives* | • To apply gentle, prolonged stretch to the contracted PIP capsule and ligaments to promote growth of the shortened tissues and restore extension range of motion |
| *Indications* | • Flexion contracture of a PIP joint |
| *Rationale* | • See Chapter 2, "Promoting Tissue Growth to Reduce Contractures." |
| *Disadvantages of This Design* | • The hand base immobilizes the MCP of the affected finger(s).<br>• The tube outrigger projects above the hand, making it conspicuous, which has a negative impact on compliance.[20]<br>• The outrigger requires rebending as the extension range improves. |
| *Materials* | • Category C or D thermoplastic—$\frac{1}{16}$ or $\frac{3}{32}$ in. (1.6 or 2.4 mm) thick<br>• Orfitube[7] or $\frac{3}{8}$ in. (9.5 mm) wide Aquatube[12] or ThermoTube[21]<br>• Wrapped elastic cord<br>• Self-adhesive hook Velcro<br>• Loop Velcro<br>• Finger loop |
| *Equipment and Tools* | • Heating pan     • For the pattern: paper towel or flexible clear plastic<br>• Heat gun          with permanent marker and straight pins, stapler,<br>• Scissors          or tape |
| *Joint Position* | • Positions the MCP of the affected digit(s) in flexion to promote function |
| *Pattern* | • Figure 11-13*b* |
| *Fabrication* | 1. Cut out the pattern.<br>2. Heat, check the temperature, and mold the hand base over the dorsum of the hand with a volar opening.<br>3. Attach the strap across the volar opening.<br>4. To shape the tube outrigger, Aquatubes and ThermoTubes must be moist heated to shape, whereas Orfitubes can be bent without heating.<br>5. Bond the Aquatube or ThermoTube to the hand base with solvent or alcohol and dry heat. To attach an Orfitube, cut two strips of thermoplastic and secure the tube to the hand base with solvent and dry heat.<br>6. Ensure that the distal end of the tube is centered over the middle phalanx when the PIP is maximally extended, with a 90°angle of pull to the long axis of the bone.<br>7. Tie the elastic cord to the finger sling, slip the finger sling around the middle phalanx, and then thread the cord through the tube and out the proximal end.<br>8. Adjust the tension in the elastic cord until the client feels a gentle stretch that can be tolerated for several hours.<br>9. Heat a scrap of thermoplastic or a $\frac{1}{4}$ in. ($\frac{1}{2}$ cm) length of Aquatube or ThermoTube and adhere to the proximal end of the elastic cord, creating a bead stop. |
| *Adjustment* | • As the PIP extension range improves, shorten the elastic cord and reshape the tube to relign its distal opening to maintain the 90° angle of pull. |
| *Wearing Regimen* | • At night and several hours per day to maintain prolonged stretch. |

| | |
|---|---|
| *Option* | • To apply corrective-extension force to the DIP, modify the design to immobilize the PIP as well as the MCP and place the finger sling around the distal phalanx. |
| *Alternatives* | • See Figure 3-11<br>• Three-point finger-based dynamic joint-aligned coil-spring PIP corrective-extension orthosis<br>• Other custom thermoplastic designs[22,23] |

●●●●●●●●●●●●●●●●●●●●●●●●●●●●●●●●●●●●●●●●●●●●●●●●

### ● Name: Circumferential Nonarticular Proximal Phalanx–Stabilizing Orthosis (Fig. 11-14*a*)

Developed by Kim Oxford, OTR, and David Hildreth, MD, University of Texas Health Science Center.[24]

| | |
|---|---|
| *Common Name* | Proximal phalanx fracture brace |
| *SCS Name* | Nonarticular splint—proximal phalanx |
| *Objectives* | • To stabilize a phalangeal fracture to promote healing, without immobilizing any joints |
| *Indications*[24] | • For a stable fracture of the proximal phalanx that requires no fixation—apply immediately.<br>• For a fracture that requires screw fixation—apply 3 to 5 days postoperatively.<br>• For a fracture that requires pinning—apply 1 to 2 weeks postoperatively, depending on fracture stability. |
| *Rationale* | • Applies circumferential compression to maintain fracture alignment.<br>• See Chapter 2, "Fractures of Long Bones." |

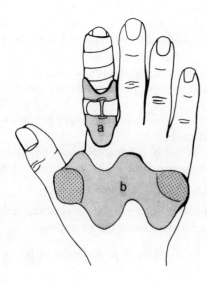

**FIGURE 11-14.** Circumferential nonarticular proximal phalanx-stabilizing orthosis. (*a*) Dorsal view showing D-ring closure and Coban wrapping under the orthosis to control edema. (*b*) Pattern. Stippling shows where the thermoplastic overlaps on the lateral side of the phalanx.

| | |
|---|---|
| *Materials* | • Category C or D thermoplastic—$\frac{1}{16}$ in. (1.6 mm) thick<br>• $\frac{1}{2}$ in. (1.3 cm) wide hook Velcro<br>• $\frac{1}{2}$ in. (1.3 cm) wide R-Thin or Extra-Thin loop Velcro<br>• $\frac{1}{2}$ in. (1.3 cm) wide D-ring (optional) |
| *Equipment and Tools* | • Heating pan      • Scissors      • Sewing machine |
| *Pattern* | • Figure 11-14*b* |
| *Fabrication* | 1. Heat and mold the thermoplastic around the proximal phalanx, overlapping the stippled areas in Figure 11-14*b*.<br>2. Apply an overlap or D-ring strap. |
| *Wearing Regimen* | • Worn at all times and removed carefully for bathing when the fracture is stable as per the physician's recommendations<br>• Can be worn over a compressive bandage wrap applied from the tip to the base of the finger, or a finger sleeve, to control edema |
| *Precautions* | • Encourage active range of motion of MCP and IPs. |
| *Options* | • For a more proximal fracture, extend the pattern proximally to support the MCP dorsally and volarly.<br>• For a more distal fracture, extend the pattern distally to stabilize the PIP with lateral supports.<br>• The orthosis in Figure 11-14*a* and the pattern in Figure 11-14*b* combine both the proximal and distal extensions. |
| *Alternatives* | • A static volar or circumferential finger orthosis, immobilizing the IPs and sometimes also the MCP |

## Name: Circumferential Finger-Based MCP Extension-Blocking Buddy Orthosis[25] (Fig. 11-15)

In this figure, the middle finger (D3) is the affected digit. However, the orthosis can also be molded to block MCP extension of the ring finger.

| | |
|---|---|
| *Common Name* | None |
| *SCS Name* | Not classified |
| *Objective* | • To block MCP extension to promote active PIP extension |
| *Indication* | • PIP extension lag with flexible or stiff PIP of D3 or D4 |
| *Rationale* | • MCP extension of the affected finger is blocked when the unaffected fingers adjacent to affected finger flex at the MCPs. As a result, active extension force is focused on the affected PIP. |
| *Materials* | • Category C or D thermoplastic—$\frac{1}{16}$ in. (1.6 mm) thick<br>• Thin self-adhesive foam or gel padding (optional)<br>• Solvent or alcohol |

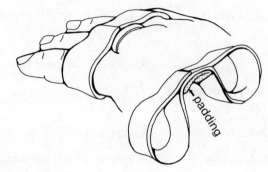

**FIGURE 11-15.** Circumferential finger-based D3 MCP extension-blocking buddy orthosis. Stippling shows gel padding against the dorsum of affected middle finger.

| | | |
|---|---|---|
| *Equipment and Tools* | • Heating pan | • Heat gun |

*Pattern*
 • A strip of thermoplastic, the width of the proximal phalanx and about 7 in. (18 cm) long

*Fabrication*
 1. If desired, apply padding to the dorsum of the affected proximal phalanx.
 2. Mold over the dorsum of the affected finger and around proximal phalanx of each adjacent finger.
 3. Bond the ends to the thermoplastic over the affected finger, using solvent or alcohol and a heat gun.
 4. Trim on the volar side to prevent pinching (Fig. 11-7c).
 5. Transfer the padding to the inside of the orthosis.

---

⬛⭕ **Name:** **Circumferential Finger-Based PIP-Stabilizing Buddy Straps** (Fig. 11-16a and b)

*Common Names*
 Buddy splint; trapper

*SCS Name*
 Not classified

*Objectives*
 • To strap an affected finger to an unaffected finger at the proximal and middle phalanges
 • To stabilize the finger joints, preventing deviation and rotation
 • To promote passive joint motion of an affected finger though active motion of an adjacent unaffected finger

*Indications*
 • PIP collateral ligament injury
 • Introduced at week 3 after a staged flexor tendon reconstruction[26]
 • Introduced at week 3 after a PIP dislocation if the joint is stable[27]

*Materials*
 • 1 in. (2.5 cm) wide nonadhesive hook and loop Velcro

*Equipment and Tools*
 • Sewing machine
 • Scissors

*Pattern*
 • For each strap:
   ○ Hook Velcro about 5 in. (12.5 cm) long

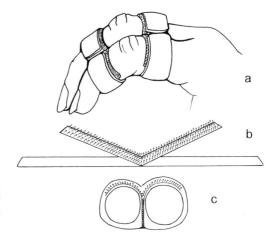

**FIGURE 11-16.** *(a)* Circumferential finger-based nonarticular D2-3 PIP-stabilizing buddy straps. *(b)* Single strap showing hook Velcro sewn on top of the loop Velcro. *(c)* Cross-sectional view.

○ Loop Velcro about 7 in. (17.5 cm) long

| | |
|---|---|
| *Fabrication* | 1. For each strap, center the hook Velcro face up on top of the loop Velcro, also face up. |
| | 2. Sew them together through their midpoints (Fig. 11-16*b*). |
| | 3. Apply and trim the straps over the volar aspect as required to ensure unimpeded IP flexion. |
| *Application* | • Apply each strap with the hook Velcro wrapping over the dorsum of the phalanges (hook side up) while the loop Velcro wraps around from the volar side and fastens to the hook Velcro over the dorsum (Fig. 11-16*c*). |
| *Options* | • Use alone or in conjunction with a hand-based orthosis such as the circumferential nonarticular metacarpal-stabilizing orthosis (described previously). |
| *Alternatives* | • Tape the corresponding phalanges together with adhesive or cohesive tape—this is called buddy taping. |
| | • Prefabricated version.[12] |
| | • Use thin thermoplastic (optionally lined with gel padding) over the volar aspect of phalanges.[28] |
| | • For PIP collateral ligament injury, custom[29] or prefabricated Rolyan® PIP Ligament Repair Splint.[12] |

○ ● ● ● ● ● ● ● ● ● ● ● ● ● ● ● ● ● ● ● ● ● ● ● ● ● ● ● ● ● ● ● ● ● ● ● ● ● ● ● ●

**Name:** **Spiral Finger-Based Static PIP Extension-Blocking Orthosis** (Fig. 11-17*a* through *c*)

| | |
|---|---|
| *Common Names* | • Swan-neck (deformity) splint; PIP hyperextension splint; Figure-eight splint |
| *SCS Name* | • Index finger PIP extension restriction; type 0[1] |

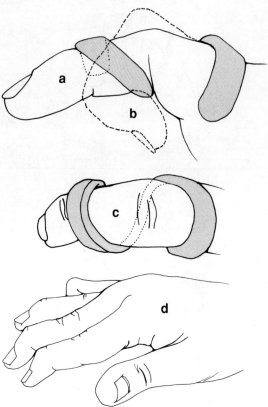

**FIGURE 11-17.** Spiral finger-based static (D2) PIP extension-blocking orthosis. *(a)* Solid line: the PIP is extended to the limit of the block. *(b)* Broken line: PIP flexion is unrestricted. *(c)* Dorsal view. *(d)* Swan-neck deformity: PIP hyperextension with MCP and DIP flexion.

---

| *Indications* | *Objectives and Rationale* |
|---|---|

- Swan-neck deformity (Fig. 11-17*d*) caused by
  - Rheumatoid arthritis causing MCP or PIP synovitis[4]
  - Intrinsic muscle tightness or contracture
  - Dorsal migration of the lateral bands of the extensor mechanism
  - Trauma causing PIP volar plate injury
- Trigger finger

- When PIP is blocked in a few degrees of flexion, the joint cannot lock in hyperextension. Early intervention prevents progression of the deformity and promotes restabilization of the lateral bands and healing of the volar plate.

- To block PIP extension to limit excursion of the long finger flexor tendons. This prevents tendon triggering at the A1 pulley, which occurs when the finger extends fully.
- By eliminating irritation that occurs when the tendon nodule catches on the A1 pulley, inflammation and triggering subside.

*Advantages of This Design*

- Easy to make; mobility of the PIP promotes hand function; there are no folds to create dirt-catching crevices; easy to achieve full PIP flexion; the noncircumferential design is easy to apply even if the PIP becomes effused.

*Materials*

- Category B, C, or D thermoplastic—⅛ in. (3.2 mm) thick, or 1/16 in. (1.6 mm) folded double

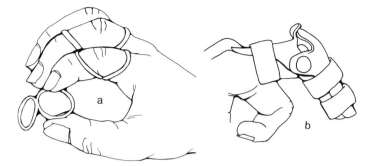

**FIGURE 11-18.** Alternate designs for PIP extension block. *(a)* Custom Siris Swan-neck Silver Ring Splint,[31] *(b)* Rolyan® PIP Extension Blocking Splint.[12] Patent No. 5,232,436.

| | |
|---|---|
| ***Equipment and Tools*** | • Heating pan      • Scissors |
| ***Joint Positions*** | • The thermoplastic over the dorsum of the proximal and middle phalanges limits extension to about 15° flexion (Fig. 11-17*a*).<br>• Full active PIP flexion is permitted (Fig. 11-17*b*). |
| ***Pattern*** | • Strip of thermoplastic ¼ in. (½ cm) wide, long enough to spiral around the finger—i.e., about 5 or 6 in. (12.5 or 15 cm) long |
| ***Fabrication*** | 1. Heat the thermoplastic, check the temperature, and mold it spirally around the finger.<br>2. The thermoplastic should course along the PIP joint crease to ensure that PIP flexion is unrestricted (Fig. 11-17*c*).<br>3. While the material cools, hold the PIP in slight flexion. |
| ***Wearing Regimen*** | • Ideally, at all times |
| ***Precautions*** | • Minimize the bulk of the thermoplastic under the PIP to ensure unrestricted PIP flexion.<br>• Position the thermoplastic over the dorsum of the finger as close to the MCP and DIP joints as possible to maximize the lever arms. |
| ***Alternatives*** | • Other custom thermoplastic designs,[30] e.g., "buttonhole" style[2,4]<br>• Prefabricated Murphy ring splints[6,12]<br>• Custom-fabricated Siris Swan-neck Silver Ring Splint[31] (Fig. 11-18*a*)<br>• Prefabricated Rolyan® PIP Extension Blocking Splint[12] (Fig. 11-18*b*) |

 **Name:** **Three-Point Finger-Based Dynamic Joint-Aligned Coil-Spring PIP Corrective-Extension Orthosis**
(Fig. 11-19*a*)

| | |
|---|---|
| ***Common Names*** | Capener splint; dynamic spring wire splint for PIP extension |
| ***SCS Name*** | Index finger PIP extension mobilization; type 0[1] |
| ***General Objective*** | • To passively extend the PIP while permitting active IP flexion |

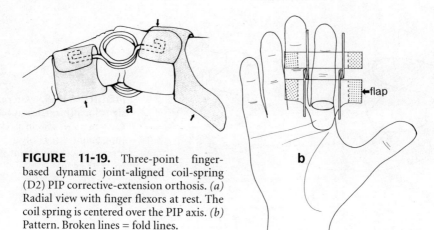

**FIGURE 11-19.** Three-point finger-based dynamic joint-aligned coil-spring (D2) PIP corrective-extension orthosis. *(a)* Radial view with finger flexors at rest. The coil spring is centered over the PIP axis. *(b)* Pattern. Broken lines = fold lines.

## Indications

- PIP flexion contracture[32]
- PIP dorsal dislocation
- Volar plate injury
- Flexor tendon repair with resulting PIP flexion contracture
- Partial or complete tear of the collateral ligament
- Boutonnière deformity

- Surgical repair of a lacerated/ruptured central slip of the extensor mechanism, with or without involvement of the lateral bands, i.e., extensor tendon injury in zone 3 (over the PIP) or zone 4 (over the proximal phalanx)

## Objectives and Rationale

- To apply gentle, prolonged stretch to a contracted PIP capsule and ligaments to promote growth of shortened tissues and restore extension range (see Chapter 2, "Promoting Tissue Growth to Reduce Contractures").
- To provide lateral stability to PIP.

- To promote restabilization of the lateral bands and prevent rupture of the central slip (see Chapter 2, "Promoting Tissue Resorption").
- To promote early protected motion and tendon excursion for optimal tendon healing with minimal range-restricting adhesions or risk of rupture (see Chapter 2, "Tendon Injuries").

| | |
|---|---|
| ***Advantages of This Design*** | • This orthosis has "no profile," minimizing its visual presence, which has a positive effect on compliance.[20] |
| ***Materials*** | • Category C or D thermoplastic—1⁄16 in. (1.6 mm) thick<br>• Two prefabricated joint jack coil springs (0.7 mm gauge)[7,10] (see Fig. 4-4a)—or substitute knuckle bender coil springs (0.9 mm gauge) (see Fig. 4-4b) or make custom coil springs formed from 0.9 mm gauge spring wire<br>• Solvent or alcohol |
| ***Equipment and Tools*** | • Heating pan<br>• Heat gun<br>• Two pairs of pliers—flat or needle nose<br>• Wire cutter<br><br>• Wire-bending jig (or round-nose pliers) to make custom coil spring from spring wire if prefabricated coil springs are unavailable |
| ***Pattern*** | • Figure 11-19b |

| | |
|---|---|
| *Fabrication* | 1. Heat the proximal piece, check the temperature, and slip the finger through the hole, molding it to the volar surface of the MC head and the dorsum of the proximal phalanx (Fig. 11-19*a*).<br>2. Heat the distal piece, check the temperature, and mold it to the volar surface of the middle phalanx.<br>3. Align the coil springs with the axis of the PIP. Bend the ends and cut off the extra wire. Mark the location of the wire bends on the proximal and distal pieces.<br>4. Heat the ends of the bent wire over the heat gun nozzle and embed them into the thermoplastic.<br>5. Apply solvent or alcohol, dry heat the flaps, and fold them over the ends of the wire and seal. Blend in all the edges for a firm bond and to eliminate dirt-collecting crevices. |
| *Wearing Regimen* | • As appropriate for the situation. |
| *Precautions* | • Guard against excessive extension force that could overstress tissue and cause inflammation.[33]<br>• To prevent injury from a piece of flying wire, cut the wire under a towel, pillowcase, or sheet. |
| *Option* | • Attach a Velcro strap over the dorsum of the middle phalanx. |
| *Alternatives* | • See Figures 1-10 and 3-11<br>• Figures 11-13, 11-20*a* and *b*<br>• Other custom thermoplastic designs[34,35]<br>• Plaster of Paris casting[36,37]<br>• Prefabricated finger-based dynamic PIP corrective-extension splints (e.g., foam-coated wire)[12,13]<br>• Prefabricated Rolyan® Dynamic Digit Extension Tube Splint[12]—neoprene tube with rubber spring |

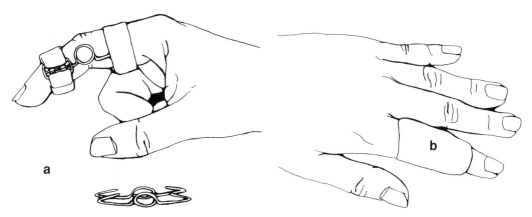

**FIGURE 11-20.** Alternate designs for PIP corrective-extension. (*a*) Rolyan® P.I.P.E. (*P*roximal *I*nterphalangeal *E*xtension) Splint[12] uses 5 pairs of interchangeable graded coil springs; as extension range improves, springs are replaced with another pair having greater torque. (*b*) Circumferential finger-based plaster of Paris serial-static PIP-corrective extension cast. Every few days the plaster cast is removed and replaced with a new one that positions the PIP in slightly more extension to accommodate the growth in the soft tissues.

● ● ● ● ● ● ● ● ● ● ● ● ● ● ● ● ● ● ● ● ● ● ● ● ● ● ● ● ● ● ● ● ● ● ● ● ● ● ● ● ● ●

## ◯ Name:   Circumferential Thumb-Based Static Thumb-MCP Orthosis (Fig. 11-21*a* and *b*)

| | |
|---|---|
| *Common Name* | Thumb splint |
| *SCS Name* | Thumb MP extension immobilization; type 0[1] |
| *Objective* | • To stabilize the thumb MCP to reduce pain and inflammation, promote healing, and prevent undue joint stress<br>• To permit thumb CMC movement |
| *Indications* | • MCP inflammation, injury, or instability associated with rheumatoid arthritis, trauma, or occupational overuse (e.g., physical or massage therapist)<br>• Gamekeeper's thumb or skier's thumb—sprain of ulnar collateral ligament of the first MCP<br>• Sprain of first MCP radial collateral ligament |
| *Materials* | • Category C or D thermoplastic—¹⁄₁₆ in. (1.6 mm) thick<br>• 1 in. (2.5 cm) nonadhesive hook Velcro<br>• 1 in. (2.5 cm) elasticized loop Velcro<br>• Hand cream<br>• Solvent or alcohol |
| *Equipment and Tools* | • Heating pan<br>• Scissors<br>• Sewing machine |

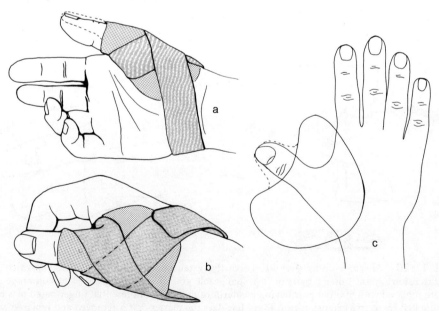

**FIGURE 11-21.**   Circumferential thumb-based static thumb-MCP orthosis. *(a)* Volar view. The broken line shows an optional dorsal extension to block the IP if desired. *(b)* Radial view. *(c)* Pattern. The broken line represents the optional dorsal extension.

| | |
|---|---|
| *Joint Position* | • Position the MCP in slight flexion to facilitate opposition. |
| *Pattern* | • Figure 11-21*c* |
| *Fabrication* | 1. Apply hand cream to the thumb. |
| | 2. Mold circumferentially around the first MCP, with the distal edge at the PIP crease, overlapping the thermoplastic in the web space. The overlap can be temporarily bonded during molding and snapped open to remove when the thermoplastic has cooled. |
| | 3. Gently flare the distal thumb edge by running a pencil or pen under it (see Fig. 10-10*e*). |
| | 4. Gently flare the proximal edge. |
| | 5. The overlap can be left unbonded to ensure easy removal over the distal phalanx and to accommodate future IP swelling. Alternatively, the overlap can be bonded with solvent or alcohol and dry heat. |
| | 6. Cut a length of elasticized loop Velcro to form a figure-eight strap (Fig. 11-21*a* and *b*). Sew a tab of hook Velcro to one end. |
| *Wearing Regimen* | • All the time or during activities that stress the joint |
| *Precautions* | • When using thermoplastics with memory, the thermoplastic around the proximal phalanx contracts as it cools, and it may be difficult to slip off over the more bulbous distal phalanx. Gently flare the distal edge to avoid this problem. |
| | • Wrist, thumb IP, and finger MCP motions should be unrestricted unless restriction is desired. |
| *Option* | • Extend the thermoplastic over the dorsum of the distal phalanx to stabilize the IP and block hyperextension (Fig. 11-21*a* and *c*). |
| *Alternatives* | • Preformed orthoses |
| | • Other custom thermoplastic designs[38–41] |

---

**Names:** **Circumferential Hand-Based Static Thumb-CMC-MCP Orthosis** (Fig. 11-22*a* and *b*)
**Circumferential Hand-Based Serial-Static Thumb-CMC-MCP Corrective-Abduction Orthosis**

| | |
|---|---|
| *Common Names* | Short opponens (splint); short thumb spica |
| *SCS Name* | Thumb CMC palmar abduction immobilization (or mobilization); type 1[2] |
| *Objectives* | • To relieve CMC pain |
| | • To immobilize the first CMC and MCP |
| | • To position the thumb in functional opposition |
| | • To prevent or serially correct a first web space contracture |
| *Indications* | • Inflammation (e.g., osteoarthritis) or injury of the first CMC joint, with or without involvement of the MCP |

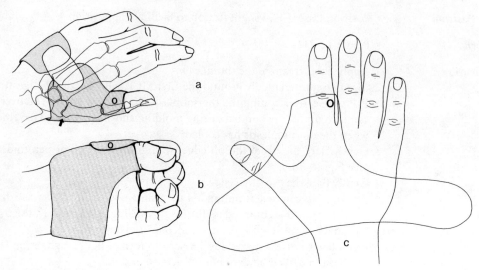

**FIGURE 11-22.** Circumferential hand-based static thumb-CMC-MCP orthosis. *(a)* Dorsal view showing the underlying bones. The arrow points to the arthritic CMC. "O" identifies the overlap. *(b)* Volar view. *(c)* Pattern. "O" identifies the overlap.

- CMC arthroplasty[42]
- Median nerve injury causing paralysis of the thenar muscles resulting in the loss of thumb opposition (see Fig. 2-17*e*)
- Quadriplegia[43–46]

*Rationale of This Design*
- Thumb CMC motion is effectively restricted because the thermoplastic extends around the ulnar border of the hand.

*Materials*
- Category C or D thermoplastic—1/16 in. (1.6 mm) thick
- 1 in. (2.5 cm) wide self-adhesive hook Velcro
- 1 in. (2.5 cm) wide loop Velcro
- Hand cream
- Solvent or alcohol

*Equipment and Tools*
- Heating pan
- Heat gun
- Scissors
- For the pattern: paper towel or flexible clear plastic with permanent marker and straight pins, stapler, or tape

*Joint Positions*
- The thumb is positioned to promote easy opposition (see Fig. 2-25*b*).
- The IP is unrestricted.

*Pattern*
- Figure 11-22*c*.
- The opening can be dorsal (as shown), ulnar, or volar.

*Fabrication*
1. When using translucent low-temperature thermoplastics (LTTs) with memory, wrap the thumb with 1/16 in. (1.6 mm) self-stick foam to prevent excessive shrinkage as the LTT cools, or apply hand cream to client's thumb.
2. Heat the thermoplastic and mold it to the palm and then around the dorsum of the hand.
3. Pull tab "O" from volar to dorsal through the first web space (Fig. 11-22*a* through *c*). The overlap can be temporarily bonded during molding and snapped open to remove the orthosis when the thermoplastic has cooled.

4. Gently flare the distal thumb edge by running a pencil or pen under it (see Fig. 10-10*e*).
5. Gently flare the proximal edge.
6. As the thermoplastic cools, keep the thumb positioned in opposition with the tips of the index and middle fingers (see Fig. 2-25*b*).
7. The overlap can be left unbonded to ensure easy removal over the distal phalanx and to accommodate future IP swelling. Alternatively, the overlap can be bonded with solvent or alcohol and dry heat.
8. Trim to clear the thumb IP, finger MCPs, and wrist.
9. Attach strap.

| | |
|---|---|
| ***Wearing Regimen*** | • All the time or as required to relieve pain and stress or to promote hand function. |
| ***Precautions*** | • When using thermoplastics with memory, the thermoplastic around the proximal phalanx contracts as it cools, and it may be difficult to slip off over the more bulbous distal phalanx. Gentle flaring of the distal edge can avoid this problem. If the orthosis will not slide over the distal phalanx, apply lotion to the skin and allow the client to pull the orthosis off. |
| | • Wrist, thumb IP, and finger MCP motions should be unrestricted unless restriction is desired. |
| | • Ensure unrestricted thumb opposition (see Fig. 2-25*b*). If you observe that the finger MCPs need to radially deviate for the middle finger to oppose the thumb, insufficient opposition was achieved. Remold to correct the thumb position. |
| ***Options*** | • Trim proximal to the thumb MCP to leave it free to move. However, this results in some loss of stabilization at the CMC. |
| | • Extend distally to block thumb IP motion as in Figure 11-21*a* and *c*. The thermoplastic extension can be restricted to the dorsal surface to stabilize IP, allowing IP flexion but limiting extension or blocking hyperextension; the volar surface of the distal phalanx is left uncovered. |
| | • Attach a writing tool for a client with quadriplegia. |
| ***Alternatives*** | • Soft prefabricated orthoses |
| | • Circumferential wrist-based dynamic thumb-opposition strap (Fig. 11-23*a*) |
| | • Other custom thermoplastic designs[47,48] |

## Names: **Circumferential Wrist-Based Dynamic Thumb-Opposition Strap** (Fig. 11-23*a*)
## **Circumferential Wrist-Based Dynamic Thumb–Radial Abduction Strap** (Fig. 11-23*b*)

| | |
|---|---|
| ***Common Name*** | Dynamic thumb opposition splint; thumb abduction splint |
| ***SCS Names*** | Thumb CMC palmer abduction mobilization; type 0[1] (Fig. 11-23*a*) |
| | Thumb CMC radial abduction mobilization; type 0[1] (Fig. 11-23*b*) |

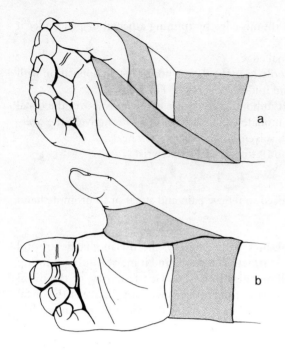

**FIGURE 11-23.** *(a)* Circumferential wrist-based dynamic thumb-opposition strap. *(b)* Circumferential wrist-based dynamic thumb-radial abduction strap.

| *Indications* | *Objectives* |
|---|---|
| • Weakness or paralysis of the thenar muscles (e.g., median nerve injury) | • To position the thumb in palmar abduction, in line with index and middle fingers, to facilitate opposition |
| • Adducted thumb position associated with high tone of a central nervous system disorder | • To position the thumb in radial abduction to to break up the pattern of flexor spasticity |

*Materials*
- For the wrist cuff:
  - ◦ 1½ in. (4 cm) wide webbing or neoprene—long enough to wrap around the wrist, plus an extra 1 in. (2.5 cm) if using webbing to sew under the cut edges.
  - ◦ 1 in. (1.5 cm) wide hook and loop Velcro
  - ◦ Foam or gel padding to prevent rotation or migration
- For the thumb loop: 1 in. (2.5 cm) wide elastic or neoprene—long enough to wrap around the base of the thumb and attach to the wrist cuff

*Equipment and Tools*
- Sewing machine
- Scissors

*Fabrication*
1. If using webbing, sew under each cut edge ½ in. (1 cm) and sew hook and loop Velcro at the closure.
2. When using neoprene, sew hook Velcro to only one edge.
3. Sew the elastic or neoprene into a loop that surrounds the base of the thumb, with about 4 in. (10 cm) extending from the loop.
4. To promote thumb opposition, sew the thumb loop to the wrist cuff adjacent to the pisiform bone (Fig. 11-23*a*).

5. To promote radial abduction, sew the thumb loop adjacent to the anatomical snuffbox (Fig. 11-23*b*).

**Precaution**

- The thumb loop should encircle the MC shaft to direct its force to the CMC without stressing the first MCP.

**Alternative**

- Prefabricated thumb loop[12]

## ● References

1. Schultz, KH: Hand-based metacarpal fracture brace and forearm ulnar or radius fracture brace. J Hand Ther 5:158, 1992.
2. Smith & Nephew Inc.: Smith & Nephew: Splinting Guidelines. Smith & Nephew Inc., Quebec, 1986.
3. Rennie HJ: Evaluation of the effectiveness of a metacarpophalangeal ulnar deviation orthosis. J Hand Ther 9:371, 1996.
4. Melvin, JL: Rheumatic Disease in the Adult and Child, Occupational Therapy and Rehabilitation, ed 3. FA Davis, Philadelphia, 1989.
5. Evans, RB, Hunter, JM, and Burkhalter, WE: Conservative management of the trigger finger: A new approach. J Hand Ther 1:59, 1988.
6. Eaton, R: Entrapment syndrome in musicians. J Hand Ther 5:91, 1992.
7. Orfit Industries: Orthotic Products Catalogue. Wiynegem, Belgium, 1992.
8. Gilbert-Lenef, L: Soft ulnar deviation splint. J Hand Ther 7:29, 1994.
9. Orfit Industries: Orfit Splinting Guide, Antwerp, 1990.
10. North Coast Medical, Inc.: Orfit Splinting Material Instruction Manual. North Coast Medical, Inc.: San Jose, CA, 1995.
11. Ziegler, EM: Current Concepts in Orthotics. Rolyan® Medical Products, Germantown, WI, 1984.
12. Smith & Nephew Inc. Rehabilitation Division Catalogue, 1997. (Rolyan® is a trademark of Smith & Nephew Inc.)
13. Alimed Inc.: Orthopedic Rehabilitation Products, 1997–98.
14. Dovelle, S, Heeter, PK, and Tuyet, V: A dynamic finger flexion loop. Am J Occup Ther 42:535, 1988.
15. Van Veldhoven, G: The proximal IP swing traction splint. J Hand Ther 8:265, 1995.
16. May, EJ, and Silfverskiold, KL: A new power source in dynamic splinting: Experimental studies. J Hand Ther 2:164, 1989.
17. Ottheirs, J: A hand glove splint for attachment of dynamic components. J Hand Ther 8:36, 1995.
18. Paynter, P, and Schindeler-Grasse, P: Techniques for improving distal interphalangeal motion. J Hand Ther 6:216, 1993.
19. Lang, A: Finger-based PIP flexion and extension assist splints. J Hand Ther 4:189, 1991.
20. Prosser, R: Splinting in the management of proximal IP joint flexion contracture. J Hand Ther 9:378, 1996.
21. North Coast Medical Hand Therapy Catalog, 1997.
22. Van Veldhoven, G: A device for tension adjustment on dynamic splints. J Hand Ther 9:405, 1996.
23. Otthiers, J: A hand glove splint for attachment of dynamic components. J Hand Ther 8:36, 1995.
24. Oxford, K, and Hildreth, D: Fracture bracing for proximal phalanx fractures. J Hand Ther 9:404, 1996.
25. Muhleman, C: Simple treatment for PIP joint extensor lag. J Hand Ther 4:21, 1991.
26. Stewart, K: Tendon injuries. In Stanley, BG, and Tribuzi, SM (eds): Concepts in Hand Rehabilitation. FA Davis, Philadelphia, 1992.
27. Mannarino, SL: Skeletal injuries. In Stanley, BG, and Tribuzi, SM (eds): Concepts in Hand Rehabilitation. FA Davis, Philadelphia, 1992.
28. Lamey, G: Buddy splint. J Hand Ther 7:30, 1994.
29. Mignardi, MM: Dynamic PIP stabilizing splint. J Hand Ther 7:31, 1994.
30. Wong, S: Combination splint for distal interphalangeal joint stability and protected proximal interphalangeal joint mobility. J Hand Ther 8:69, 1995.
31. Silver Ring Splint Company Catalog, Charlottesville, VA, 1996.
32. Prosser, R, and Connolly, WB: Complications following surgical treatment for Dupuytren's contracture. J Hand Ther 9:344, 1996.
33. Fess, EE: Force magnitude of commercial spring-coil and spring-wire splints designed to extend the proximal interphalangeal joint. J Hand Ther 1:86, 1988.
34. Callahan, AD, and McEntee, P: Splinting proximal interphalangeal joint flexion contracture: A new design. Am J Occup Ther 40:408, 1986.
35. Lang, A: Finger-based PIP flexion and extension assist splints. J Hand Ther 4:189, 1991.
36. Bell, J: Plaster casting for the remodeling of soft tissue. In Fess, EE, and Philips, CA: Hand Splinting Principles and Methods. Mosby, St. Louis, 1987.
37. Colditz, JC, and Schneider, AM: Modification of the digital serial plaster casting technique. J Hand Ther 8:215, 1995.
38. Moore, JW, and Braverman, SE: Splinting for radial instability of the thumb MCP joint. J Hand Ther 3:202, 1990.
39. Diaz, J: Three-point static splint for chronic volar subluxation of the thumb MP joint. J Hand Ther 7:195, 1994.
40. Allen, KD, Flegle, JH, and Watson, TS: A thermoplastic thumb post for the treatment of thumb-sucking. Am J Occup Ther 46:552, 1992.
41. Barrett, KP, Parks, BJ, and Voss, K: The use of Hexcelite in splinting the thumb. Am J Occup Ther 37:266, 1983.
42. Tenney, CG, and Lisak, JM: Atlas of Hand Splinting. Little, Brown, Boston, 1986.
43. Fishwick, G, and Sellers, JN, Jr: Occupational therapy for patients with cervical cord injury. In Pierce, DS, and Nickel, VH (eds): The Total Care of Spinal Cord Injuries. Little, Brown, Boston, 1977, p 205.
44. Linden, CA, and Trombly, CA: Orthoses: Kinds and purposes. In Trombly, CA (ed): Occupational Therapy for Physical Dysfunction, ed 4. Williams & Wilkins, Baltimore, 1995, p 551.
45. Fess, EE, and Philips, CA: Hand Splinting: Principles and Methods, ed 2. Mosby, St. Louis, 1987, p 353.

46. Malick, MH, and Meyer, CMH: Manual on the Management of the Quadriplegic Upper Extremity. Maude H Malick, Pittsburgh, 1978, p 54.
47. Goodman, G, and Bazyk, S: The effects of a short thumb opponens splint on hand function in cerebral palsy: A single-subject study. Am J Occup Ther 45:726, 1991.
48. Johnson, C: Splinting the injured musician. J Hand Ther 5:107, 1992.

# Lower Extremity Orthoses

## Chapter Outline

This chapter describes the fabrication process for eight lower extremity orthoses. The orthoses are organized from proximal to distal; as the chapter progresses, the orthoses incorporate more distal limb joints. Some of these orthoses are large and elaborate, requiring the assistance of a second person to manage large pieces of thermoplastic and position the client's joints.

For some orthoses, the design can be used to achieve more than one objective. When this is the case, no objective is included in the name, for example for the posterior static knee orthosis, which could be stabilizing or protective (to prevent knee contracture). When the orthosis is made for the client, the pertinent objective can be inserted into the name.

An evaluation form for lower extremity orthoses can be found at the end of Chapter 7. It can be used as a guideline for designing, fabricating, and evaluating many of the orthoses in Chapter 12. Refer to the introduction to Chapter 8 for more information.

● ● ● ● ● ● ● ● ● ● ● ● ● ● ● ● ● ● ● ● ● ● ● ● ● ● ● ● ● ● ● ● ● ● ● ● ● ● ● ● ● ● ● ● ● ●

⬤ **Name:**     **Static Plastazote Hip-Stabilizing Orthosis for Congenital Dysplasia of the Hip (CDH)** (Fig. 12-1)

| | |
|---|---|
| *Common Name* | Plastazote diaper, CDH splint |
| *Objective* | • To maintain baby's hips in 90° flexion and 45° to 60° abduction to keep the femoral head in the acetabulum, allowing ligaments and capsule to tighten and stabilize the hip joint as per the physician's protocol[1] |
| *Indication* | • Congenital hip dysplasia (unilateral or bilateral) |
| *Materials* | • ½ in. (1.2 cm) thick, perforated foam thermoplastic—#1 pink Plastazote or 4E AliPlast<br>• 1 in. (2.5 cm) wide self-adhesive hook Velcro—approximately 15 in. (37 cm) long<br>• 1 in. (2.5 cm) wide nonadhesive loop Velcro straps—approximately 18 in. (45 cm) long |
| *Equipment and Tools* | • Kitchen or splinting oven with good ventilation<br>• Metal tray lined with release paper, cornstarch, or talcum powder<br>• Measuring tape<br>• Scissors<br>• Belt sander, bench, or hand grinder<br>• Large-diameter rolling pin<br>• Heat gun |

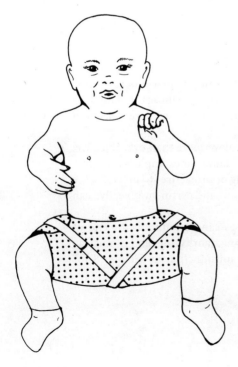

**FIGURE 12-1.**   Static Plastazote hip-stabilizing orthosis for congenital dysplasia of the hip (CDH).

| | |
|---|---|
| ***Client's Position*** | • Supine on an elevated plinth at a comfortable work height for the therapist |
| | • Hips in 90° flexion and 45° to 60° abduction[1] |
| ***Therapist's Position*** | • Standing at the feet of the baby |
| ***Pattern*** | • Figure 12-2*a* |
| ***Fabrication*** | 1. Preheat oven to 250°F (140°C). |
| | 2. Cut the pattern from Plastazote/AliPlast. |
| | 3. Bevel the outer edges with scissors and then smooth with a sander or grinder (Fig. 12-2*b*). |
| | 4. Heat Plastazote until pliable and then mold it around a rolling pin to form a cylinder, bringing the back corners over the front corners, creating front and back overlapping flaps. Remove when cool. |
| | 5. Check the fit on the baby. Ensure about 1 in. (2.5 cm) clearance between each knee crease and the edge of the orthosis. Mark and trim if necessary. |
| | 6. Warm the adhesive backing of the two strips of hook Velcro with the heat gun and attach to the orthosis in a criss-cross fashion (Fig. 12-2*a*). |
| | 7. Attach two strips of loop Velcro to the hook Velcro (Fig. 12-2*a*). |
| | 8. Apply the orthosis to the baby, bringing the back flaps over the front flaps and securing the loop Velcro straps. |
| ***Wearing Regimen*** | • Worn over diapers; removed only for diaper changes and bathing. |
| | • Cloth diapers should be square folded; disposable diapers should be fully expanded. |

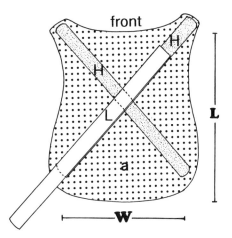

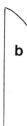

**FIGURE 12-2.** *(a)* Outside view of orthosis for CDH in its unmolded form. L = length from the navel to waist level at back; W = width—distance between the knee creases (when the hips are abducted and flexed) less 1 in. (2.5 cm) on each side; H = self-adhesive hook Velcro straps; L = one of two loop Velcro straps. *(b)* Cross section of edge showing material removed (shaded) to create bevel.

*Precautions*
- Joint damage may result if the orthosis applies excessive force to a contracted hip. If the legs do not readily abduct to the desired position, mold the orthosis directly to the baby and remold as hip abduction range improves.
- Do not move the hips out of position when the orthosis is off.
- Replace with a larger orthosis as required to accommodate growth.

*Variations*
- Prefabricated version: pediatric hip abduction orthosis[2]
- Prefabricated Pavlik harness[2,3]

---

● **Name:**   **Spiral Dynamic Hip-Knee-Ankle-Foot Rotation Strap**
(Fig. 12-3)

*Common Name*   Prefabricated Rolyan® Lower Extremity TAP™ (*Tone and Positioning*) Splint[4]

*Objectives*
- Depending on the direction in which the strap is wrapped, the orthosis will promote either hip external rotation and foot inversion while supporting the medial longitudinal arch or hip internal rotation and foot eversion. Knee and ankle motion is unrestricted.
- To assist hypotonic muscles.
- To reduce the tone of hypertonic muscles.
- To improve the gait pattern.
- To help secure the head of the femur in the acetabulum.

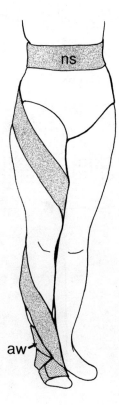

**FIGURE 12-3.** Spiral dynamic hip-knee-ankle-foot rotation strap composed of neoprene strap (ns) and ankle wrap (aw).

| | |
|---|---|
| *Indications* | • Head injury<br>• Spina bifida<br>• Cerebral palsy<br>• Multiple sclerosis<br>• Cerebrovascular accident<br>• Lower extremity paralysis or weakness<br>• Mild hip joint subluxation after hip replacement |
| *Materials* | • This prefabricated orthosis consists of an elastic ankle wrap and a neoprene strap—3 in. (7.5 cm) wide for adults; 2 in. (5 cm) wide for children.<br>• The ankle wrap does not replace an ankle-foot orthosis (AFO); however, an AFO can be used in combination with the rotation strap. |
| *Client's Position* | • Sitting to apply the ankle wrap and then standing to apply the strap. |
| *Therapist's Position* | • Seated or standing beside the client |
| *Application* | • To promote external rotation, wrap the strap around the limb as shown in Figure 12-3.<br>• To promote internal rotation, reverse the direction of the wrapping. |

● ● ● ● ● ● ● ● ● ● ● ● ● ● ● ● ● ● ● ● ● ● ● ● ● ● ● ● ● ● ● ● ● ● ● ● ● ● ● ● ● ● ●

⬤ **Name:** **Posterior Static (or Serial-Static) Knee Orthosis (Posterior KO)** (Fig. 12-4*a*)

| | |
|---|---|
| *Common Names* | Posterior slab knee splint; knee extension splint; resting knee splint |
| *Objectives* | • To prevent or reduce knee flexion contracture<br>• To stabilize the knee during ambulation<br>• To rest the knee to relieve inflammation and pain |

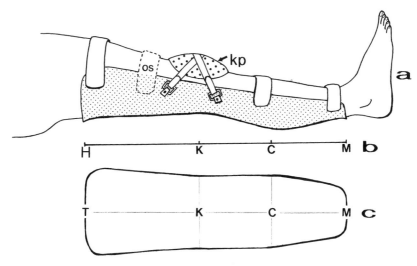

**FIGURE 12-4.** (*a*) Posterior static (or serial-static) knee orthosis. kp = knee pad; os = optional strap for a long limb. (*b*) Location of measurements for pattern. (*c*) Pattern. H/T = upper thigh near hip; K = knee; C = widest part of calf; M = 2 in. (5 cm) above malleoli.

| | |
|---|---|
| ***Indications*** | • Whenever knee stabilization or immobilization is required because of |

• Whenever knee stabilization or immobilization is required because of
  ◦ Burns
  ◦ Knee Surgery
  ◦ Patellar fracture
  ◦ Ligament injuries
  ◦ Distal femoral or proximal tibial fracture (although a circumferential orthosis is generally preferred)
  ◦ Knee effusion (arthritis)
  ◦ Transtibial (below-knee) amputation
• Flexion contracture of the knee requiring serial reduction

***Materials***

• ⅛ in. (3.2 mm) thick thermoplastic—preferably perforated
  ◦ For gravity-resisted molding, use opaque A or Ezeform
  ◦ For gravity-assisted molding, use Ezeform or translucent B
  ◦ For serial-static, use a thermoplastic with memory
• ⅛ in. (3.2 mm) self-adhesive foam or gel padding (optional)
• For the knee pad
  ◦ ½ in. (1.2 cm) thick, perforated foam thermoplastic—#1 pink Plastazote or 4E AliPlast
  ◦ Four D-rings
  ◦ 1 in. (2.5 cm) wide self-adhesive hook Velcro
  ◦ 1 in. (2.5 cm) wide loop Velcro
  ◦ Four Chicago screws/nylon screws/rapid rivets
• For the straps:
  ◦ 2 or 3 in. (5 or 7.5 cm) wide self-adhesive hook Velcro, depending on size of limb
  ◦ 2 or 3 in. (5 or 7.5 cm) wide loop Velcro or padded alternative

***Equipment and Tools***

• Large heating pan (alternatively, use oven for isoprene-based category A materials)
• Oven or heat gun for knee pad
• Sewing machine
• For gravity-resisted molding: elastic bandage/Thera-Band/Orfiband—choose from 2 in. (5 cm) to 6 in. (15 cm) wide, depending on the size of the limb
• Scissors
• Measuring tape
• Hammer and anvil if using rapid rivets

***Client's Position***

• For gravity-resisted molding:
  ◦ Ideal position is sitting on an elevated plinth or high stool with the leg at a comfortable work height for the therapist. The limb should be supported at the buttock and heel, leaving the posterior surface free for molding.
  ◦ Alternate positions: lying supine with foot elevated or with the limb resting on soft foam.
• For gravity-assisted molding: lying prone on a plinth or bed.
• The knee should be not quite fully extended. Full extension places the knee in its close-packed position and may stress the ligaments and cartilage.

***Therapist's Position***

• Standing beside the client.

| | |
|---|---|
| *Pattern* | 1. Measure the distances between H, K, C, and M (Fig. 12-4*b*). |
| | 2. Take three fifths of the circumference at H, K, C, and M so that the trough will extend slightly more than halfway around the sides. |
| | 3. Lay out the pattern (Fig. 12-4*c*). The midline of the orthosis is one-half of T. |
| | 4. Cut out a circle of foam thermoplastic to cover the anterior knee. Bevel the outer edges (see Fig. 12-2*b*). |
| | 5. For a transtibial amputation, adjust the measurements and pattern accordingly. |

| | |
|---|---|
| *Fabrication* | 1. If desired, apply padding to the malleoli and calcaneal (Achilles) tendon. |
| | 2. Heat and cut out the pattern. |
| | 3. Check temperature of the thermoplastic on your skin and then on the client's skin. |
| | 4. Place the warm thermoplastic against the posterior surface of the limb. |
| | 5. For gravity-resisted molding use elastic bandage, Thera-Band, or Orfiband and spiral wrap it around the thermoplastic from distal to proximal. Guard against twisting of the material with this technique. Assistance from a second therapist may be necessary to elevate the limb when the client is supine. Alternatively, if the client is lying supine on a soft bed, use a series of 6 in. (15 cm) wide elastic bandages tied around the warm thermoplastic to conform it to the contours. |
| | 6. For gravity-assisted molding, firmly stroke the thermoplastic into the contours of the limb. Assistance from a second therapist may be helpful. |
| | 7. Flare the distal edge away from the malleoli and calcaneal tendon and flare the proximal edge posteriorly, but not medially. A medial flare will irritate the other thigh. |
| | 8. When the material is almost cool, unwrap the bandage, mark the trim lines, remove the orthosis, and trim. |
| | 9. Transfer the padding to the inside of the orthosis or discard. |
| | 10. Attach the straps (Fig. 12-4*a*). |
| | 11. Construct the knee pad and attach D-ring anchors (see Fig. 9-12). |

| | |
|---|---|
| *Wearing Regimen* | • As appropriate for the situation |

| | |
|---|---|
| *Precautions* | • Monitor carefully for pressure points or impaired circulation, especially if the client lacks full sensation in the lower extremity. |

| | |
|---|---|
| *Options* | • If the knee pad cannot be tolerated, substitute 2 in. (5 cm) wide straps above and below the patella. |
| | • Delete the straps and knee pad and secure with either sterile gauze bandage (for acute burns) or elastic bandage (for edema). |
| | • For a serial-static design, reheat and remold the thermoplastic as the contracture is reduced. |

| | |
|---|---|
| *Alternatives* | • Other custom thermoplastic orthoses (Fig. 12-5) |
| | • Circumferential precuts—QuickCast[5,6] or Dynacast Rapide Knee Splint[4] or Orfizip Kneesplint[7] |
| | • Numerous prefabricated designs[2] |
| | • Prefabricated circumferential Rolyan® Progressive Knee Splint[4] (original design courtesy of Lynn Swedberg, MS, OTR)—soft foam/plush wash- |

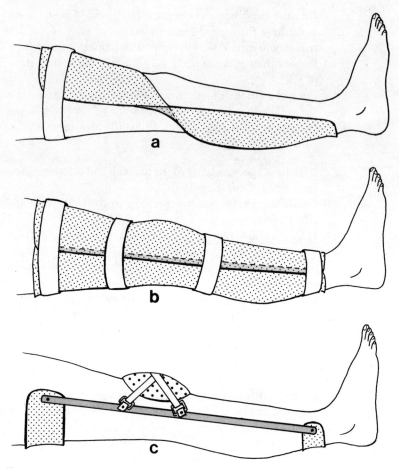

**FIGURE 12-5.** Alternate custom designs for knee orthoses. *(a)* Bisurfaced—shaded area beside knee shows overlapped thermoplastic. *(b)* Bivalved—anterior and posterior slabs overlap at the sides; overlap is shaded. *(c)* Three-point.

able orthosis with remoldable Ezeform insert; especially good for long-term care

⬤ **Name:**      **Circumferential (Nonarticular) Tibia-Stabilizing Orthosis** (Fig. 12-6)

Figure 12-6 shows the orthosis with an optional heel cup, which limits leg rotation by restricting inversion and eversion at the subtalar joint. When the heel cup is excluded, the orthosis is nonarticular; when it is included, it is articular and does not fit into the design categories identified in Chapter 1.

*Common Names*      Tibial fracture/functional brace; Sarmiento tibial brace

*Objectives*
- To stabilize fracture to promote healing, without immobilizing any joints
- To protect fragile bones from fracture

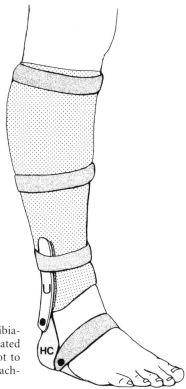

**FIGURE 12-6.**   Nonarticular circumferential tibia-stabilizing orthosis. HC = optional prefabricated heel cup to block inversion and eversion of foot to prevent leg rotation; U = upright with Velcro attachment to orthosis.

| | |
|---|---|
| *Indications* | • Midshaft tibial fractures, with or without fibular fracture—usually applied 1 to 3 weeks after fracture, although the time varies with the physician and the type of fracture<br>• **Osteogenesis imperfecta** |
| *Rationale* | • Applies circumferential compression to soft tissues of the leg to maintain alignment of the fracture site.<br>• See Chapter 2, "Fractures of Long Bones." |
| *Materials* | • ⅛ in. (3.2 mm) thick perforated thermoplastic<br>  ○ Opaque category A or C (opaque B may become too rigid when cool)<br>  ○ Translucent category B or C<br>• For the posterior insert—⅟₁₆ in. (1.6 mm) thick thermoplastic, category B or C—about 2 in. (5 cm) wide and 20 in. (50 cm) long<br>• 3 Velcro overlap or plastic (radiolucent) D-ring straps, 1 in. (2.5 cm) wide<br>• Stockinette or Tubigrip<br>• ⅛ in. (3.2 mm) thick self-adhesive foam or gel padding<br>• Solvent or 100 percent isopropyl alcohol<br>• Prefabricated heel cup (optional—used to limit leg rotation)[2,4] |
| *Equipment and Tools* | • Heating pan<br>• For the pattern: measuring tape or flexible clear plastic with permanent marker and straight pins, stapler, or tape<br>• Scissors |

**Client's Position**
- Sitting on a table, plinth, or stool with thighs fully supported and both legs hanging over the edge (Fig. 12-7). If desired, support the foot on a stool.

**Therapist's Position**
- Seated at a lower level in front of the client (Fig. 12-7).

**Pattern**
- Follow the steps in Fig. 12-8.
- Alternatively, make a pattern using flexible clear plastic, secured with pins, staples, or tape along the posterior midline. Using a permanent marker, mark the following:
  ○ Posterior midline
  ○ Upper and lower borders
- Remove plastic, cut along pattern lines, and add 1½ in. (3 cm) to each side.
- Lay out the pattern, heat, and cut out.

**Fabrication[8,9]**
1. Apply padding to the malleoli and the calcaneal (Achilles) tendon.
2. Posterior insert: Heat and mold the thermoplastic against the skin at the location of the posterior opening (Fig. 12-9).
3. Apply a layer of Stockinette or Tubigrip over the molded insert. Because of shrinkage, use two layers if using a material with memory.
4. Heat the thermoplastic and align the proximal edge at the level of the femoral condyles.
5. While the client or an assistant holds the proximal edge, mold the thermoplastic around the limb from distal to proximal. Use both hands to stretch the thermoplastic from the anterior midline around to the posterior midline and then squeeze together, flush with the limb (see Fig. 9-9*c*).
6. Cut off the excess material along the posterior midline while the material is warm, creating a closed seam (see Fig. 9-9*c*).
7. Mold into the contours of the patellar tendon, tibial condyles, and calcaneal tendon.
8. Mark the trim lines around the knee to ensure unrestricted flexion and around the ankle to permit full plantar flexion and dorsiflexion.

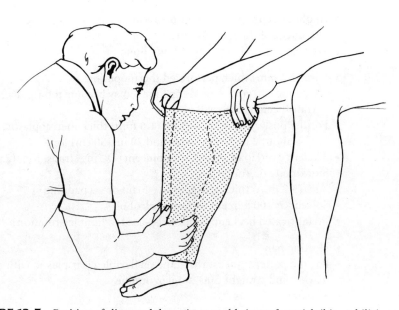

**FIGURE 12-7.** Position of client and therapist to mold circumferential tibia-stabilizing orthosis.

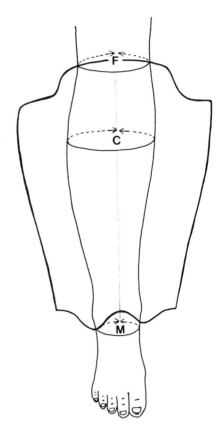

**FIGURE 12-8.** Pattern for circumferential non-articular tibia-stabilizing orthosis. Measure the distances between the femoral condyles (F), widest part of the calf (C), and below the malleoli (M). Take circumferences at F, C, and M, then add 3 in. (7.5 cm) to each. The midline of the orthosis is half of circumference at C, plus 1½ in. (3.75 cm).

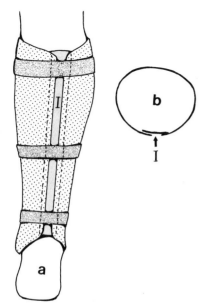

**FIGURE 12-9.** (*a*) Posterior view of circumferential nonarticular tibia-stabilizing orthosis showing posterior opening and insert (I) to prevent pinching of the skin. The insert is adhered to one side of the posterior opening. Heel cup is not shown. (*b*) Superior view.

9. Snap apart the posterior seam and remove the orthosis. If it has adhered to the Stockinette, cut through the Stockinette to remove the orthosis.
10. Once the orthosis is off the leg, the Stockinette can be peeled away.
11. Trim with scissors and flare the upper and lower edges.
12. Transfer the malleolar pads to the orthosis or discard. Remove and discard the calcaneal tendon pad.
13. Cut along the trim lines and remove ½ in. (1 cm) from each side of the posterior opening.
14. Adhere the insert to one inside edge using solvent or alcohol and dry heat (Fig. 12-9).
15. Apply the orthosis and attach three overlap or D-ring straps with center patches of hook Velcro (Fig. 12-6).
16. With the orthosis in place, confirm fracture alignment with an x-ray.

**Wearing Regimen**
- To be worn at all times and removed carefully for bathing as per the physician's recommendations.
- Continue with the orthosis until fracture healing is complete.

**Application and Removal**
- May require the assistance of another person to hold the cylinder open.

**Precautions**
- If edema develops in the foot because of compression around the leg, apply two layers of Tubigrip over the foot or use a knee-high support stocking before applying the orthosis. Encourage elevation of the foot while sitting (see Chapter 3, "Edema").
- The client progresses from non–weight bearing to partial weight bearing to full weight bearing, as directed by the therapist or physician.
- Circumferential orthoses can be difficult to apply and may require assistance from another person to hold the sides open.

**Options**
- An optional heel cup can be added to prevent leg rotation by blocking inversion and eversion at the subtalar joint. Prefabricated heel cups[4,7] have bilateral uprights with self-adhesive Velcro strips for attachment to the orthosis. When a heel cup is used, wrap the lower strap over the uprights (Fig. 12-6).

**Alternatives**
- Precuts,[4,7] including Rolyan® AquaForm Tibial Fracture Brace[4] with zipper closure
- Preformed low-temperature thermoplastic or high-temperature plastic tibial fracture braces[2,4]

---

⬤ **Name:**   **Posterior Static (or Static-Progressive or Serial-Static) Ankle-Foot Orthosis (Posterior AFO)**
(Figs. 12-10 and 12-11)

**Common Names**   Foot drop splint, ankle-foot orthosis

**Objectives**
- To rest the ankle to relieve pain
- To immobilize the ankle to promote healing
- To prevent or correct ankle contractures

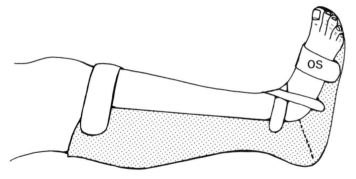

**FIGURE 12-10.** Posterior static (or serial-static) ankle-foot orthosis (AFO) with a seamless heel created during gravity-assisted molding using a category C thermoplastic, shown with side patch straps. The broken line represents an alternate heel design using a mitered seam that is pinched together and cut off when warm. The mitered seam should be reinforced with a strip of bonded thermoplastic (not shown).

**Indications**

For *non–weight-bearing* situations when the client is in bed, sitting, or walking with crutches or walker:

- Mild to moderate spastic hemiparesis
- Post repair of calcaneal/Achilles tendon
- Musculoskeletal injuries of the distal tibia/fibula or ankle
- Unconscious client at risk of developing ankle flexion contractures
- Congenital deformities of the foot (e.g., clubfoot)—see "Options" for more details
- Acute burns
- Skin grafting
- Cerebral palsy
- Flaccid hemiparesis
- Soft tissue ankle injuries
- Peroneal nerve lesions
- Painful joint inflammation
- **Plantar fasciitis**[10-12]—night use

**Materials**

- ⅛ in. (3.2 mm) thick perforated thermoplastic—for a small child, choose a thinner thermoplastic
  ○ For gravity-resisted molding, use category A or B
  ○ For gravity-assisted molding, use category C
  ○ For serial-static, use category B with memory
- 2 in. (5 cm) wide self-adhesive hook Velcro
- 2 in. (5 cm) wide loop Velcro or padded alternative
- ⅛ or ¼ in. (3.2 or 6.4 mm) thick self-adhesive foam or gel padding (use the thicker padding if the client is recumbent most of the time)

**Equipment and Tools**

- Heating pan—alternatively, use oven for isoprene-based materials
- Measuring tape

**FIGURE 12-11.** Posterior static-progressive ankle-foot orthosis with open heel seam and tension-adjustable straps (shaded) spanning from the toes to the upper calf. Increasing the tension in these straps increases ankle dorsiflexion. This heel design is the easiest to make and is adjustable.

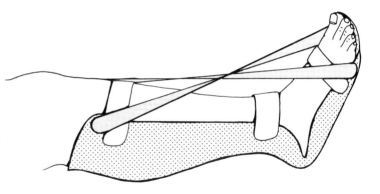

- For gravity-resisted molding, 3 in. (7.5 cm) wide elastic bandage or Thera-Band/Orfiband
- Scissors

**Client's Position**

- For gravity-resisted molding, supine or sitting with the heel supported and the knee extended, preferably on an elevated plinth at a comfortable work height for the therapist.
- For gravity-assisted molding, prone with the foot extending over the edge of a plinth or bed, allowing 0° to 5° of dorsiflexion—use this position to create a seamless heel.
- For plantar fasciitis, 5° of dorsiflexion prevents shortening of the plantar fascia when non–weight bearing overnight.[10] Initially, if less than 5° of dorsiflexion can be tolerated, choose the open-seam heel design and increase dorsiflexion gradually, using tension-adjustable straps and a static-progressive approach (Fig. 12-11).

**Therapist's Position**

- If the client is on a plinth, the therapist stands beside the plinth.
- If the client is sitting on a chair, the therapist squats beside the chair.

**Pattern**

- Select a heel design: seamless or mitered seam for static or serial-static designs (Fig. 12-10) or an open seam for static-progressive design (Fig. 12-11).
- Make a pattern following the steps in Figure 12-12.
- Lay out the pattern, heat, and cut out.

**Fabrication**

1. Apply padding to the heel region and malleoli.
2. Heat the thermoplastic and check the temperature on your skin and then on the client's skin.
3. For gravity-resisted molding, apply the warm thermoplastic to the posterior surface, and then wrap the foot with elastic bandage or Thera-Band/Orfiband. Position ankle in neutral, pinch and cut to form a mitered seam (see Fig. 9-5*a* and *b*), and then proceed with wrapping up the leg.
4. For gravity-assisted molding, stretch the material over the heel to avoid a seam.
5. Apply any necessary corrective forces to position the ankle.
6. Flare the proximal edge of the material posteriorly.

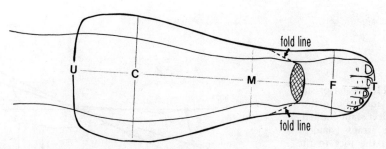

**FIGURE 12-12.** Pattern for posterior AFO and bisurfaced AFO. Measure the distances between the upper leg (U), widest part of the calf (C), above the malleoli (M), forefoot (F), and end of toes (T). Take three-fifths of the circumferences at U, C, M, and F so that the trough will extend slightly more than halfway around the sides. The hole (cross-hatched) is cut out for the bisurfaced AFO only and the fold lines are used only for the bisurfaced AFO.

7. When the thermoplastic is set but still partially warm, unwrap, mark the trim lines, remove the orthosis, and cut, ensuring unrestricted knee flexion. Trim the sides along the midline of the malleoli.
8. To reinforce the mitered heal seam, bond a piece of thermoplastic over the seam (see Fig. 9-5*c*).
9. For a static-progressive open seam, snap open the mitered seam and cut away about ½ in. (1 cm) from each side of the seam (Fig. 12-11).
10. Transfer the heel and malleolar pads to the inside of the orthosis, or discard them to leave space. The thicker the pads used, the greater the space created.
11. Apply straps (Fig. 12-10 or 12-11). These figures show side-patch straps, which are easier for the client to fasten and unfasten but are less durable than center-patch straps.

*Wearing Regimen*  • As appropriate for the situation.

*Precautions*  • Monitor closely for pressure points over the heel or malleoli.

*Options*
- For clubfoot, mold the thermoplastic to the medial side of the foot and calf rather than the posterior surface.
- Delete the straps and secure with either sterile gauze bandage (for acute burns) or elastic bandage (for edema).
- For the recumbent client, add medial and lateral antirotation side extensions to control hip rotation and knee flexion (Fig. 12-13). Cut a 3 in. (7.5 cm) wide strip of thermoplastic, heat, and bond to the orthosis using sol-

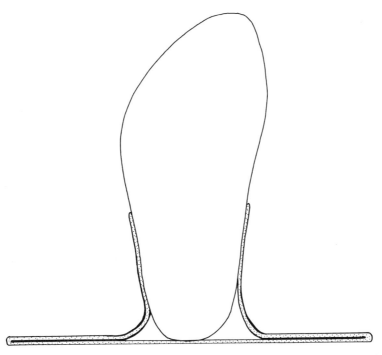

**FIGURE 12-13.** Plantar view of posterior AFO with antirotation side extensions. For the client positioned supine in bed, the extensions control medial and lateral limb rotation; also, knee flexion is inhibited.

vent or alcohol, or scrape to remove the surface coating (see Chapter 7, "Thermoplastic Bonding").

- To prevent wrinkling or shrinkage of a skin graft over the dorsum of the foot, mold the thermoplastic to the anterior surface over an elastomer insert.

*Alternatives*

- Custom bisurfaced AFO (described below).
- Custom dynamic AFO (described later).
- Extend the proximal end to the upper thigh to support the knee, creating a knee-ankle-foot orthosis.
- Circumferential precut Dynacast Rapide[4] or QuickCast[5,6] Foot Splints.
- Preformed low-temperature thermoplastic ankle-foot splints.[4]
- Prefabricated ankle-positioning orthoses[4] for the client supine in bed (e.g., Orfit's TTL (Total Transfer Layer) Anti-decubitus Splint Kit[7]).

---

 **Name:**   **Bisurfaced Static (or Serial-Static) Ankle-Foot Orthosis (Bisurfaced AFO)[14]**   (Fig. 12-14)

*Common Name*

(Antispastic) foot drop splint

*Objectives*

- To prevent or reduce ankle flexion contracture
- To relieve pain
- In weight-bearing applications, helps clear the toes during the swing phase of gait

*Indications*

- Non–weight-bearing indications: see posterior AFO
- Weight-bearing indications: weak or paralyzed ankle dorsiflexors

*Advantages over Posterior AFO*

- Uses gravity-assisted molding; therefore no bandage wrapping is required.
- The heel is uncovered.
- When applying, leverage helps to dorsiflex the ankle (see Fig. 1-16).

*Materials*

- ⅛ in. (3.2 mm) thick perforated thermoplastic—category B or C.
- For weight-bearing applications,[15] use Aquaplast Resilient T or Orfit Stiff.
- For serial-static applications, use material with memory.
- 2 in. (5 cm) wide self-adhesive hook Velcro.
- 2 in. (5 cm) wide loop Velcro or padded alternative.
- ⅛ in. (3.2 mm) thick self-adhesive foam or gel padding.
- Solvent or alcohol.

*Equipment and Tools*

- Heating pan
- Scissors

*Client's Position*

- Supine or sitting on an elevated plinth at a comfortable work height for the therapist, with the heel supported, the knee extended, and the sole of the foot at the end of the plinth

*Therapist's Position*

- Standing facing the sole of the client's foot

*Pattern*

- Figure 12-12.
- Cut out the cross-hatched hole over the anterior surface of the ankle.

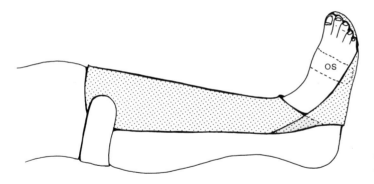

**FIGURE 12-14.** Birsurfaced static (or serial-static) AFO. OS = optional strap over forefoot.

*Fabrication*

1. Apply padding to the malleoli. For weight-bearing applications, also pad the tibial crest.
2. Heat the thermoplastic and slip the foot through the hole so that the material drapes over the anterior leg and the heel of the foot is uncovered.
3. Mold to the sole of the foot.
4. While you lean your abdomen against the sole of the foot to push the ankle into a neutral dorsiflexed position, fold the wings upward along the fold lines (Fig. 12-12), pressing them firmly against the thermoplastic anterior to the malleoli. For weight-bearing applications, place the ankle in about 5° of dorsiflexion to assist toe clearance during gait.
5. Gently flare the edges above the ankle and anterior to the heel on the sole of the foot.
6. Mark the trim lines, remove the orthosis, and trim while the material is still partially warm.
7. For static design, use solvent or alcohol and a heat gun to seal the folded wings to eliminate any crevices. For serial-static design, do not seal the wings, so that the ankle position can be changed when the thermoplastic is reheated later.
8. Remove the padding from the client's skin and transfer to the inside of the orthosis or discard.
9. Attach the straps (Fig. 12-14*a*).

*Wearing Regimen*

• As appropriate for the situation.

*Precautions*

• Monitor carefully for pressure points, especially if used for weight bearing.

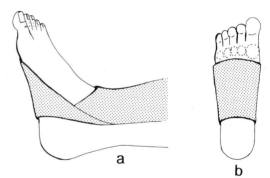

**FIGURE 12-15.** Bisurfaced static AFO for weight bearing. *(a)* Plantar view. *(b)* Lateral view. Broken outlines represent the MT heads.

a

b

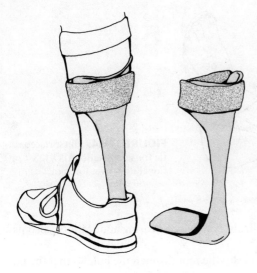

**FIGURE 12-16.** Prefabricated Rolyan® Posterior Leaf Splint fabricated from high-temperature plastic.[4]

| | |
|---|---|
| *Adjustments* | • For serial-static design, reheat the entire orthosis, unseal the folds, and re-mold, positioning the ankle in more dorsiflexion. |
| *Options* | • For weight-bearing applications:<br>  ○ Trim away from the sides of metatarsal heads so that the foot and or-thosis will fit into shoe (Fig. 12-15*a*)<br>  ○ Trim the distal edge just proximal to the metatarsal heads (Fig. 12-15*b*)<br>• Select a wide-fitting lace-up shoe; remove the insole to create space for the orthosis. An extra-depth shoe is ideal because there is more room in the front of the shoe and it has a removable insole. |
| *Alternatives* | • Precuts[7]<br>• Custom[1] or prefabricated[2,4] high-temperature plastic AFOs designed for weight bearing (also called posterior leaf splints) (Fig. 12-16)<br>• Posterior AFO (above)<br>• Circumferential calf-based dynamic ankle assistive-dorsiflexion orthosis (described next) |

 **Name:** **Circumferential Calf-Based Dynamic Ankle Assistive-Dorsiflexion Orthosis** (Fig. 12-17)[16]

| | |
|---|---|
| *Common Names* | Dynamic foot drop splint; ankle extension assist; dorsiflexion splint |
| *Objectives* | To passively dorsiflex the ankle to clear the toes when walking, while allow-ing active plantar flexion |
| *Indications* | • Weak or paralyzed ankle dorsiflexors caused by<br>  ○ Cerebral palsy<br>  ○ Flaccid hemiplegia<br>  ○ Peroneal nerve injury |

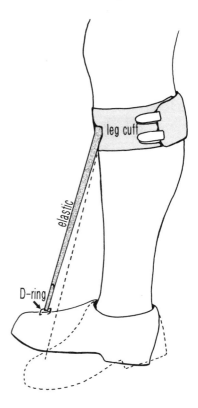

**FIGURE 12-17.** Circumferential calf-based dynamic ankle assistive-dorsiflexion orthosis. Solid lines show the passively dorsiflexed position created by tension in the elastic. Broken lines show the effect of active ankle plantar flexion against the resistance of the elastic.

| | |
|---|---|
| ***Advantages over Bisurfaced AFO*** | • Quick and easy to make without thermoplastic molding<br>• Mounted to the outside of the shoe |
| ***Materials*** | • *A—Leg cuff:*<br>  ○ 2 or 3 in. (5 or 7.5 cm) wide heavy cotton webbing or neoprene<br>  ○ ½₂ in. (.8 mm) thick self-adhesive gel padding (e.g., Krystal Gel)<br>  ○ 1 in. (2.5 cm) wide nonadhesive hook and loop Velcro, two pieces of each, 4 in. (10 cm) long<br>• *B—Shoe attachment:*<br>  ○ Supportive, lace-up shoe with a nonslip, broad sole<br>  ○ Metal D-ring—1 or 1½ in. (2.5 or 3.8 cm) wide<br>• *C—Dynamic component:*<br>  ○ Elastic—1 or 1½ in. (2.5 or 3.8 cm) wide (same as D-ring) and about 20 in. (50 cm) long<br>  ○ 1 in. (2.5 cm) wide nonadhesive hook and elastic loop Velcro—one piece of each, 3 in. (7.5 cm) long |
| ***Equipment and Tools*** | • Sewing machine   • Two pairs of pliers<br>• Scissors |
| ***Client's Position*** | • Sitting with the foot supported in a neutral ankle position |
| ***Therapist's Position*** | • Squatting on the floor or sitting on a footstool |
| ***Fabrication*** | *Shoe D-ring:*<br>1. Attach the D-ring to a lace-up shoe. One method is to pry open the metal D-ring and insert through the two distal lace holes. |

*Leg cuff:*

2. Measure the circumference immediately below the tibial tuberosity. Add 3 in. (7.5 cm) and cut the webbing to this length, or add 2 in. and cut the neoprene to this length.
3. Fold over and sew ½ in. (1 cm) at each end to finish the edges (unnecessary with neoprene).
4. Sew loop and hook Velcro strips to the webbing/neoprene.
5. Sew elastic to the front of the leg cuff.
6. Line the inside of the left cuff with foam or gel padding to cushion and prevent distal migration.
7. Apply the leg cuff to the client's calf.

*Dynamic component:*

8. Slip the elastic through the shoe D-ring, adjusting the length until the tension can overcome the weight of the foot to dorsiflex the ankle.
9. Cut the elastic to this length plus 3 in. (7.5 cm).
10. Sew hook Velcro over the distal 3 in. (7.5 cm) of the elastic.
11. Sew elastic loop Velcro over the next 3 in. (7.5 cm) of the elastic.

**Wearing Regimen**

• Whenever walking

**Precautions**

• Circulation below the leg cuff will be compromised if the leg cuff is too tight.

**Alternatives**

Prefabricated version: calf-based toe lifter[5]
Custom bisurfaced ankle orthosis[15]
Custom or prefabricated polyethylene/polypropylene ankle-foot orthoses (Fig. 12-16)

## ● Foot Orthoses

The foot orthosis is the most common category of orthosis dispensed. Prefabricated styles are numerous and can be purchased without prescription or professional recommendation from shoe stores, shoe repair kiosks, drug stores, and home health care outlets. Therapists can order prefabricated foot orthoses or stock components (contoured footbed and arch pads) available from rehabilitation suppliers[2,4] to fabricate customized supports.

Custom foot orthoses can be created by numerous techniques, including direct molding of a low-temperature thermoplastic, forming high-temperature thermoplastic to a positive plaster mold, and computer-controlled shaping of rubber. This is a highly specialized area of orthotic intervention, dominated by orthotists, pedorthists, podiatrists, and chiropodists. Occupational therapists and physical therapists who have pursued postgraduate training to learn about the biomechanics of weight bearing and gait can also become specialists in managing foot disorders and fabricating foot orthoses. Suitable thermoplastics include isoprene-based materials such as San-Splint and translucent materials such as Aquaplast T, which are direct molded to the non–weight-bearing boot. However, fabrication instructions for thermoplastic foot orthoses are not provided here in recognition of the extensive training required before fitting orthoses that influence biomechanics and joint alignment. An ill-fitting corrective foot orthosis can disrupt lower extremity alignment and gait and cause injury. In contrast, the accommodative Plastazote/PPT foot orthosis described next is soft and can do little harm. It is designed to cushion inflamed joints, compensate for atrophied fat pads, and protect fragile skin.

A foot orthosis functions in combination with a compatible, supportive shoe. In some cases, foot orthoses are unnecessary and client education and supportive footwear relieve symptoms. Footwear is discussed at the end of this chapter.

⬤ **Name:** **Plantar Static Plastazote/PPT Foot Protective Orthosis** (Fig. 12-18)

PPT is the name of the foam sheeting material. Its name is derived from *Professional Protective Technology*, the name of the manufacturer.

*Common Names* Arch support; insole

*Objectives*
- To provide cushioning and mild support, relieving pain during weight bearing
- To transfer weight off painful metatarsal heads
- To improve the alignment of the metatarsophalangeal joints and the medial longitudinal arch
- To protect fragile skin
- To promote healing of ulcerated skin
Note: This orthosis is protective, *not* corrective

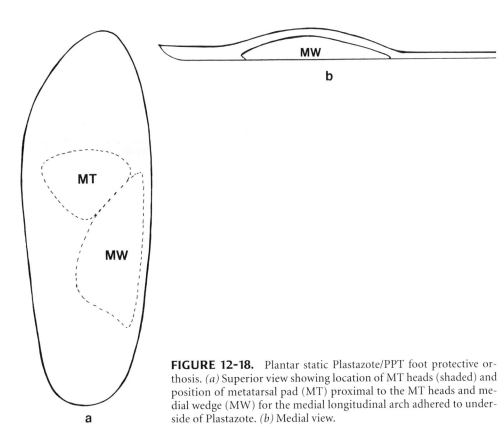

**FIGURE 12-18.** Plantar static Plastazote/PPT foot protective orthosis. *(a)* Superior view showing location of MT heads (shaded) and position of metatarsal pad (MT) proximal to the MT heads and medial wedge (MW) for the medial longitudinal arch adhered to underside of Plastazote. *(b)* Medial view.

**TABLE 12-1.   Features of Supportive Footwear**

| Component or Characteristic | Recommended Characteristics | Special Considerations |
|---|---|---|
| Weight | • Lightweight to minimize fatigue. | • Especially important for persons who are elderly or have lower extremity weakness. |
| Upper material (Fig. 12-19a) | • Porous material<br>• Stretches to mold to contours of foot.<br>• Natural materials (leather, suede) and some synthetic materials. | • For fragile skin, especially for client with diabetes or other peripheral vascular disease, the inside should be smooth and seamless with soft material (e.g., deerskin, glove leather, soft suede, or Plastazote). |
| Upper edge around ankle (Fig. 12-19a) | • Terminate just below the malleoli to provide adequate support to the medial border of foot. | • For ankle instability, severe pronation, patellofemoral syndrome, etc., consider an ankle boot that comes up over the malleoli. |
| Heel counter—the reinforcement around the sides of the heel (Fig. 12-19a) | • Snug fitting, firm. | • The more severe the hindfoot pronation, the greater the need for a strong heel counter that extends farther along the medial side of the shoe. |
| Toe box—the front of the shoe enclosing the toes (Fig. 12-19a) | • Adequate width and depth that allow room for the toes to move.<br>• The forefoot should not hang over the outer sole.<br>• Avoid shoes with pointed toes—they promote hallux valgus and bunions. | • For sensitive skin, hallux valgus, hammer/cock-up/claw toes, select extra-depth shoes (Fig. 12-19b), which feature extra-high toeboxes and one or two removable insoles. |
| Closure | • Laces ensure a secure fit through the midfoot and support to the medial longitudinal arch (MLA).<br>• Slip-on shoes may be acceptable if they have a firm heel counter and there is no foot problem. | • The more pronated the foot, the greater the need for laces or alternate form of closure.<br>• Elastic laces are a common alternative for persons unable to lace their shoes; however, they convert the shoe to a slip-on style, which may not provide adequate support to the MLA; instead use Velcro and D-ring closure.<br>• Lace-up shoes or alternatives are essential for individuals with foot orthoses that feature metatarsal contours that occupy extra room in the shoe. |
| Outer sole Material (Fig. 12-19a) | • Nonslip, shock-absorbing material. | • For elderly persons who walk with a shuffling gait (e.g., those with Parkinson's disease), the sole of the shoe should not be too sticky; otherwise, the person may fall forward. |

*(continued)*

| | |
|---|---|
| ***Indications*** | • Joint inflammation (e.g., rheumatoid arthritis)<br>• Atrophied fat pads<br>• Metatarsalgia (forefoot pain)<br>• Diabetes |
| ***Materials*** | • Diab-A-Sheet[2]—a laminate of ⅛ in. (3.2 mm) PPT and ⅛ in. (3.2 mm) #1 Plastazote.<br>• Birkenstock cork pads[17] or PPT pads[2]:<br> ○ One splayfoot pad or one metatarsal pad |

## TABLE 12-1. Features of Supportive Footwear (Continued)

| Component or Characteristic | Recommended Characteristics | Special Considerations |
| --- | --- | --- |
| Steel shank (Fig. 12-19c and d) | • This is a steel strip positioned deep in the outersole to reinforce the shoe and help it retain its shape and stability.<br>• It runs the length of the sole from the heel to the metatarsophalangeal joints.<br>• Test for its presence by bending the shoe in half; the shoe should not bend proximal to the MTP joints; if the shoe can be curved into a circle, there is no steel shank. | |
| Heel width | • Avoid narrow heels.<br>• A wide base of support under the heel is desirable. | • If ankle instability and tendency to sprain the ankle are chronic problems, consider a wide, outflared heel (Fig. 12-19d); in addition, a shoe with high sides provides extra support for an unstable ankle. |
| Heel height (the difference between the height of the heel and toes) | • Ideally ½ to 1 in. (2 to 2.5 cm) high.<br>• Greater than 1 in. (2.5 cm) promotes hammer/cock-up/claw toes, equinus (short calcaneal tendon), forefoot pain, and lumbar lordosis. | • Higher heels are unsuitable for clients with forefoot disorders.<br>• A 1 in. (2.5 cm) high heel helps take the tension off the plantar fascia, which may help relieve plantar fasciitis.<br>• Avoid negative heels, in which the heel is lower than the toes; this creates undue tension in the plantar fascia. |
| Insole (arch supports) (Fig. 12-19d) | • Ideally the insole is cushioned and contoured to support the medial arch.<br>• Extra-depth shoes and the better-constructed athletic shoes have contoured insoles that are removable. | • Especially important for persons with hindfoot pronation (i.e., flat foot; fallen arch).<br>• Plastazote insoles are recommended for individuals with fragile or ulcerated skin. |

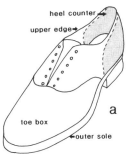

**FIGURE 12-19.** Features of supportive footwear. (*a*) The heel counter is the reinforcing material positioned between the inner and outer layers of the upper materials. (*b*) The solid line represents the standard shape of a toe box. The broken line represents a toe box with extra depth. (*c*) A view of the underside of the shoe shows the reinforcing shank, which is located between the outer sole (removed in this figure) and the insole. (*d*) A cross section through the heel region of the shoe. The broken line shows the shape of an outflare heel, which is flared on both the medial and lateral sides to provide extra stability and prevent ankle sprains.

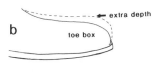

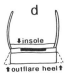

    ○ One medial wedge/pad (for medial longitudinal arch)
- Double-sided tape, hot melt glue stick, or solvent-free contract cement for attachment of PPT pads.
- The orthosis occupies space in the shoe. Select a lace-up shoe with a deep toebox (i.e., extra-depth shoe with a removable insole) or a shoe one-half size larger than usual. Ensure that the fitting is not too tight.

*Durability*

- Plastazote will bottom out after 6 months to 1 year, depending on the weight of the client and the amount of walking.

*Equipment and Tools*

- Scissors
- For attachment of cork pads—heat gun
- For attachment of PPT pads—hot glue gun unless tape or contact cement is used

*Client's Position*

- Seated on a chair, ideally on a raised platform so that the client's foot is at table height and the therapist does not need to bend down to floor level.

*Therapist's Position*

- Ideally, standing if the client is seated on a raised platform. If the client's foot is at floor level, the therapist must squat or sit on a footstool.

*Pattern*

- Cut out a piece of Diab-A-Sheet to fit the inside of the shoe with the Plastazote surface against the foot (Fig. 12-18).

*Fabrication (Fig. 12-18a)*

1. While holding the Diab-A-Sheet cutout against the sole of the foot, palpate through the material to locate the metatarsal heads and mark the position of the metatarsal (MT) pad proximal to MT heads (Fig. 12-18).
2. Mark the position of the medial wedge under the medial longitudinal arch.
3. Attach the pads to the underside of the Diab-A-Sheet, against the PPT surface. Cork pads are impregnated with adhesive that is activated with a heat gun. The PPT pads can be attached with double-sided tape, hot-melt glue, or contact cement.
4. Remove the insole from the shoe to make room for the orthosis or use an extra-depth shoe.
5. Apply the shoe and orthosis and have the client walk. Trim sides or grind the underside to achieve a comfortable fit.
6. Over the first few days of use, the Plastazote will automold to the contours of the foot with weight bearing.

*Wearing Regimen*

- Whenever weight bearing.

*Precautions*

- Ensure that pads are well adhered to the orthosis.
- This orthosis provides little correction of biomechanical malalignment.
- If the foot problem is unilateral, we recommend providing a foot orthosis for both feet to keep the pelvis level.

*Options*

- To reduce the space occupied by the ¼ in. (6.4 mm) thickness, use ³⁄₁₆ in. (4.8 mm) thick Diab-A-Sheet.
- Replace the Diab-A-Sheet with ¼ in. (6.5 mm) #1 or #2 Plastazote, heat in an oven, and mold to the foot when weight bearing on a foam block.
- If the medial wedge is not high enough (because of a very high medial arch), attach a second pad on top of the other during the initial fabrication or later.

- If either pad is too high, use a grinder to make it thinner.
- The shape of the pads can be modified with scissors, grinder, or razor knife.

*Alternatives*
- Prefabricated resilient foot orthoses[2,4]

# Footwear

Footwear ranges from styles that are ideally supportive to those that are injurious. Many biomechanical disorders can be attributed to injurious footwear. In such circumstances, correction of footwear may be all that is necessary to relieve the symptoms. Therapists should advise their clients about the footwear features to meet their individual needs (Table 12-1).

# References

1. Webber, D (ed): Clinical Aspects of Lower Extremity Orthotics. Elgin Enterprises, Oakville, Canada, in conjunction with the Canadian Association of Prosthetists and Orthotists, 1990.
2. AliMed Inc.: Orthopedic Rehabilitation Products 1997–98. AliMed Inc., Dedham, MA, 1997.
3. Speers, A, and Speers, M: Care of the infant in a Pavlik harness. Pediatr Nurs 18:229, 1992.
4. Smith & Nephew, Inc. Rehabilitation Division: International Catalogue. Germantown, WI, 1997. (Rolyan and Progressive are trademarks of Smith & Nephew, Inc.)
5. Sammons Preston Catalog. Bolingbrook, IL, 1997.
6. North Coast Medical, Hand Therapy Catalog. San Jose, CA, 1997.
7. Orfit Industries: Orthotic Products Catalogue. Wijnegem, Belgium, 1992.
8. Orfit Industries: Tibial Fracture Bracing (video). Orfit Industries, Wijnegem, Belgium.
9. Van Leeuwen, W: Functional Treatment of Tibial Fractures. Orfit Industries, Wijnegem, Belgium.
10. Wapner, KL, and Sharkey, PF: The use of night splints for treatment of recalcitrant plantar fasciitis. Foot Ankle 12:135, 1991.
11. Pezullo, DJ: Using night splints in the treatment of plantar fasciitis in the athlete. J Sport Rehabil 2:287, 1993.
12. Batt, ME, and Tanji, JL: Management options for plantar fasciitis. Physician Sportsmed 23:77, 1995.
13. Ryan, J: Use of posterior night splint in the treatment of plantar fasciitis. Am Fam Phys 52:891, 1995.
14. Orfit Industries: Orfit Splinting Guide, Antwerp, 1990.
15. Wu, SH: An anterior direct molding ankle-foot orthosis. J Occup Ther Assoc ROC 10:75, 1992.
16. Bruckner, J: Design for a soft orthosis. Am J Phys Ther 65:1522, 1985.
17. Serum International Inc., Montreal, Canada. (See Appendix D.)

# *Orthotic Materials*

All tables in this appendix refer to characteristics and applications of orthotic materials and products discussed in Chapter 4. In Tables 1 and 2, materials in the same category column can be used interchangeably (see Chapter 4 "Conformability Characteristics").

---

**TABLE 1.  Translucent-When-Heated Thermoplastics**

|  | Category | | | |
|---|---|---|---|---|
|  | A | B | C | D |
| Handling and finishing characteristics | Low <------------------------------CONFORMABILITY ------------------------------> High | | | |
|  | Low <--------------------------------STRETCHINESS --------------------------------> High | | | |
|  | High <---------------------------THERAPIST'S CONTROL---------------------------> Low | | | |
|  | Requires careful cutting or grinding<---------EDGE FINISHING ---------> Smooths with heat | | | |
| General applications | Gravity-resisted molding<-------------------------------------->Gravity-assisted molding | | | |
|  | Large, low-conforming orthoses<------------------------>Small, high-conforming orthoses | | | |
|  | Suitable for the novice or experienced fabricator<------------------------------------------->the novice fabricator | | | Can be challenging for |

| Supplier | A | B | C | D |
|---|---|---|---|---|
| Smith & Nephew Inc. |  | Aquaplast Watercolors (1986)* | Aquaplast Original (1975) |  |
|  |  | Aquaplast Resilient T (formerly Green Stripe Aquaplast) (1977) | Aquaplast T (1978) | Aquaplast Prodrape T (formerly Blue Strip Aquaplast) (1979) |
| NCM†(USA) and Vaillancourt (Canada) |  | Orfit Classic Stiff (1985) | Orfit Classic Soft (1985) |  |
| Vaillancourt (Canada) | Orfilined (1996) | Orfit NS (Non-Stick) Stiff (1996) Colorfit (1995) | Orfit NS (Non-Stick) Soft (1996) |  |
| NCM (USA) AliMed Ortho-Dynactive (USA) Physio E.R.P. (Canada) |  | Prism (1995) | Encore (1996) Turbocast (1989) | Multiform Clear |
| Sammons Preston Larson Products |  |  | KayPlast (1997) New Wave Memory |  |

*Date (19XX) is the year the material was introduced.
†NCM—North Coast Medical.

**TABLE 2.  Opaque-When-Heated Thermoplastics—Current and Discontinued Materials**

**Category***

Handling and finishing characteristics:

- Low <————————————— CONFORMABILITY —————————————> High
- Low <————————————— STRETCHINESS —————————————> High
- High <————————————— THERAPIST'S CONTROL —————————————> Low
- Low <————————————— SURFACE IMPRESSIONABILITY —————————————> High
- Requires careful cutting or grinding <————— EDGE FINISHING —————> Smooths with heat

General applications:

- Gravity-resisted molding <—————————————————> Gravity-assisted molding
- Large, low-conforming orthoses <—————————————————> Small, high-conforming orthoses
- Suitable for the novice or experienced fabricator <—————————————————> Challenging for the unskilled therapist
- OK to use elastic bandage when molding ————————— Do not use elastic bandage when molding

| Supplier | A 1 (Isoprene rubber base) | A 2 | B 1 (Opaque materials with memory) | B 2 | C 1 (Rebound because of partial memory) | C 2 | D 1 | D 2 |
|---|---|---|---|---|---|---|---|---|
| Smith & Nephew Inc. | San-Splint (also called Polysplint A) (mid-1960s)[*] | Synergy (1988) | | Ezeform (1984 granular when stretched) | | Polyflex II (also called San-Splint XR) (1979) | Polyform (1975) | |
| *(Kay-Splint — shaded)* | | | | Kay-Splint Series 3 (1984–95)[†] | | Kay-Splint Isoprene (1979–95) | | Kay-Splint Series 1 (1975–95)[‡] |
| Sammons Preston | Orthoplast (mid-1960s) | | | | | Orthoplast II | | |
| *(Kay-Splint)* | KayPrene (1997) | Kay-Splint Basic IV (1997) | Kay-Splint Basic III (1996) | | | Kay-Splint Basic II (1996) | Kay-Splint Basic I (1996) | |
| Remington Medical (beginning 1996) | Orthoform (1996) | | | | Thermoflex (1996) | Thermosplint (1996) | Thermoform (1996) | Thermoform Plus (1996) |
| Larson Products, Inc. | Orthoprene | | Ortho-Eze (1997) | | New Wave Universal | | New Wave Precision | |

*(continued)*

**TABLE 2.  Opaque-When-Heated Thermoplastics—Current and Discontinued Materials (Continued)**

| Supplier | A | | B | | C | | D | |
|---|---|---|---|---|---|---|---|---|
| | *Isoprene rubber base* | | *Opaque materials with memory* | | | *Rebound because of partial memory* | | ‡ |
| | 1 | 2 | 1 | 2 | 1 | 2 | 1 | 2 |
| North Coast Medical | NCM Omega Plus (1997) (with memory) | | NCM Omega Max (1997) (formerly Omega) (1994) | | NCM Spectrum (1988) | NCM Preferred (1988) | NCM Clinic (1988) | NCM Clinic D (1990) |
| Polymed (1986–92), Zimmer Canada (1986–89), Remington Medical (1989–96) | | | Ultra Splint (1986–88) (formerly MR 2000) | | Custom Splint Plus (1988–96) | Custom Splint (1986–96) (formerly JU 1000) | Precision Splint (1986–96) (formerly RS 3000) | Precision Splint Plus (1990–96) |
| Jobst (1984–86) | | | MR 2000 (1985–86) | | | JU 1000 (1984–86) (formerly Polysplint II) | RS 3000 (1984–86) (formerly Polysplint I) | |
| Polymed (1982–84) | | | | | | Polysplint II (1982–84) | Polysplint I (1982–84) | |
| PhysioE.R.P. (Canada) and Ortho-Dynactive (USA) | | | Spina (1990s) | | | | | |
| AliMed | Multiform Isoprene | | | | | | Multiform Plastic | |
| Vaillancourt (Canada) | | | Easy Fit (1994) | | Soft-Fit (1990s) | | | |

*Categories A through D are subdivided (1, 2) to demonstrate the eight degrees of conformability in opaque thermoplastics, ranging from low to high (A1 is low; D2 is high).
†Single date (19XX) represents the year the material was introduced.
§Date range (19XX–XX) represents the year the material was introduced and the year it was discontinued.
‡Shaded boxes represent discontinued materials.

**TABLE 3. Recommended Applications for Different Thicknesses of Low-Temperature Thermoplastics**

| Thickness* | 1/32 in. (0.8 mm) | 1/16 in. (1.6 mm) | 3/32 in. (2.4 mm) | 1/8 in. (3.2 mm) |
|---|---|---|---|---|
| Working time | Short<-------------------------------------------------------------------------->Long |
| Conformability | More<-------------------------------------------------------------------------->Less |
| Flexibility | Maximum flexibility<-------------------------------------------------->Maximum rigidity |
| Size of orthosis | Small<-------------------------------------------------------------------------->Large |
| Weight | Minimum<-------------------------------------------------------------------->Maximum |
| Applications | • To finish edges of maxi-perforated orthoses | • Finger-based orthoses | • Forearm-based wrist orthoses<br>• Forearm-based wrist-MCP orthoses<br>• Forearm-based wrist-thumb orthoses<br>• Multiple-joint orthoses for infants or small children<br>• In-shoe foot orthoses<br>• Orthoses for clients with arthritis<br>• Hand-based orthoses | • Forearm-based wrist-hand orthoses | • Circumferential stabilizing orthoses<br>• Elbow, knee, shoulder, ankle orthoses<br>• Inserts for lumbar orthoses<br>• Bases for dynamic orthoses with embedded wire(s) |

*3/16 in. (4.8 mm) thickness is also available in some low-temperature thermoplastics but is rarely used by therapists.

**TABLE 4. Low-Temperature Thermoplastics (LTTs) Color Availability**

| Flesh tones | Pastels | Peach | Vibrant Colors | White |
|---|---|---|---|---|
| Kay-Splint Basics II and III | Aquaplast<br>Colorfit<br>Turbocast<br>Opaque LTTs | Orfit<br>Orfilined<br>Turbocast | Aquaplast<br>Colorfit<br>Prism | Aquaplast<br>Easy-Fit<br>Soft-Fit<br>Prism<br>Opaque LTTs |

**TABLE 5. Foam Thermoplastics, Available Thicknesses, Shore A Firmness, and Common Applications in Orthotics**

| Foam Thermoplastic | Available Thicknesses | Firmness Category* | Shore A Firmness Scale† | Common Applications in Orthotics |
|---|---|---|---|---|
| **Plastazote** | 1/16, 1/8, 3/16, 1/4, 1/2, 3/4, 1 in. | #1 medium pink | 20 | |
| cross-linked polyethylene | 1/8, 3/16, 1/4, 1/2 in. | #1 medium pink perforated | 20 | • 1/2 in.—cervical collars; knee or elbow pads |
| | 1/16, 1/8, 3/16, 1/4, 3/8, 1/2, 3/4, 1 in. | #1 medium white | 20 | • 1/4 in.—insoles; cervical collars for children; pressure conformers for pressure sores or sensitive diabetic skin |
| | 1/16, 1/8, 3/16, 1/4, 3/8, 1/2, 3/4, 1 in. | #2 firm white | 35 | |
| | 1/8, 1/4, 1/2 in. | #2.5 black | unknown | |
| | 1/8, 1/4, 1/2 in. | #3 black | 69 | • Outersoles |
| **AliPlast** | 3/16 in. | 2E | 15 | |
| cross-linked polyethylene | 1/8, 3/16, 1/4, 1/2 in. | 4E | 23 | • 1/2 in.—cervical collars; knee or elbow pads |
| | 1/8, 1/4 in. | 6A | 34 | • 1/4 in.—insoles |
| | 1/8 in. | 10 | 60 | |
| | 3/16, 3/8, 9/16 in. | XPE | 68 | • Outersoles |
| **AliSoft** | 1/8 in. | AliPlast 10 with durable, blue nylon fabric | 60 | • Low-conforming hand orthoses—especially radial wrist-thumb |
| **NickelPlast** | 3/16, 3/8 in. | Lite | 42 | • 3/16 in.—insoles |
| alloy of ethylene vinyl acetate and polyethylene; resistant to bottoming out | 1/8, 3/16, 1/4, 3/16 in. | S | 45 | |
| | 1/8, 3/16, 1/4, 3/8, 1/2 in. | X-Firm | 55 | • Outersoles |
| **PE LITE** | unknown | Soft | 14 | |
| | unknown | Medium | 37 | |
| | 3/16 in. | Firm | 45 | |

*The firmness category indicates the suppliers' terms used to describe the degree of firmness. There is no consistency between firmness categories for different materials. However, the Shore A Firmness Scale does provide a reliable comparison to compare the firmness of different materials.

†The lower the number, the greater the conformability. Information from Alimed Inc: Orthopedic Rehabilitation Products catalog, 1996–97.

‡Conversion of inches to millimeters: 1/16 (1.6), 1/8 (3.2), 3/16 (4.8), 1/4 (6.4), 3/8 (9.6), 1/2 (12.8), 9/16 (14.4), 3/4 (19.2), and 1 (25.6).

**TABLE 6. Zipper Precuts**

| Made from Orfit Classic (OC) | | Made from Aquaplast-T | Applications |
|---|---|---|---|
| From Vaillancourt (Canada only) or Orfit Industries | From North Coast Medical (US only) | From Smith & Nephew, Inc. | |
| Orfizip Corset | | Rolyan® Aquaform Corset (uses Velcro D-ring closure instead of a zipper) | • Conditions requiring secure immobilization of lumbar spine<br>• Vertebral fractures<br>• Spondylolisthesis |
| Orfizip Knee Splint<br>1/12 in. (2 mm) thick mini-perforated or 1/8 in. (3 mm) thick mini-perforated OC | | | • Postsurgical immobilization<br>• Correction of knee contractures |
| | | Rolyan® Aquaform Zippered Tibial Fracture Brace 1/8 in. (3.2 mm) thick 4% perforated | • Midshaft fractures of the tibia |
| | Orfizip Wrist Splint<br>1/12 in. (2 mm) thick maxi-perforated or 1/8 in. (3 mm) thick mini-perforated OC | Rolyan® AquaForm Zippered Wrist Splint 3/32 in. (2.4 mm) thick 4% perforated<br>a. Short (two thirds up forearm)<br>b. Long (up to the elbow) | • Presurgical assessment before wrist fusion<br>• Carpal bone instability<br>• Forearm fractures |
| | Orfizip Wrist and Thumb Splint<br>1/12 in. (2 mm) thick maxi-perforated or 1/8 in. (3 mm) thick mini-perforated OC | Rolyan® AquaForm Zippered Wrist and Thumb Spica Splint 3/32 in. (2.4 mm) thick 4% perforated<br>a. Short (two thirds up forearm)<br>b. Long (up to the elbow) | • Fractures of scaphoid or thumb MCP<br>• Posttrapeziotomy<br>• Post–thumb MCP reconstruction |

**TABLE 7.  Closed-Cell, Heat Moldable, Self-Stick, Foam Linings and Paddings—Rank Ordered According to Firmness, Based on Suppliers' Catalog Information**

| Product and Features | Thickness | Shore A Firmness Rating* |
|---|---|---|
| Soft Sponge [1] | ⅛ or ¼ in. (3.2 or 6.4 mm) | 6 |
| AliBrite—bright, solid colors [1] | ⅛ in. (3.2 mm) | 12 |
| QuickStick [1,2] | ³⁄₁₆ in. (4.8 mm) | 15 |
| Plastazote #1 [1,2,3] | ¹⁄₁₆, ⅛, ³⁄₁₆, or ¼ in. (1.6, 3.2, 4.8, or 6.4 mm) | 20 (medium) |
| AliPlast Self-stick (4E) [1] | ⅛ in. (3.2 mm) | 23 |
| Kushionflex [2]—resists bottoming out | ¹⁄₁₆, ⅛, or ½ in. (1.6, 3.2, or 12.8 mm) | unknown |
| Polycushion [1,2] | ⅛ in. (3.2 mm) | unknown |
| Luxafoam [4,5,6] | ⅛ in. (3.2 mm) | Medium |
| SplintCushion [4]—regular, low tack, stretch | ⅛ or ¼ in. (3.2 or 6.4 mm) | Medium |
| Firm Foam Padding [4] | ³⁄₁₆ in. (4.8 mm) | High |
| NickelPlast [1] | ⅛ or ³⁄₁₆ in. (3.2 or 4.8 mm) | 48 |

*Information from AliMed, Inc.: Orthopedic Rehabilitation Products catalog, 1996–97.

**TABLE 8.  Open-Cell, Self-stick, Nonmoldable Foam Linings**

| Product | Thickness | Density | Color | Distinctive features |
|---|---|---|---|---|
| BioPad [4] | ½ in. (1.2 cm) | • Low | • White | |
| Reston Foam [1] | ⅞ in. (2.2 cm) | • Low | • White | • Readily compresses, fast rebound |
| Rolyan® Foam Padding [2] | ½ in. (1.2 cm) | • Low | • White | |
| | ⅜ in. (1 cm) | • Extra low | • Tan | • Slow rebound |
| T Foam [1] | 1 in. (2.5 cm) | • Low | • Pink | • Self-contouring to body contours |
| | ⅜ or 1 in. (1 or 2.5 cm) | • Medium | • Blue | |
| Contour Foam [6] | ⅜ in. (1 cm) | • Low | • Pink | • Total contact and uniform cushioning |
| PPT™ (from Professional Protective Technology) [2] | ⅜ or 1 in. (1 or 2.5 cm) | • Medium | • Blue | |
| | ⅛ in. (3.2 mm) | • High | • Blue | • Extremely durable shock absorber, will not bottom out, no contourability |

*Bracketed numbers in Tables 7 and 8 refer to the following suppliers: 1, AliMed; 2, Smith & Nephew, Inc.; 3, Sammons Preston; 4, North Coast Medical; 5, Orfit Industries; 6, Vaillancourt (Canada only).

**TABLE 9. Conforming Materials for Scar Management**

| Category | Supplier | Product | Size | Adherent to the Skin | Moisturizes Skin |
|---|---|---|---|---|---|
| Silicone elastomer | AliMed | • Silastomer (RTV Silicone Elastometer) | 454 g (16 oz) | No | Yes |
| | | • Otoform K/c | 790 g (28 oz) | No | Yes |
| | | • AliMed Putty #2 | 680 g (24 oz) | No | Yes |
| | | • Pediplast | 250 g (8.8 oz) | No | Yes |
| | North Coast Medical | • Elastomer 121—liquid style | Set of two—237 ml (8 oz) tubes | No | Yes |
| | | • Otoform K—putty style | 170 g (6 oz) or 800 g (16 oz) | No | Yes |
| | | • Soft Putty Elastomer | 340 or 907 g (12 or 32 oz) | No | Yes |
| | | • Putty Elastomer | 340 or 907 g (12 or 32 oz) | No | Yes |
| | Sammons Preston | • Rose-gel Silicone Elastomer—putty style | Not specified | No | Yes |
| | | • Sammons Preston Elastomer—liquid style | 456g (16 oz) | No | Yes |
| | Smith & Nephew Inc. | • Rolyan Silicone Elastomer Sheets | 0.47 × 23 × 36 cm (0.18 × 9 × 14 in.) sheets | No | Yes |
| | | • Silicone Elastomer | | | |
| | | • Liquid style | 450 g or 2260 g (15.8 or 80 oz) | No | Yes |
| | | • Ezemix putty style | 220 g or 858 g (7.76 or 30.26 oz) | No | Yes |
| | | • 50/50 | 240 g or 847 g (8.5 or 29.8 oz) | No | Yes |
| Prosthetic foam | AliMed or Smith & Nephew, Inc. | • Prosthetic Foam | 454 g (16 oz) | No | No |
| Silicon gel sheeting | Smith & Nephew, Inc. | Cica Care (sterile) | 12 × 15 cm (4¾ × 6 in.) or 12 × 6 cm (4¾ × 2.4 in.) sheets | Yes | Yes |
| | North Coast Medical | TopiGel (sterile) | 12 × 14 cm (4¾ × 5½ in.) sheets 0.35 cm (⅛ in.) thick—30 × 4 cm (12 × 1¾ in.) strips 0.35 cm (⅛ in.) thick—5 × 6 cm (2 × 2½ in.) patches | Yes | Yes |
| | Smith & Nephew, Inc. or AliMed | Spenco | 0.32 × 10 × 10 cm (⅛ × 4 × 4 in.) pads | No | unknown |
| | Ped-a-Ligne | Silipos WonderFlex (can be sterilized repeatedly) | 0.2/0.3/0.5 cm (0.08/0.12/0.2 in.) × 27 × 37.5 cm (11 × 15 in.) sheets | No | Yes |

*(continued)*

**TABLE 9. Conforming Materials for Scar Management (Continued)**

| Category | Supplier | Product | Size | Clings to the Skin | Moisturizes Skin |
|---|---|---|---|---|---|
| Polymer gel (hydro gel) sheeting | Ped-a-Ligne | Silipos Scar Care —sheets/squares/ dots/body sleeves, tubes, caps, gloves | 0.4 cm thick—20 × 20, 30 × 40, 40 × 51 cm (⅛ in. thick—8 × 8 in., 12 × 16 in., 16 × 20 in.) sheets | No | Yes |
| | | | 0.3 × 10 × 10 cm (⅛ × 4 × 4 in.) squares | Yes/No | Yes |
| | | | 0.3 cm thick × 2.5 cm diameter (⅛ × 1 in.) dots | Yes/No | Yes |
| | | | 10 or 20 × 91 cm (4 or 8 × 36 in.) sheets | Yes/No | Yes |
| | Sammons Preston or Alimed | Silipos Thero-Gel Scar Care—discs, dots, sheets, body tubes, finger caps, sleeves | 0.35 cm (⅛ in.) thick—0.5 or 1 cm (2¼ or 4 in.) discs | Yes | Yes |
| | | | 0.35 cm (⅛ in.) thick—2.5 cm (1 in.) diameter flat or concave dots | Yes | Yes |
| | | | 0.35 cm (⅛ in.) thick—10 cm (4 in.) square patches | Yes | Yes |
| | North Coast Medical | Silipos Thero-Gel Scar Care—sheets/ discs/body sleeves | 10 × 10 cm (4 × 4 in.) sheets | Yes | Yes |
| | | | 6.4 × 10 cm (2½ or 4 in.) disks | Yes | Yes |
| | Ped-a-Ligne or North Coast Medical | Krystal Gel sheeting (also called Adhesive Gel Liner) | 0.8 mm (1/32 in.) thick 10 cm (4 in.) or 20 cm (8 in.) wide—91 cm (36 in.) roll (can be applied to LTT before immersing in hot water; however, it has minimal stretch and reduces the conformability of the thermoplastic) | Yes | Yes |
| | Smith & Nephew, Inc. | Elasto-gel Cast and Splint Pads | 0.35 cm (⅛ in.) thick 10 × 10 cm (4 × 4 in.) 15 × 20 cm (6 × 8 in.) 30 × 30 cm (12 × 12 in.) pads | No | Yes |
| | North Coast Medical | Second Skin Dressing (sterile) | 8 × 10 cm (3 × 4 in.) sheet | No | Yes |
| | | Elasto-gel Occlusive Dressing (sterile) | 10 × 10 cm (4 × 4 in.) or 15 × 20 cm (6 × 8 in.) pads | No | Yes |
| | Beiersdorf-Jobst | Cutinova Hydro/Thin | 0.32 or 0.16 cm thick—5 × 7.5, 10 × 10, 10 × 15 cm (⅛ or 1/16 in. thick—2 × 3, 4 × 4, 4 × 6 in.) squares | Yes | Yes |

# *Glossary*

**active range of motion:** The range through which a joint can move voluntarily, without assistance or resistance; measured in degrees of a circle.

**adhesions:** Abnormal fibrous strands that adhere together tissue structures that are normally separate; they develop secondary to inflammation or injury.

**anesthesia:** Partial or complete loss of sensation resulting from disease, injury, or administration of an anesthetic agent.

**ankylosis:** An abnormal bony or fibrous fusion of a joint. The condition may be congenital or it may result from disease, trauma, surgery, or contractures resulting from immobility.

**ankylosis takedown:** Surgical removal of range-restricting bone at the margins of a joint.

**annular ligament:** Circular or ring-shaped ligament.

**antagonistic muscle:** A muscle whose action is the direct opposite to that of another muscle.

**ape-hand deformity:** The hand posture resulting from a median nerve injury in which the thenar muscles are paralyzed and become atrophied and thumb opposition is lost.

**arthritis:** Inflammation of joints.

**arthroplasty:** Surgical reconstruction of a damaged or malformed joint to alleviate pain and improve joint mobility. An artificial joint (prosthesis) may or may not be used.

**assistive:** A type of passive force applied by an orthosis to facilitate movement when muscles are weak or paralyzed.

**atrophy:** Wasting or decrease in size of a tissue, organ, or entire body resulting from death and resorption of cells, and diminished cellular proliferation due to disuse, pressure, ischemia, malnutrition, denervation, decreased activity, or hormonal changes.

**autonomic dysreflexia:** A syndrome affecting persons with lesions of the spinal cord above the midthoracic level; characterized by sudden elevation of blood pressure, slowed heart rate, excessive sweating, facial flushing, nasal congestion, and headache. It is due to an exaggerated autonomic response to such stimuli as distention of the rectum or bladder.

**avascular:** Absence of blood supply.

**blood plasma:** The fluid in which cellular elements of the blood are suspended.

**capsular tightness:** Tightness of the saclike envelope enclosing the cavity of a synovial joint, causing restricted joint range of motion.

**carpal tunnel syndrome:** Compression of the median nerve in the carpal tunnel, located on the volar side of the wrist. Initial symptoms are pain, tingling, or numbness in the median nerve distribution of the hand (i.e., palmar side of the thumb, index, middle finger, and radial half of the ring finger) that may radiate into the arm. Prolonged compression/entrapment leads to weakness and atrophy of the thenar muscles. It may be attributed to elevated pressure in the carpal tunnel because of pregnancy, cumulative trauma, poor wrist positioning, or wrist fracture.

**cerebral palsy (CP):** Defect of motor power and coordination caused by maldevelopment of the brain.

**cerebrovascular accident (CVA):** Brain damage resulting from a sudden interruption in blood supply because of a blood clot or hemorrhage.

**circumferential:** Encircling.

**clawhand deformity:** Hand posture resulting from paralysis of the intrinsic muscles of the hand, resulting from a combined median and ulnar nerve lesion, causing hyperextension of the MCPs, flexion of the IPs, and adduction of the thumb.

**CMC:** Carpometacarpal (joint).

**cock-up splint:** A static splint designed to immobilize the wrist in extension.

**collagen:** A strong, fibrous insoluble protein found in connective tissues, including the dermis, tendons, ligaments, deep fascia, bone, and cartilage.

**Colles' fracture:** A transverse fracture of the distal end of the radius (just proximal to the wrist) with displacement of the hand backward. Often the ulnar head becomes more prominent postfracture.

**cone-style:** A feature of a hand orthosis in which the thermoplastic against the volar surface of the palm and fingers is molded into a cone shape that is flared toward the ulnar side of the hand.

**conformability:** Pertains to the ease with which a warm thermoplastic molds to the contours of the body.

**conformer:** A piece of thermoplastic, elastomer, prosthetic foam, or other material that has been formed to the contours of the body. When set, it is firmly secured in place to apply evenly distributed compression to soften and flatten scarred skin.

**congenital dysplasia of the hip:** Abnormal fetal development of the acetabulum and head of the femur, causing instability, subluxation, or dislocation of the hip joint after birth.

**contracted:** Shortened.

**contracture:** Abnormal shortening of connective or muscle tissue causing restricted joint mobility.

**corrective:** A type of passive force applied by an orthosis to promote growth of shortened tissues to improve range of motion.

**cosmesis:** Appearance.

**craniotomy:** Surgical opening of the skull.

**cryotherapy:** Therapeutic use of cold.

**cumulative trauma:** Injury resulting from the cumulative effect of repeated application of low stress, when tissues are not allowed sufficient time to recover.

**custom:** Pertaining to an orthosis made specifically for an individual and his or her body dimensions.

**deformity:** Distortion of any part or general disfigurement of the body. It may be acquired or congenital.

**denervated:** Loss of nerve supply to muscle or skin, resulting in paralysis or loss of sensation, respectively.

**de Quervain's tenosynovitis (stenosing tenosynovitis):** Inflammation of the tendons of abductor pollicus longus and extensor pollicus brevis in their synovial sheaths in extensor tunnel 1.

**DIP:** Distal interphalangeal (joint).

**dislocation:** Complete loss of joint alignment occurring when the bone ends forming the joint lose all contact with each other.

**dorsal:** Pertaining to the back or posterior.

**drapability:** Pertains to the ease with which a warm thermoplastic molds to the contours of the body.

**DTA:** Distal transverse arch of the hand.

**Dupuytren's contracture:** Shortening and fibrosis of the palmar fascia usually causing the ring and little fingers to bend into the palm so that they cannot be extended.

**edema:** Accumulation of excess fluid in soft tissues, causing swelling.

**effusion:** Excess synovial fluid causing painful swelling of the joint.

**end feel:** The sensation transmitted to the evaluator's hands at the extreme end of passive range of motion. The nature of the sensation indicates the structures that are limiting the range of motion. It is interpreted as abnormal when the quality of the feel is different from the normal response at that joint.

**entrapment:** Compression of a nerve or vessel by adjacent tissue, such as the walls of a fibrous or osseofibrous tunnel, muscle, tendon, or other tissue.

**epicondylitis:** Inflammation of tissues attaching to the lateral or medial epicondyle of the humerus.

**epithelialization:** Regrowth of the epithelial layer of the skin to close a wound.

**ergonomics:** The science relating to humans and their work, embodying the anatomic, physiologic, psychologic, and mechanical principles affecting the efficient use of human energy.

**excursion:** Movement of a tendon through a fibrous sheath.

**fibroblast:** A connective tissue cell that produces collagen, elastin, and reticular fibers.

**fibrosis:** Formation of abnormal fibrous tissue.

**fibrotic:** Marked by, or pertaining to, fibrosis.

**filtrate:** Fluid that has been passed through a filter.

**fixation:** A method by which an orthosis is kept in place on the body. The most common method of fixation uses Velcro straps.

**flaccid:** Lacking muscle tone, causing floppy paralysis.

**flexorplasty:** Surgical transfer of a shoulder muscle (usually pectoralis major) or a wrist muscle to provide active elbow flexion.

**foot drop (drop foot):** Plantar flexed posture of the foot caused by paralysis of the ankle dorsiflexors.

**force:** An action that tends to change the state of rest or motion of a body to which it is applied.

**gamekeeper's thumb:** A cumulative trauma injury of the ulnar collateral ligament of the thumb MCP. This injury was common among gamekeepers because of the repetitive strain of killing birds by twisting their necks.

**gauntlet:** A circumferential support conforming to the contours of the forearm and hand.

**gutter:** A term pertaining to the semicircular or U-shaped trough of half-shell orthoses. The term is often applied to the half-shell that is molded to the ulnar or radial side of the forearm and hand. Sometimes it is used in reference to volar half-shell orthoses for the fingers.

**half-shell:** The style of an orthosis that encloses half of the limb, in contrast to a circumferential orthosis that encloses the limb.

**hemiparesis:** Muscle weakness or partial paralysis affecting one side of the body.

**hemiplegia:** Paralysis of one side of the body.

**hemophilia:** A hereditary blood disease marked by greatly prolonged coagulation time, with consequent failure of the blood to clot and abnormal bleeding, sometimes accompanied by swelling of the joints.

**heterotopic ossification:** The formation of new bone in tissues that normally do not ossify, for example, joint capsule or ligaments of a joint. Its formation is associated with severe circumferential burns around the affected joint, spinal cord injury, head injury, CVA, or musculoskeletal trauma. It can interfere with joint range of motion.

**high profile:** A type of extension outrigger in which the outrigger acts as the anchor for the traction force.

**histology:** The study of the microscopic structure (cells and fibers) of tissues.

**homeostasis:** A state of balance or equilibrium in the body with respect to various functions, and the chemical compositions of the fluids and tissues.

**hypersensitivity:** An exaggerated sensitivity to a stimulus of any kind in which the response to the stimulus is excessive.

**hypertonic:** A state of greater than normal tension or incomplete relaxation, in muscle; the opposite of hypotonic.

**hypertrophic:** Pertaining to, or marked by, hypertrophy.

**hypertrophic scar:** Excessive regeneration of the dermal layer of the skin after a burn, injury, or incision, forming a thickened, raised scar with a tendency to shrink (contract), causing tight skin that can limit joint range of motion.

**hypertrophy:** An increase in the size of a tissue, structure, or organ of the body, owing to growth rather than tumor formation. The opposite of atrophy.

**hyposensitivity:** Having a reduced ability to respond to stimuli.

**hypotonic:** A state of less than normal muscle tone.

**impressionability:** The degree to which the surface of a warm thermoplastic material becomes marked by fingerprints or other textures.

**inflammation:** A localized response, elicited by injury or destruction of tissues, which is the body's attempt to protect the injured tissues. It is characterized by redness, swelling, and pain.

**interstitial fluid (tissue fluid):** The fluid found among the cellular and fibrous elements of tissues.

**intra-articular:** Within a joint.

**intrinsic minus position:** Extension or hyperextension of the MCPs with flexion of the IPs, often caused by paralysis or weakness of the intrinsic hand muscles.

**intrinsic tightness:** Contracture of the intrinsic hand muscles causing limited finger IP flexion when the respective MCP is passively extended.

**IP:** Interphalangeal (joint).

**ischemia:** A local, temporary deficiency of blood supply caused by the obstruction of circulation to the part.

**Kirschner wire (K-wire):** A wire designed for skeletal traction that is useful for the fabrication of some orthoses.

**kyphotic:** Abnormally increased convexity in the curvature of the thoracic spine as viewed from the side.

**laminectomy:** Removal of the posterior arch of a vertebra, composed of the spinous process and both adjacent laminae. The procedure is performed to permit access to the disk or nerve roots. The term is often inappropriately used for a hemilaminectomy (removal of only one lamina) or laminotomy (formation of a hole in the lamina). The latter is the most common approach to a herniated disk.

**lax:** Without tension; loose; slack.

**lesion:** A circumscribed area of pathologically altered tissue; an injury or wound.

**lever arm:** The perpendicular distance from the axis of rotation to the line of application of the force.

**leverage:** The mechanical advantage gained by a lever.

**low profile:** A type of extension outrigger in which the outrigger acts as a pulley to redirect the traction force. Compared with a high-profile outrigger, it has a lower profile because the outrigger is closer to the hand.

**LTT:** Low-temperature thermoplastic.

**lysis:** Dissolution of tissue; decomposition; release of scar tissue or adhesions.

**maceration:** Softening or loss of surface tissue (e.g., skin) caused by prolonged exposure to moisture.

**magnitude:** Size, extent, or dimensions.

**mallet finger deformity:** Ruptured or lacerated extensor tendon of the DIP, causing loss of active DIP extension and a flexion posture that becomes fixed without intervention.

**MC:** Metacarpal.

**MCP:** Metacarpophalangeal (joint).

**MERiT:** A prefabricated thumb screw to attach to a static-progressive orthosis to control and adjust the amount of corrective force.

**microstomia:** Literally means "small opening"; refers to restriction of the mouth opening because of tight perioral scar tissue, usually caused by facial burns.

**motion blocking:** The design element of an orthosis that limits active joint motion without immobilizing the joint.

**MT:** Metatarsal.

**MTP:** Metatarsophalangeal (joint).

**multiple sclerosis:** Slowly progressive disease of the nervous system in which scattered areas of myelin degeneration occur, usually in the spinal cord; cause unknown.

**muscle tone:** Degree of tension within a muscle.

**myotome:** A group of muscles innervated by a single spinal segment (nerve root).

**neutral position:** A joint position that is essentially 0°, without any measurable flexion, extension, deviation, or rotation.

**nonarticular:** An orthotic design that crosses no joints, thus having no direct influence on joint mobility.

**opaque:** Impervious to light; not transparent or translucent. Pertains to a type of thermoplastic material.

**orthosis:** A device applied to the body to stabilize or immobilize, prevent or correct deformity, protect against injury, promote healing, or assist function. Orthotic devices may be made from a variety of materials, including rubber, leather, metal, canvas, rubber synthetics, and plastic.

**osteoarthritis:** A type of arthritis marked by progressive cartilage deterioration in the synovial joints and new bone formation around the joint. Risk factors include aging, obesity, trauma, and overuse or abuse of joints caused by sports or strenuous occupations.

**osteogenesis imperfecta:** An inherited disorder of the connective tissue causing excessively brittle bones, which are prone to fractures.

**osteoporotic:** A general term describing any disease process that results in reduction in the mass of bone per unit of volume. The reduction is sufficient to interfere with the mechanical support function of bone, causing susceptibility to fractures.

**O.T.(C):** Designation for an occupational therapist who has the qualifications to practice occupational therapy in Canada.

**OTR:** Designation for an occupational therapist who has the qualifications to practice occupational therapy in the United States.

**outrigger:** A component of dynamic and static-progressive orthoses, attached to the thermoplastic base, acting as a pulley to redirect a traction force (as in a low-profile or tube outrigger) or as the attachment site for the force (as in a high-profile outrigger).

**palmar:** Concerning the palm of the hand.

**paralysis:** Loss or impairment of voluntary muscle function; palsy.

**paresthesia:** Abnormal sensations such as numbness, tingling, burning, or prickling; experienced in central and peripheral nerve lesions.

**passive range of motion:** The range through which a joint can be moved by an external force; measured in degrees of a circle.

**pathogenic:** Causing disease or disorder.

**pathomechanics:** Mechanisms that tend to promote pathology or joint distortion.

**perioral:** Around the mouth.

**peritendinous:** Around a tendon.

**PIP:** Proximal interphalangeal (joint).

**plantar fasciitis:** Inflammation of the deep fascia of the sole of the foot at its attachment to the calcaneus.

**precut:** Thermoplastic material that has been previously cut by a rehabilitation supply company to a standard shape and size to be molded into a specific style of orthosis.

**prefabricated:** Mass-produced.

**preformed:** Thermoplastic material that has been previously cut and formed by a rehabilitation supply company to a specific style of orthosis.

**prehension:** The primary function of the hand; includes pinching, grasping, and manipulation of objects.

**prone:** Horizontal body position with the face downward; opposite of supine.

**prophylactically:** Type of action undertaken to prevent an undesirable outcome.

**prosthesis:** A device used to replace or augment a missing body part, or an artificial organ or joint.

**protective:** An orthotic design characteristic that affords protection to susceptible tissues or structures to prevent injury and promote optimal healing.

**proximal:** Closer to the trunk of the body or point of origin; the opposite of distal.

**quadriplegia:** Partial or complete paralysis of all four extremities and the trunk muscles, caused by injury to the spinal cord in the cervical spine. The higher the injury, the less function that is available in the arms.

**RA:** Rheumatoid arthritis.

**ray:** The phalanges of a single digit and the corresponding metacarpal or metatarsal.

**remodeling:** The reshaping or reconstruction of body tissues by surgical intervention or by natural physiologic processes that are influenced by internal and external forces and the individual's inherent healing capacity.

**replantation:** Surgical reattachment of a body part (e.g., finger, hand, limb) that has been traumatically amputated.

**resection:** Removal or excision of a tissue or body part.

**resorb:** To reabsorb.

**resorption:** The process of reabsorbing.

**rheumatoid arthritis:** A chronic, progressive, systemic disease marked by inflammation and tendency toward deformity of synovial joints.

**rigidity:** Tenseness; immovability; stiffness; inability to bend or be bent.

**ROM:** Range of motion.

**scleroderma:** A chronic manifestation of progressive systemic sclerosis, often used synonymously with that name, in which the skin becomes taut, firm, and edematous, limiting movement.

**SCS:** Splint Classification System.

**skier's thumb:** A traumatic injury of the ulnar collateral ligament of the thumb, caused by the force of a ski pole during a fall while skiing.

**skin graft:** Using the skin from another part of the body to repair a defect or trauma of the skin.

**slack:** Loose or lax tissues or other structures.

**spasticity:** A state of increased muscle tone with exaggerated tendon reflexes, causing rigidity of the body part and limited or absent voluntary muscle control; the result of an upper motor neuron lesion.

**spica:** A style of orthosis or cast that immobilizes an appendage by incorporating the body part proximal to the appendage. The most common spica orthoses and casts are for the thumb, shoulder, and hip.

**spina bifida:** A congenital defect, usually in the lumbosacral region, caused by incomplete development of the posterior neural arch, leaving a portion of the spinal cord without bony protection. Depending on the degree of damage to the spinal nerve roots in the area, the impact ranges from no impairment to complete lower extremity paralysis.

**spinal cord injury:** An acute traumatic injury of the spinal cord, causing loss of sensation and muscle function in the trunk and extremities. The extent of the deficits depends on the level of the injury on the spinal cord. Injury in the thoracic or lumbar regions causes paraplegia; injury in the cervical region causes quadriplegia.

**splint:** An appliance made of plastic, wood, metal, or plaster of Paris; used for the fixation, union, or protection of an injured part of the body.

**spondylolisthesis:** Any forward slipping of one vertebra on the one below it.

**stasis:** Decreased or absent flow of fluids, such as blood.

**stenosing:** Narrowing or constricting of a passage or opening.

**stress:** The result produced when forces act on a structure, system, or organism, disrupting equilibrium or producing strain.

**sublux:** To cause partial loss of joint alignment.

**subluxation:** Partial loss of joint alignment.

**supinated:** The position of the hand or foot with the palm or sole facing upward.

**supine:** Lying on the back with the face upward; the opposite of prone.

**swan-neck deformity:** A finger deformity commonly seen in rheumatoid arthritis, marked by flexion of the DIP, hyperextension of the PIP, and flexion of the MCP.

**synergistic muscle:** A muscle that aids or cooperates with another.

**synovectomy:** Excision of diseased synovial membrane.

**synovitis:** Inflammation of a synovial membrane lining a joint capsule or tendon sheath, causing excess production of synovial fluid, which in turn causes joint swelling and pain.

**synthesis:** Formation, composition.

**tendinitis:** Inflammation of a tendon.

**tennis elbow:** Inflammation of the origin of the wrist extensors at the outer elbow. Also called lateral epicondylitis.

**tenosynovitis:** Inflammation of a synovial tendon sheath.

**tensile:** Refers to distraction/traction forces acting on bones, joints, tendons, or ligaments.

**tension:** The force created in a tissue or structure when traction is applied.

**thermoplastic:** A rubber or plastic-based material that softens and becomes pliable when heated, allowing for shaping. After a few minutes it hardens and returns to its previous rigid state, retaining the new contours.

**tone reducing:** A type of passive force applied by an orthosis to relax the sustained, involuntary contraction of spastic muscles.

**torque (moment of force):** The extent to which a force tends to cause rotation of an object (body part) about an axis; the product of force multiplied by the lever arm.

**torticollis:** A deformity of the neck caused by shortening of muscles on one side of the neck, causing the head to tilt to the affected side with the chin pointing to the other side. It may be congenital or acquired. The muscles affected are principally those supplied by the spinal accessory nerve.

**traction:** The act of exerting a pulling force, as along the long axis of a structure.

**translucent:** Transmitting light, but diffusing it so that objects beyond are not clearly distinguished. Pertains to a type of thermoplastic material.

**trigger finger (stenosing tenosynovitis):** A condition that temporarily stops flexion or extension of a digit because of a swelling on a finger flexor tendon that catches on the flexor digital sheath. When sufficient force is generated, the finger snaps into extension or flexion, causing a trigger action of the finger. Any finger may be involved, but the ring or middle finger is most commonly affected.

**trough:** The semicylindrical part of a half-shell orthosis. It often refers to the forearm component of a forearm-based orthosis.

**ulnar drift:** Subluxation at the MCP characterized by ulnar deviation of the proximal phalanx on the head of the metacarpal, commonly seen in rheumatoid arthritis.

**unilateral neglect:** The state in which an individual is perceptually unaware of and inattentive to one side of the body because of cerebral damage from a head injury or CVA.

**vascular:** Pertaining to, or composed of, blood vessels.

**vascularity:** The condition of being vascular. The extent to which a tissue is nourished by a blood supply.

**vasoconstriction:** A decrease in the caliber of a blood vessel leading to decreased blood flow to the tissues it supplies.

**vasodilation:** An increase in the caliber of a blood vessel leading to increased blood flow to the tissues it supplies.

**vertigo:** The abnormal sensation of moving around in space or of having objects move about the person. Vertigo is sometimes used as a synonym for dizziness, light-headedness, or giddiness.

**vinculum (singular), vinculi (plural):** Narrow bands of connective tissue transmitting blood vessels to the finger flexor tendons.

**volar:** Refers to the palm of the hand or front of the forearm. Alternate terms for reference to the palm of the hand are palmar and palmaris.

**wrist drop:** A condition in which the hand is flexed at the wrist and cannot be actively extended; commonly caused by injury of the radial nerve, causing paralysis of the wrist extensors.

**yield point:** The point of stress on the load deformation curve that separates the elastic range from the plastic range, at which point increased load causes residual deformation of the tissues after the load is removed.

## References

Berkow, R (ed): The Merck Manual, ed 16. Merck, New Jersey, 1992.

Dorland's Illustrated Medical Dictionary, ed 28. WB Saunders, Philadelphia, 1994.

Sloane, SB: Medical Abbreviations and Eponyms. WB Saunders, Philadelphia, 1985.

Taliaferro Blauvelt, C, and Nelson, FRT: A Manual of Orthopaedic Terminology, ed 5. Mosby, St. Louis, 1994.

Thomas, CL (ed): Taber's Cyclopedic Medical Dictionary, ed 18. FA Davis, Philadelphia, 1997.

# Case Studies

Answers begin on page 323.

## CASE 1

Two months ago, 32-year-old Malini began an office job comprising primarily computer data entry and answering the telephone. Within a couple of weeks, she began to develop symptoms of pain, tingling, and numbness in the palm of her hands. After 4 weeks, she consulted a physician because the symptoms had progressively worsened and were interfering with her work activities. She was diagnosed with carpal tunnel syndrome and referred for custom wrist orthoses.

1. Should the therapist provide custom wrist orthoses as per the physician's order, or should another course of action be undertaken?

2. If the therapist decides to provide orthoses, what are the objectives of the orthotic intervention?

3. Identify the desirable qualities of the orthotic design.

4. Describe the categories and thicknesses of suitable thermoplastics for custom wrist orthoses.

5. Outline an appropriate wearing regimen for this client.

## CASE 2

Cory, a 24-year-old graphic artist, sustained a fracture of the right humerus in a car accident. The fracture healed, but damage to the radial nerve resulted in lack of active wrist extension (wrist drop), MCP extension, thumb abduction and extension, and weakened forearm supination. His hand had a wrist drop posture. These deficits caused a weak grasp and interfered with his ability to position his hand and manipulate his art tools. Nerve conduction tests revealed that the radial nerve was regenerating and the paralyzed muscles would eventually be reinnervated.

1. What is the rationale for orthotic intervention in this situation, when the motor deficit is temporary?

2. (a) What orthotic designs should be considered for this client, and what factors would influence the selection of design(s)? (b) What if the client was an active 10-year-old child?

3. How should the wrist be positioned in an orthosis?

4. What would be an appropriate wearing regimen?

5. As the radial nerve regenerates, active wrist extension returns before active MCP extension. What impact does this have on orthotic intervention during the recovery period?

## CASE 3

Shelley, a 3-year-old girl, sustained a deep partial thickness circumferential burn to her left arm, caused when the sleeve of her shirt caught fire. The skin was not grafted, but rather allowed to re-epithelialize on its own. She was discharged to her home in a remote area of northern Ontario, without follow-up for scar control. When she was seen 2 months later, hypertrophic scar tissue was pronounced and her elbow lacked 65° of extension and 50° of flexion. These restrictions interfered with feeding herself and play activities. Consequently, she was adapting to these limitations by developing unilateral hand skills, which promoted disuse of the affected arm. She was referred to a therapist for intervention to manage the scarring and the contracture.

1. What orthotic designs should be considered?

2. What would be an appropriate wearing regimen?

3. Describe the thickness and categories of suitable thermoplastics.

4. What scar management products could be considered, and what is the rationale for providing them?

## CASE 4

George, a 58-year-old man, underwent a left trans-tibial (below-knee) amputation because he had developed gangrene in a diabetic ulcer on his left foot. He is a good candidate for prosthetic fitting.

1. Describe orthotic intervention designed to prevent (or correct) a knee flexion contracture in the residual limb.

2. Describe the thickness and categories of suitable thermoplastics for his orthosis.

3. Describe the features of recommended footwear to protect the skin of George's right foot and to enhance stability when walking.

## CASE 5

Maria, a 76-year-old female, sustained a right CVA (stroke) resulting in left upper extremity spasticity and unilateral neglect. Her left arm developed a flexor synergy pattern. The therapist provided her with a custom bisurfaced forearm-based static wrist-hand tone-reducing orthosis (see Fig. 10-19).

1. Explain the rationale for providing a bisurfaced design.

2. What strategies would facilitate the molding of the orthosis?

3. What position should the joints be placed in?

4. Given that Maria is an inpatient and has unilateral neglect, how would thermoplastic color choice and strapping techniques be affected?

5. Identify alternative orthoses to reduce spasticity in the hand.


## CASE 6

Razak, a 45-year-old man, lacerated his finger flexor tendons at the level of the PIP (in zone 2) of his index finger when the knife he was using to cut an apple slipped. After the surgical repair, the healing tendon was protected with a dorsal forearm-based dynamic D2 MCP-IP protective-flexion and MCP extension-blocking orthosis (see Fig. 10-23). After 6 weeks, when the orthosis was discontinued, the therapist observed restricted index PIP extension.

1. What orthotic intervention would be appropriate if the restricted range was caused by shortened finger flexors resulting from prolonged positioning of the wrist, MCPs, and IPs in flexion during the previous 6 weeks? How should the joints be positioned?

2. What orthotic intervention would be appropriate if the restricted range was caused by contracture of the PIP joint capsule?

3. What precautions should be observed when attempting to reduce the flexion contracture?


## CASE 7

Jeff, a 17-year-old male, developed osteomyelitis (infected bone) of the skull caused by an abscess that developed when an infected sinus burst. A 2 in. (5 cm) diameter section of infected bone was removed from the temporal-occipital region of the skull. The surgeon delayed inserting a protective plastic plate for several months until antibiotic therapy had eradicated the infection and the cut edge of the bone had healed. During the interim, a bicycle or baseball helmet was recommended to provide protection to the area of skull deficit to prevent brain injury. The client rejected this suggestion because he desired a more discrete protective device and sought out an alternative form of protection.

1. Suggest an orthotic design that would provide protection but be inconspicuous, taking into consideration that Jeff likes to wear a baseball hat or toque. What materials would be appropriate for a protective orthotic device and why?

2. How would the orthosis be fabricated?

3. How could this device be secured in place?

## CASE 8

Elizabeth, a 43-year-old woman with a 16-year history of rheumatoid arthritis, noticed that the MCPs of her index through little fingers of her right (dominant) hand were becoming progressively more ulnarly deviated. She worked as a nurse in a hospital and wanted an orthosis that would not interfere with her work activities, to stop the progression of the deformity, and, if possible, correct it. Her wrists were not deformed and were rarely actively inflamed.

1. What styles of orthoses should be considered and why?

2. How should the incorporated joints be positioned?

3. What is the recommended wearing regimen and why?

4. What thickness, category, and color of material would be best suited for her custom thermoplastic orthosis?

## CASE 9

Gordie, an 8-year-old child, was struck by a car while riding his bicycle to school. He wasn't wearing a helmet and sustained severe head injuries. Among the numerous physical consequences of the injury, he had marked plantar flexion spasticity of his right foot, which interfered with his ability to walk.

1. What are the objectives of orthotic intervention for this problem?

2. What types of orthoses should be considered and why?

3. How would orthotic intervention differ if the ankle plantar flexion was caused by a peripheral nerve injury, causing flaccid paralysis (drop foot)?

## CASE 10

Anne is a 62-year-old woman who acquired poliomyelitis when she was 13 years old. Although she regained much of her strength over the 2 years after the onset, recently she has noticed progressive muscle weakness and fatigue. Anne was diagnosed with the late effects of polio (post-polio syndrome). One of the manifestations is weak neck extensors, making it difficult for her to hold up her head. In addition, she often has pain and tingling radiating down her arms.

1. What are the objectives of orthotic intervention for Anne?

2. What neck orthoses can be offered for Anne to consider?

3. Is a collar required for night use?

# ● Answers to Case Studies

## CASE 1

1. First, the therapist should investigate the factors causing the carpal tunnel syndrome, in particular, the ergonomic risk factors in the setup of the work environment, especially the position of the wrist when using the keyboard and the location of the mouse. In addition, activities outside of work might be aggravating the problem. Modification of the work environment and activities may relieve the symptoms, and orthoses may not be required. Another consideration is that most wrist orthoses are likely to interfere with keyboarding because they are designed to block the offending wrist postures that are required to position the fingers over the keys of a standard keyboard.

2. To position the wrist as close to neutral as possible, without excessive restriction of hand function, to minimize the pressure in the carpal tunnel and alleviate compression of the median nerve (see Chapter 2, "Carpal Tunnel Syndrome"). To immobilize the wrist as little as possible while meeting these objectives.

3. Because complete wrist immobilization is usually unnecessary and undesirable, consider a design that blocks harmful wrist flexion, such as the Prefabricated Daytimer Carpal Tunnel Support (see Fig. 10-6) or a semiflexible circumferential prefabricated wrist orthosis. If a custom orthosis is fabricated, the design can be either volar (see Fig. 10-2) or dorsal (see Fig. 10-3).

4. Some flexibility is desirable, and the thinner the material, the more flexible the orthosis. For a volar orthosis, select a category C thermoplastic, preferably perforated for comfort, $\frac{1}{16}$ or $\frac{3}{32}$ in. (1.6 or 2.4 mm) thick. For a dorsal orthosis, select a category B or C thermoplastic, $\frac{3}{32}$ or $\frac{1}{8}$ in (2.4 or 3.2 mm) thick. Alternatively, a flexible material such as Kushionsplint can be used, but the orthosis will be bulky because the material is $\frac{1}{4}$ in. (6.4 mm) thick.

5. Wear the orthosis during activities that tend to promote wrist flexion or deviation, to ensure a neutral wrist position. Night wear is appropriate if inadvertent ill positioning of the wrist when sleeping causes symptoms at night or on waking in the morning.

## CASE 2

1. To prevent contracture of the innervated wrist and MCP flexors and MCP collateral ligaments and prevent overstretching of the paralyzed wrist and MCP extensors from the sustained drop wrist posture. To promote prehension of the hand by substituting for the paralyzed muscles.

2. (a) A variety of static wrist or dynamic hand orthoses— custom or prefabricated—can be offered for the client to consider (see Table 7-2). The most functional orthosis provides dynamic extension assist to the wrist, finger MCPs, and thumb; however, it is more conspicuous because of the outrigger mechanism. Therefore a static wrist orthosis may be preferable for some social situations. Another consideration is that spring wire is susceptible to becoming bent out of shape and thus is not appropriate for vigorous activities. For some clients, it may

be appropriate to fabricate two or more styles of orthoses because one may not be adequate for all applications. (b) A static orthosis will probably be more durable than a dynamic orthosis for an active child. Using brightly colored thermoplastic or allowing the child to decorate the orthosis with stickers or splint markers might enhance compliance.

3. If the orthosis immobilizes the wrist and Cory needs gross grasp or a power grip, the wrist should be positioned in functional extension, ranging from 15° to 30°, depending on the requirements of most tasks (see Fig. 2-20). The therapist should observe the amount of wrist extension that naturally occurs for the client during a power grasp and replicate it during the molding process. When molding an orthosis to promote a power grasp, the naturally occurring deviation should be incorporated into the wrist positioning, along with the appropriate degree of wrist extension (see Fig. 2-21).

   In contrast, precision function often requires neutral or slight flexion of the wrist to position the fingers to pick up and manipulate objects (see Fig. 2-24a). Consider the best-compromise position in which to immobilize the wrist—extension to promote a power grasp, or neutral to slight flexion to promote precision function.

4. Generally, an orthosis is required at all times. A static design is preferable when sleeping, for occasions when an inconspicuous orthosis is desirable, and during vigorous activities that could damage an outrigger. Use a dynamic orthosis during activities that require finger dexterity.

5. The orthotic design can be changed from a forearm-based style to hand-based style to provide dynamic assistive extension to the MCPs and thumb only, leaving the wrist free to move (see Fig. 11-4).

## CASE 3

1. An anterior serial-static elbow corrective-extension orthosis can be used to gradually correct the elbow flexion contracture while applying compression to the scar tissue over the anterior surface of the arm, elbow, and forearm (see Fig. 9-11). To correct the extension contracture, use a static-progressive elbow-flexion harness (see Fig. 9-16). During the day, alternate between the anterior elbow orthosis and the elbow-flexion harness every 3 to 4 hours, with gentle active range-of-motion exercises in between. During the night, use either the orthosis or the harness depending on which range is more limited.

2. For the anterior elbow orthosis, use a ⅛ in (3.2 mm) thick category C thermoplastic (category B for a larger limb) that has memory, with ½ in. (1.2 cm) thick Plastazote or AliPlast for the elbow pad.

3. To soften and flatten the hypertrophic scar tissue, Shelley should wear elastic bandages, Lycra compression garments (e.g., Jobst) or cohesive tape under the orthosis to apply continuous pressure. Consider adding highly conforming rubberlike insert formed from silicone elastomer under bandages, garment, or orthosis. Alternatively, gel sheeting can be applied over the scar tissue. See Chapter 2, "Scar Management," for the rationale. See Table 9 in Appendix A.

# CASE 4

1. Fabricate a posterior static (or serial-static) knee orthosis, with a Plastazote or AliPlast kneepad, to be worn all the time, except for bathing and knee range-of-motion exercises. Mold it over the customary stump bandaging. As the limb atrophies, it may be necessary to remold the orthosis to accommodate the diminished limb girth. When George is in a wheelchair, provide a seat extension to support the underside of the residual limb. Once he starts to walk with a prosthesis, the knee orthosis can probably be discontinued.

2. Select a lightly perforated category A or B thermoplastic, ⅛ in. (3.2 mm) thick.

3. The footwear should be lightweight, with porous upper material that has a smooth seamless lining such as deerskin, glove leather, soft suede, or, better yet, Plastazote. The sole should be shock absorbing and nonslip to ensure stability when walking and it should have a steel shank reinforcement. The shoe should have laces or an alternate form of closure rather than be slip-on. Ensure that the heel is no higher than 1 in. (2.5 cm) above the toes. The toe box should be extra deep to prevent any irritation to the sensitive skin of the toes. Avoid pointed toes and narrow heels; a wide base of support under the heel is desirable. Plastazote insoles are recommended to protect fragile or ulcerated skin of the intact foot.

# CASE 5

1. This design uses leverage when it is put on to extend the wrist (see Fig. 1-16). Theoretically, the thermoplastic molded to the volar surface of the fingers and thumb applies pressure on the tendon insertions to inhibit the flexor muscle tone. See Chapter 2, "Spasticity," for more discussion.

2. Before molding, use tone-inhibiting techniques to suppress flexor tone. The assistance of a second person may be helpful to position the joints during the molding process.

3. While keeping the finger MCPs moderately flexed and the IPs slightly flexed, position the wrist in submaximal extension, avoiding excessive tension within the wrist flexors that could stimulate flexor muscle tone. Position the thumb in a comfortable amount of abduction to help break up the flexor spasticity.

4. Consider a brightly colored thermoplastic to help distinguish the orthosis from the bed linens and thus prevent inadvertent laundering or loss of the orthosis. Furthermore, bright colors serve as a visual attraction to help counteract the tendency toward unilateral neglect. Detachable loop Velcro straps can also be lost in the white linen of the hospital bed. To minimize this possibility, use brightly colored Velcro straps. Alternatively, secure the loop Velcro to one side of the orthosis as described in Chapter 7.

5. • Volar forearm-based static C-bar wrist-hand orthosis (see Fig. 10-18).
   • The volar hand portion can be wider and molded to abduct the fingers and thumb, forming a "ball splint" to break up the flexor spasticity (see Fig. 7-7d).
   • Hand-based versions of the ball splint.
   • Soft prefabricated orthoses (e.g., Rolyan® Progressive Palm Protector, Fig. 10-20).

- Hand-based versions of the Palm Protector.
- Ulnar forearm-based static wrist-hand cone-style tone-reducing orthosis (see Fig. 10-21).

## CASE 6

1. A volar or bisurfaced forearm-based serial-static wrist-hand orthosis (see Figs. 10-18 and 10-19), excluding the thumb. The wrist, MCPs, and IPs of all fingers should be positioned to create a gentle, prolonged extension force to promote growth and elongation of the contracted flexors. The orthosis requires remolding every few days as the contracture is reduced to maintain the desired amount of tension in the contracted tissues.

2. A finger-based orthosis, either prefabricated or custom fabricated, such as the three-point finger-based dynamic joint-aligned coil-spring PIP corrective-extension orthosis (see Fig. 11-19). Alternatively, provide a hand-based orthosis as shown in Figures 3-11*a* through *c*.

3. Ensure that the corrective force is within the elastic range, which is sufficient to stimulate growth but too low to promote inflammation of the stretched tissues (see Chapter 2, "Promoting Tissue Growth to Reduce Contractures"). Monitor the joint range of motion to ensure that the prolonged application of extension force does not lead to loss of flexion range. Advise the client to remove the orthosis periodically for active and passive range-of-motion exercises.

## CASE 7

1. Use ½ in. (1.2 cm) thick Plastazote or AliPlast, cut into a pattern that extends about 1 in. (2.5 cm) beyond the edge of the skull defect over the intact bone. This will form a resilient, shock-absorbing layer. Use any ⅛ in. (3.2 mm) thick unperforated thermoplastic, cut to the same pattern, to form a hard outer shell.

2. The Plastazote or AliPlast is heated and molded carefully to the head, taking care not to apply compression where there is no bone. When it has cooled, contact cement is applied to the outer surface and allowed to set. The thermoplastic is heated, dried, and then adhered to the contact cement.

3. To help the orthosis cling to the hair, apply a layer of thin, self-adhesive gel sheeting. To secure the orthosis to the baseball hat or toque, adhere a piece of self-adhesive hook Velcro to the outer surface of the orthosis. If necessary, sew a piece of loop Velcro to the inside of the hat or toque, although the orthosis might stay in place without it.

## CASE 8

- Volar (or circumferential) hand-based static D2-5 MCP-stablizing orthosis (see Fig. 11-2).
- Circumferential hand-based dynamic traction D2-5 MCP-corrective radial deviation orthosis (see Fig. 11-3).
- A prefabricated MCP-stabilizing orthosis.

1. The dynamic traction orthosis has soft, absorbent material that might be a disadvantage in her work environment because of the need to wash her hands frequently. Also this orthosis provides no stability to the volar side of the MCPs; as a result, although it should prevent further progression of the ulnar drift, it would be unlikely to promote correction of the deformity.

2. Only the finger MCPs are incorporated, and they should be positioned with neutral deviation and slight flexion to promote restabilization of the MCPs while allowing functional use of the fingers. Wrist, thumb, and IP motions should be unrestricted.

3. To help promote restabilization of the MCPs the orthosis should be worn at all times, except for washing the hands. If the client wants only to prevent progression of the deformity, the orthosis need be worn only during activities using the hands, especially those involving lateral pinch, ulnar deviating forces, and power grasp, because they promote ulnar drift.

4. Select 1/16 in. (1.6 mm) thick perforated category C or D thermoplastic. If possible, offer the client a choice of colors ranging from inconspicuous flesh tones to brightly colored thermoplastic. Elizabeth would probably prefer to have an inconspicuous orthosis.

# CASE 9

1. • To reduce the high tone of the ankle plantar flexors.
   • To prevent shortening of the calcaneal tendon.
   • To promote optimal gait.

2. The most suitable custom orthosis for Gordie is probably the bisurfaced static (or serial-static) ankle-foot orthosis (see Fig. 12-14). It uses leverage when it is applied to dorsiflex the ankle into position. If a serial-static design is desired to promote elongation of contracted plantar flexor muscles, use a thermoplastic with memory. This orthosis can be used for both weight bearing and non–weight bearing. For long-term use, a custom orthosis of high-temperature thermoplastic could be made by an orthotist and be used when walking (see Fig. 12-16). Alternatively, for non–weight-bearing applications, removable bivalved plaster of Paris casts are sometimes made to reduce muscle tone.

3. Here high tone is not a problem, so a dynamic orthosis can be substituted during gait. For example, use either a custom or prefabricated circumferential calf-based dynamic ankle assistive-dorsiflexion orthosis (see Fig. 12-17).

# CASE 10

1. • To support the weight of the head to compensate for the weak neck extensors.
   • To optimally position the cervical joints to relieve nerve root compression.
   • To provide the least amount of support that will achieve these goals to avoid unnecessary restriction of neck motion (especially rotation).

2. • A custom-molded circumferential static Plastazote stabilizing collar (see Fig. 8-6) or the prefabricated bivalved version, the Philadelphia Collar.
   • Open designs are less conspicuous and retain less heat than enclosing collars. They include the Canadian Collar (custom orthosis kit) and the prefabricated Headmaster Collar.

3. If Anne experiences pain or tingling in her arms at night, support is warranted to prevent ill positioning of the neck causing nerve root compression. The neck can be stabilized with a prefabricated soft foam collar, a hand towel (folded lengthwise in thirds, wrapped around neck, and secured with safety pins), or static cervical-stabilizing ruffs (see Fig. 8-10). If there are no symptoms at night, a collar is unnecessary.

# Addresses and Websites of Suppliers and Manufacturers

**AliMed Inc.**
http://www.alimed.com/
297 High Street, Dedham, MA 02026-9135, USA
Tel: 800-225-2610, fax: 800-437-2966

Supplier of:
Plastazote, AliPlast, NickelPlast
Multiform Plastics
Equipment and tools

**Beiersdorf-Jobst**
U.S. address:
   5825 Carnegie Blvd., Charlotte, NC 28209-4633, USA
   Tel: 800-221-7573 fax: 704-551-8581
Canadian address:
   8400 Jane St., Suite 12, Bldg. B, Concord,
   ON L4K 4L8
   Tel: 800-795-6278, fax: 800-423-2876

Manufacturer/supplier of:
Custom and prefabricated pressure
   and vascular garments
Cutinova Hydro (scar management
   gel sheeting)
Comprilan (low-tension elastic
   bandage)

**Chesapeake Medical Products Inc.**
(Previously Polymed Industries Inc.)
23 Fontana Lane, Suite 110,
   Baltimore, MD 21237, USA
Tel: 410-637-7058, fax: 410-560-1929

Manufacturer of:
Thermoplastics sold by various suppliers

**Danmar Products Inc.**
221 Jackson Industrial Dr., Ann Arbor, MI 48103, USA
Tel: 800-783-1998, fax: 313-761-8977

Supplier of:
Protective helmets

**Landec Corporation**
3603 Haven Ave., Menlo Park, CA 94025, USA
Tel: 415-306-1650, fax: 415-368-9818

Manufacturer of:
Dynacast Rapide (also called
   QuickCast)

**Larson Products, Inc.**
http://www.iwaynet.net/~larpro/about.html
2392 Charles St., Columbus, OH 43209, USA
Tel: 614-235-9100, fax: 614-235-0040

Manufacturer/supplier of:
New Wave Memory/Universal/Precision
Orthoprene

**Monarch Rubber Co., Inc.**
PO Box 188, Spencer, WV 25276, USA
Tel: 304-927-1380

Manufacturer of:
   Orthoplast and Orthoplast II

**North Coast Medical**
http://www.disprodpc.com/northcoa.htm/
187 Stauffer Blvd., San Jose, CA 95125-1042, USA
Tel: 800-821-9319, fax: 408-283-1950

U.S. supplier of:
Orfit Plastics
North American supplier of:
Prism, Encore
Omega Plus, Omega Max, Spectrum,
   Preferred, Clinic, and Clinic D
Quick Cast
Equipment and tools

**Orfit Industries**
Paul Van Lede, OT, Product Manager,
Vosveld 9A, B-2110 Winjegem, Antwerp, Belgium
Tel: 32/3/3262026, fax: 32/3/3261415

Manufacturer of:
Orfit Plastics

**Ortho-Dynactive, Inc.**
5910 Breckenridge Pkwy., Suite D,
  Tampa, FL 33610, USA
Tel: 800-230-3962, fax: 800-248-3962

**Ped A Ligne**
3542 Ashby, St-Laurent, Quebec H4R 2C1, Canada
Tel: 800-547-4767, fax: 888-638-1525

**Physio E.R.P. Ltd.**
3232, autoroute Laval Ouest,
Laval, Quebec H7T 2H6, Canada
Tel: 800-668-0425, fax: 514-687-8035


**Remington Medical**
401 Bentley St., Suit #9, Markham, ON L3R 0T2,
  Canada
Tel: 800-267-5822 or 905-470-7790, fax: 905-470-7787



**Sammons Preston Inc.**
http://www.sammonspreston.com
E-mail: sp@sammonspreston.com
U.S. address:
  4 Sammons Court, Boling Brook, IL 60440, USA
  Tel: 800-323-5547, fax: 800-547-4333
Canadian address:
  755 Queensway E., Mississauga,
  ON L4Y 4C5, Canada
  Tel: 800-665-9200, fax: 905-566-9207

**Serum International**
2375 Benjamin Sulte, Montreal, Quebec
  H3M 1R8, Canada
Tel: 800-361-7726, fax: 514-384-8011

**Silver Ring Splint Company**
Post Office Box 2856, Charlottesville,
  VA 22902-2856, USA
Tel: 804-971-4052, fax: 804-971-8828

**Smith & Nephew, Inc.**
http://www.smithnephew.com
U.S. address:
  One Quality Dr., P.O. Box 1005,
  Germantown, WI 53022, USA
  Tel: 800-228-3693 or 414-251-7840,
  fax: 414-253-3066
Canadian address:
  2100 52nd Ave.,
  Lachine, Quebec, H8T 2Y5, Canada
  Tel: 800-363-5723 or 514-636-0772,
  fax: 514-636-1684

**T Tape Company bv**
Hogebergdreff 60, 4645, EX Putte, The Netherlands
Tel: 31/164/602952, fax: 31/104/772430

**Toronto Medical Orthopaedics Ltd.**
email: tmol@www.tormed.com
901 Dillingham Rd., Pickering, ON L1W 2Y5,
  Canada
Tel: 905-420-3303, fax: 905-420-3970

U.S. supplier of:
  Turbocast Plastics
  Plastazote

Manufacturer and supplier of:
  Silipos Products, which contain
  mineral oil–based polymer gel

Canadian supplier of:
  Turbocast Thermoplastics
  Recyclocast
  Hexcelite
  Equipment and tools

Canadian supplier of:
  Transform
  Orthoform, Thermosplint Plus,
  Thermosplint,
  ThermoForm,
  Thermoform Plus, Ortho-Eze

Supplier of:
  Kay-Splint Basics
  Orthoplast and Orthoplast II
  QuickCast
  Equipment and tools

Supplier of:
  Cork pads for foot orthoses

Supplier of:
  Siris Silver Ring Splints

Manufacturer and supplier of:
  Aquaplast Plastics
  San-Splint, Synergy, Ezeform,
  San-Splint XR, Polyflex,
  Polyform
Supplier of:
  Dynacast Rapide and Hexcelite
  Equipment and tools
  Kinetec

Manufacturer of:
  Turbocast and Recyclocast

Canadian supplier of:
  Toronto Medical's Continuous
  Passive Motion (CPM)
  Devices

**OrthoLogic Corp.**
2850 South 36th Street, Phoenix, AZ 85034, USA
Tel: 602-437-5520, fax: 602-437-5524

U.S. supplier of:
   Toronto Medical's Continuous
     Passive Motion (CPM)
     Devices

**J. Vaillancourt Corp. Ltd.**
7 Rue Duvernay, Vercheres, Quebec J0L 2R0, Canada
Tel: 800-361-3317 or 514-583-3317,
fax: 514-583-6827

Canadian supplier of:
   Orfit plastics
   Equipment and tools

**Zotefoams Inc.**
http://www.biomech.com/biomech/mall/zotefoams
319 Airport Rd., Hackettstown, NJ 07840, USA
Tel: 800-362-8358 or 908-850-7250, fax: 908-850-7216

Manufacturer of:
   Plastazote

**Zotefoams plc**
675 Mitcham Road, Croydon, Surrey CR93AL, England
Tel: 44-181-684-3622, fax: 44-181-684-7571

Manufacturer of:
   Plastazote

# INDEX

Note: Pages numbers followed by an f indicate a figure and a t indicate a table.